Ciba Foundation Symposium 199

THE NATURE AND ORIGIN OF AMYLOID FIBRILS

1996

JOHN WILEY & SONS

Chichester · New York · Brisbane · Toronto · Singapore

Published in 1996 by John Wiley & Sons Ltd
Baffins Lane, Chichester
West Sussex PO19 1UD, England

Telephone National (01243) 779777
International (+44) (1243) 779777

Other Wiley Editorial Offices

John Wiley & Sons, Inc., 605 Third Avenue,
New York, NY 10158-0012, USA

Jacaranda Wiley Ltd, 33 Park Road, Milton,
Queensland 4064, Australia

John Wiley & Sons (Canada) Ltd, 22 Worcester Road,
Rexdale, Ontario M9W 1L1, Canada

John Wiley & Sons (Asia) Pte Ltd, 2 Clementi Loop #02-01,
Jin Xing Distripark, Singapore 0512

Suggested series entry for library catalogues:
Ciba Foundation Symposia

Ciba Foundation Symposium 199
xi+253 pages, 41 figures, 18 tables

Library of Congress Cataloging-in-Publication Data

The nature and origin of amyloid fibrils / [editors, Gregory R. Bock and Jamie A. Goode].
p. cm.—(CIBA Foundation symposium ; 199)
"Symposium on the nature and origin of amyloid fibrils, held at the Palácio dos Marqueses de Pombal, Oeiras, Portugal, 23–25 October 1995"—Contents p.
Includes bibliographical references and index.
ISBN 0 471 96361 5 (alk. paper)
1. Amyloid—Congresses. 2, Amyloid beta-protein—Congresses. 3. Amyloidosis—Congresses. I. Bock, Gregory. II. Goode, Jamie. III. Series.
QP552.A45N38 1996
612.8′042—dc20 96-2872
CIP

British Library Cataloguing in Publication Data

A catalogue record for this book is available from the British Library

ISBN 0 471 96361 5

Typeset in 10/12pt Times by Dobbie Typesetting Limited, Tavistock, Devon.
Printed and bound in Great Britain by Biddles Ltd, Guildford.
This book is printed on acid-free paper responsibly manufactured from sustainable forestation, for which at least two trees are planted for each one used for paper production.

Contents

Symposium on The nature and origin of amyloid fibrils, held at the Palácio dos Marqueses de Pombal, Oeiras, Portugal 23–25 October 1995

Editors: Gregory R. Bock (Organizer) and Jamie A. Goode

This symposium was based on a proposal made by Horácio Menano, Maria João Saraiva and Pedro Costa

Participants

T. Arvinte Pharmaceutical and Analytical Development Department, Ciba-Geigy Ltd, K-136.481, CH-4002 Basle, Switzerland

M. D. Benson Indiana University School of Medicine, Department of Medicine, Division of Rheumatology, c/o Veteran Affairs Medical Center (583/111Rh), 1481 West 10th Street, Indianapolis, IN 46202–2884, USA

C. C. F. Blake Laboratory of Molecular Biophysics and Oxford Centre for Molecular Sciences, University of Oxford, The Rex Richards Building, South Parks Road, Oxford OX1 3QU, UK

J. D. Buxbaum The Laboratory of Molecular and Cellular Neuroscience, The Rockefeller University, 1230 York Avenue, New York, NY 10021, USA

J. N. Buxbaum New York VA Medical Center, 423 East 23rd Street, New York 10010, USA

B. Caughey Laboratory of Persistent Viral Diseases, National Institute of Allergy and Infectious Diseases, NIH, Rocky Mountain Laboratories, Hamilton, Montana 59840, USA

P. P. Costa *(Chairman)* Centro de Estudos de Paramiloidose, Hospital de Sto. Antonio, 4100 Porto, Portugal

A. M. Damas Instituto de Ciencias Biomedicas Abel Salazar, Universidade de Porto, Largo do Prof. Abel Salazar, 4050 Porto, Portugal

B. Frangione Department of Pathology, New York University Medical Center, 550 1st Avenue TH 427, New York, NY 10016, USA

D. Goldgaber Department of Psychiatry, School of Medicine, State University of New York at Stony Brook, Stony Brook, NY 11794–8101, USA

L. Hendriks Neurogenetics Laboratory, Born-Bunge Foundation, University of Antwerp, Department of Biochemistry, Universiteitsplein 1, B-2610 Antwerp, Belgium

J. W. Kelly Department of Chemistry, Texas A&M University, College Station, TX 77843–3255, USA

D. A. Kirschner Department of Biological Sciences, University of Massachusetts at Lowell, Olsen 6, One University Avenue, Lowell, MA 01854, USA

R. Kisilevsky Department of Pathology, Queens University and The Syl and Molly Apps Research Center, Kingston General Hospital, Kingston, Ontario, Canada K7L 3N6

Q.-X. Lin *(Ciba Foundation Bursar)* Department of Pathology, The University of Melbourne, Parkville, Victoria 3052, Australia

E. Lundgren Department of Cell & Molecular Biology, University of Umeå, S-90187 Umeå, Sweden

S. Maeda Department of Biochemistry, Yamanashi Medical University, 1110 Shimogato, Tamaho-machi, Nakakoma-gun, Yamanashi 409–38, Japan

C. L. Masters Department of Pathology, The University of Melbourne, Parkville, Victoria 3052, Australia

C. P. J. Maury Department of Medicine 4, University of Helsinki, Unioninkatu 38, SF-00170 Helsinki 17, Finland

H. Menano Director, Instituto Gulbenkian de Ciência, Rua da Quinta Grande 6, Apartado 14, 2781 Oeiras Codex, Portugal

G. Merlini Hospital IRCCS S Matteo, Research Lab. Biotechnologies, Institute of Clinical Medicine 2, University of Pavia, I-27100 Pavia, Italy

J. A. Palha *(Ciba Foundation Bursar)* Centro de Estudos de Paramiloidoise, Hospital de Sto. Antonio, 4000 Porto, Portugal

M. B. Pepys Immunological Medicine Unit, Royal Postgraduate Medical School, Hammersmith Hospital, DuCane Road, London W12 0NN, UK

S. B. Prusiner Department of Neurology, Biochemistry and Biophysics, University of California, San Francisco, CA 94143, USA

M. J. M. Saraiva Centro de Estudos de Paramiloidose and Instituto de Ciências Biomédicas, Hospital de Sto. Antonio, 4100 Porto, Portugal

E. Da Cruz E Silva Laboratory of Molecular and Cellular Neuroscience, The Rockefeller University, Box 296, 1240 York Avenue, New York, NY 10021, USA

J. D. Sipe Department of Biochemistry, School of Medicine, University of Boston, K121 80 East Concord Street, Boston, MA 02118, USA

P. Westermark Department of Pathology I, University Hospital, S-581 85 Linköping, Sweden

S. P. Wood ICRF Structural Molecular Biology Unit, Department of Crystallography, Birkbeck College, Malet Street, London WC1E 7HX, UK

Preface

Although based in London, the Ciba Foundation is truly an international organization whose mission is to foster scientific cooperation globally. Most of our international symposia are held in our London headquarters but wherever possible we try to hold meetings outside the UK. In order to do this, we occasionally join forces with another organization to share the costs involved in holding the meeting outside London. The idea of holding a meeting in Portugal was originally suggested to the Ciba Foundation by Dr Horácio Menano, Director of the Gulbenkian Foundation's Institute for Science in Oeiras. Our two charitable foundations then joined forces to share the costs and the organizational work involved in preparing the meeting in Portugal. We were particularly fortunate in that the Medical Research Programme of the European Union in Brussels agreed to make a contribution to the costs of this meeting, and we gratefully acknowledge the encouragement and support of Dr Wolfgang Hebel from the Commission of the EU. The topic chosen for the meeting was one which we felt was relevant to Portuguese interests and also one where Portuguese scientists have made outstanding contributions to the progress of the field.

Gregory R. Bock
Deputy Director, The Ciba Foundation

Introduction

Pedro P. Costa

Centro de Estudos de Paramiloidose, Hospital de Sto. Antonio, 4100 Porto, Portugal

I would like to take this opportunity of welcoming you to this symposium. I would also like to thank the Ciba Foundation and the Gulbenkian Foundation for this opportunity to discuss, in Portugal, the many biological and medical issues related to the amyloid fibril.

In a sense we could say that the amyloid fibril was born in 1959, when Alan Cohen and Euan Calkins published their electron microscope observations on the fibril structure of amyloid of diverse origin (Cohen & Calkins 1959) (unfortunately, due to a sudden illness Alan cannot be here today with us, as was initially planned). For the next 12 years the fibril progressively became synonymous with amyloid itself, and isolation of the fibril from different organs became a major concern of several groups working in the field. We now had as reference a morphological entity, which was an enormous advantage. It was a time of much discussion and controversy which culminated in 1967 with the first international symposium on amyloidosis, held in Groningen (see Mandema et al 1968).

Quick progress followed and in 1971 the fibril reached the biochemical age when George Glenner and his colleagues demonstrated that in his fibril preparations the major component was, with one exception, an immunoglobulin light chain or a fragment of this (Glenner et al 1971). Only one year later, Benditt & Eriksen (1972) and Franklin et al (1972) showed that the one exception in Glenner's fibril preparations corresponded to a secondary amyloidotic fibril with a quite different amino acid sequence. Thus was confirmed what the histochemists of the 1930s always suspected—that there was a difference between the primary- and secondary-type amyloidotic substance.

The number of different amyloidotic proteins identified began to increase, starting in our laboratory in 1978 with the identification of transthyretin as the fibril protein in familial amyloidotic polyneuropathy (Costa et al 1978). So far 16 different amyloidotic proteins have been identified, according to Jean Sipe's recent review (Sipe 1994). Many of them are associated with such important pathologies as Alzheimer's disease, point mutations such as familial amyloidotic polyneuropathy, long-term haemodialysis for treatment of kidney failure, and even normal biological events such as ageing. The diversity of amyloid protein precursors in amyloidotic syndromes was thus established.

Amyloid, however, maintained a few unifying characteristics: the Congo red binding of Benhold (1922), the green birefringence of Divry (1927), and the fibrillar structure of Cohen & Calkins (1959). All these defining properties appear to be related to the secondary structure of the amyloidogenic proteins, always rich in β-pleated sheet structures, which was first demonstrated by X-ray diffraction by Eanes & Glenner in 1968. In fact, the unifying functional concept among all amyloid fibrils is the biological difficulty of disposing of protein fragments rich in β-sheet structures which tend to aggregate and are deposited in the tissues as fibrils.

During the last 12 years, amyloid has entered the molecular genetics age. We will hear a lot about this in the next few days.

The title of this symposium is 'The nature and origin of amyloid fibrils'. We now know a lot about the nature and origin of amyloid fibrils and their protein precursors. I think a major issue in the discussions will be how these precursors are processed and transformed into protein fibrils. In other words, we will be discussing fibrillogenesis. The subject of fibrillogenesis is closely related to the old question of fibril structure. In some cases, the clarification of structure has proven to be a difficult task and models are still being proposed. The protofilament of the 1967 Groningen meeting is still alive and well, as Colin Blake will tell us. Bob Kisilevsky and Mark Pepys will remind us that the amyloid fibril is one thing and that amyloid deposits are another, as these contain other constituents such as proteoglycans and P components which may well play a role in modulating the process of fibrillogenesis.

I think that we are at the point where data from different laboratories will contribute towards a better understanding of fibril formation. I do not believe that a general theory of fibrillogenesis applicable to all cases will emerge, but taking into consideration the different types of amyloidotic syndromes and physiopathological situations, it is conceivable that we will gradually clarify the different although often closely related processes involved. I hope this meeting will be a step in that direction.

I would like to end with a few words about the untimely death of George Glenner, four months ago. For me it was a personal loss: I worked for a few months with him at NIH in Bethesda in 1973, soon after a major breakthrough by his laboratory in the history of amyloid research—the identification of the immunoglobulin light chain as the major component of the immunocytic fibril. He was already thinking about leaving for San Diego and dedicating himself to the subject of amyloid in Alzheimer's disease. We all know what came out of it: the 1984 report on the characterization of amyloid β-protein in Alzheimer's disease which initiated prodigious development in the field (Glenner & Wong 1984). He was a passionate and honest scientist. He liked to address fundamental questions, leaving the collateral issues for others. He certainly was one of the top amyloidologists of this century. I would like to propose the dedication of this symposium to his memory.

References

Benditt EP, Eriksen N 1972 Chemical similarity among amyloid substances associated with long-standing inflammation. Lab Invest 26:615–625

Benhold H 1922 Eine spezifische Amyloidfarbung mit Kongorot. Munchen Med Wschr 69:1537–1538

Cohen AS, Calkins E 1959 Electron microscopic observation on a fibrous component in amyloid of diverse origins. Nature 183:1202–1203

Costa PP, Figueira AS, Bravo F 1978 Amyloid fibril protein related to prealbumin in familial amyloidotic polyneuropathy. Proc Natl Acad Sci USA 75:4499–4503

Divry P 1927 Étude histochemique des plaques séniles. J Neurol Psychiat 27:643–657

Eanes ED, Glenner GG 1968 X-ray diffraction studies on amyloid filaments. J Histochem Cytochem 16:673–677

Franklin EC, Pras M, Levin M, Frangione B 1972 The partial amino acid sequence of the major low human amyloid fibrils. FEBS Lett 22:121–123

Glenner GG, Terry W, Harada M, Ikersky C, Page D 1971 Amyloid fibril proteins: proof of homology with immunoglobulin light chains by sequence analysis. Science 172:1150–1151

Glenner GG, Wong CW 1984 Alzheimer's disease: initial report of the purification and characterization of a novel cerebrovascular amyloid protein. Biochem Biophys Res Commun 120:855–890

Mandema E, Ruinen L, Scholten JH, Cohen AS (eds) 1968 Amyloidosis. Proceedings of a symposium on amyloidosis, Groningen, 1967. Excerpta Medica, Amsterdam

Sipe JD 1994 Amyloidosis. Clin Lab Sci 31:325–354

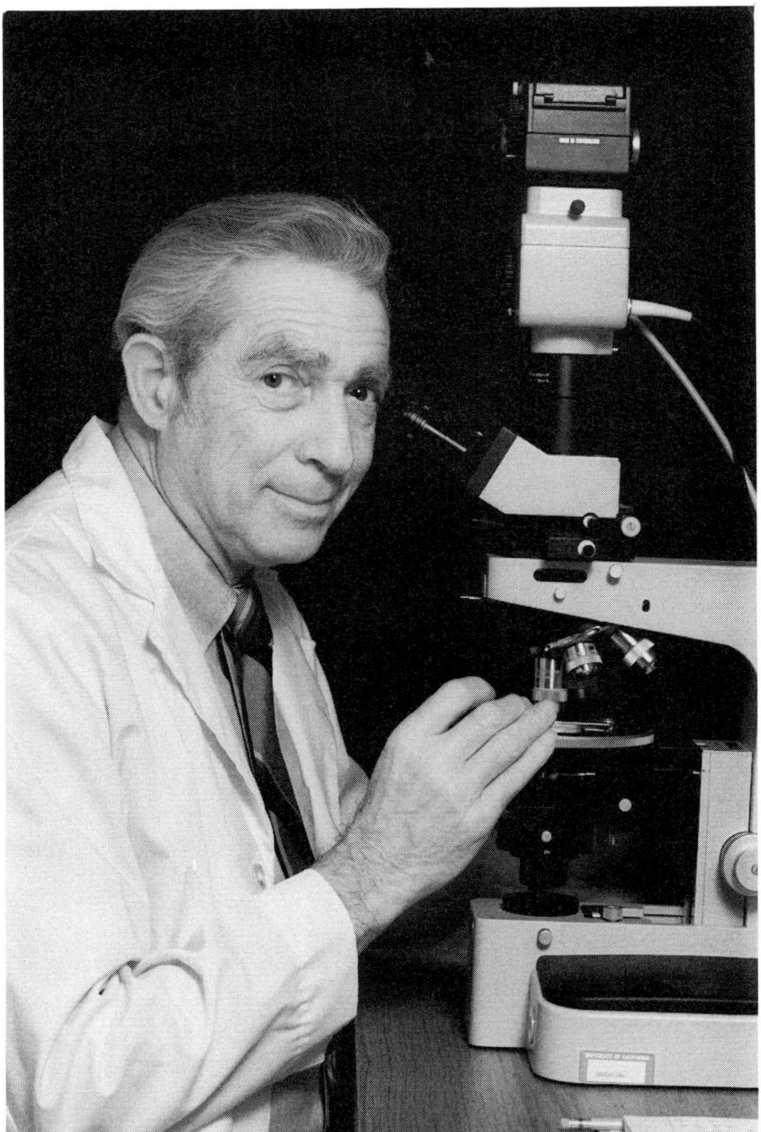

In memoriam

George Glenner died on July 12 1995 at the age of 67. He graduated at the Johns Hopkins School of Medicine in 1953. In 1958 he moved to the National Institutes of Health in Bethesda, where he was Chief of the Laboratory on Molecular Biology for 22 years. It was there that he started research on amyloidosis and produced seminal work in the field, including the demonstration of the secondary structure of the fibril protein, the identification of the immunoglobulin light chain as the major component of the 'primary type' amyloid and the creation of amyloid fibrils *in vitro*. In 1982 he moved to the San Diego School of Medicine at the University of California where he concentrated his research on the subject of amyloidosis in Alzheimer's disease. The identification of the amyloid β-protein in 1984 constituted a major breakthrough and opened an entirely new era in the study of this disease. He was an active participant in all seven international symposia on amyloidosis and many other meetings, where his brilliant mind and warm personality were deeply appreciated by his colleagues. George Glenner was also recognized for his humanitarian efforts on behalf of Alzheimer's patients and their families. In 1982, he and his wife, Joy, founded the first day care centres for Alzheimer's patients in California which have served as a national model for similar centres across the country. Among many awards, he received in 1988 a $1 million Merit Award for 10 years of research support by the National Advisory Council on Aging, National Institutes of Health. He was truly one of the great amyloidologists of this century.

P. P. Costa

A molecular model of the amyloid fibril

Colin C. F. Blake, Louise C. Serpell, Margaret Sunde, Ola Sandgren* and Erik Lundgren*

*Laboratory of Molecular Biophysics and Oxford Centre for Molecular Sciences, University of Oxford, The Rex Richards Building, South Parks Road, Oxford OX1 3QU, UK and *Department of Cell and Molecular Biology, University of Umeå, S-901 87, Umeå, Sweden*

Abstract. We have investigated the ultrastructure of the homozygous amyloid fibrils from the vitreous humour of patients with Met30 familial amyloidotic polyneuropathy (FAP) by high-resolution electron microscopy and X-ray diffraction using synchrotron radiation. Image reconstruction of thin sections of Met30 FAP fibrils shows that they are composed of four parallel protofilaments, 50–60 Å in diameter, arranged in a square around a hollow centre. The X-ray diffraction patterns are consistent with the presence in the protofilaments of a repeating unit of 24 β-strands forming a continuous β-sheet extended along the fibre axis, with the β-strands perpendicular to the axis. We have characterized this repeat unit as one turn of a β-sheet helix. This newly-described helix reconciles the classical cross-β structure of amyloid with the twisted β-sheet that is known to be the most stable form of the structure. All four β-sheets composing the protofilament twist around a single helical axis which is coincident with the axis of the protofilament. Other amyloid diffraction patterns are similar to that of FAP, suggesting that the β-sheet helix may be the generic core structure of amyloid.

1996 The nature and origin of amyloid fibrils. Wiley, Chichester (Ciba Foundation Symposium 199) p 6–21

Amyloidoses are diseases in which variants of usually soluble proteins are deposited in the form of stable, insoluble fibrils, which invade the extracellular space of essential tissues causing dysfunction (Benson & Wallace 1989, Sipe 1992). Amyloidosis accompanies and is associated with a number of medical disorders including Alzheimer's disease, late-onset diabetes and familial amyloidotic polyneuropathy (FAP). Some 16 different proteins have been identified as being amyloidogenic (Sipe 1992, Pepys et al 1993), each being associated with a specific amyloidosis. In spite of the involvement of a number of different protein molecules, there is considerable evidence that amyloid fibrils from different sources share a common ultrastructure. For example, electron microscopy shows similar long, rigid, unbranched fibrils about 100 Å in diameter, X-ray diffraction of fibrils shows a 'cross-β' pattern suggestive of a

β-sheet structure in which the β-strands are arranged perpendicular to the fibre axis, and all amyloid fibrils stain with Congo red to exhibit a characteristic green birefringence suggestive of a particular ordering and environment for the bound dye molecules. Although a common ultrastructure for amyloid fibrils is indicated by these physical characteristics, the nature of this representative structure is not clear. It is important to define amyloid structure in order to understand the molecular processes whereby globular protein molecules become incorporated into the growing fibril, as an initial step in the process of attempting to inhibit or reverse amyloid growth.

X-ray patterns from laboratory X-ray sources are usually very weak and exhibit only 4.7 Å meridional and 10 Å equatorial reflections (Eanes & Glenner 1968, Bonar et al 1969) which have been interpreted as indicating the presence of β-structure in the fibrils oriented so that the β-strands are perpendicular to the fibre axis—the so called 'cross-β' structure (Pauling & Corey 1951). The lack of more detailed X-ray patterns has so far prevented the proposal of more detailed molecular models of amyloid. In their absence, the molecular model of the cross-β structure proposed for insect silk from the egg stalk of the lacewing *Crysopa* by Geddes et al (1968) has been widely adopted for amyloid. Although its general character is probably correct, there must be some doubt about certain important details when using a protein specifically designed to form a fibrous structure as a model for fibrils derived from abnormal globular proteins. For example, the *Crysopa* silk has flat β-sheets (Geddes et al 1968) which are not normally seen in globular proteins. As Chothia (1973) has shown, the twisted β-sheet represents a low energy conformation of the polypeptide chain. Apparently, higher energy flat sheets, if they exist in fibrous proteins, may do so as a result of specific amino acid sequences, possibly rich in glycine to relax the structural constraints (Chothia 1973), which would not occur in globular amyloid precursors. A further area of uncertainty is the relationship between the current amyloid models derived from X-ray diffraction, and the hierarchy of structures (fibrils, protofilaments and sub-protofilaments) seen in electron micrographs of amyloid (Shirahama & Cohen 1967).

In an attempt to resolve some of these problems, we have carried out electron microscopy and X-ray studies of FAP amyloid fibrils. The amyloid in FAP is composed largely or entirely of the protein transthyretin (TTR) (Costa et al 1978), formerly known as prealbumin or thyroxine binding prealbumin (TBPA), a homotetramer of 55 kDa (Kanda et al 1974). The molecular structure of the protein is based on a framework consisting of a stack of four eight-stranded β-sheets (Blake et al 1974, 1978). FAP is an autosomal dominant disease affecting kindreds predominantly in Portugal, Sweden, Japan and the USA. These kindreds exhibit clinical features including peripheral neuropathy and cardiac, renal and intestinal symptomatology, and in some cases vitreous opacities. Patients with FAP secrete genetic variants of TTR, mostly corresponding to single amino acid substitutions. Forty different FAP variants of TTR have been listed by Saraiva (1995), but substitution of Met for Val30 is by far the most widely found. We have used amyloid from Swedish patients homozygous for Met30 FAP, where it is deposited in the vitreous humour of the eye (Fig. 1). The fibrils are extracted using particularly mild procedures, thus providing excellent samples for biophysical study.

Electron microscopy

Cryo-electron microscopy of homozygous Met30 FAP fibrils from the vitreous humour of the eye (Serpell et al 1995) shows that the fibrils are long, unbranched and uniform with small-scale surface features. Their diameter is about 120–130 Å. Thin transverse sections show that the fibrils have an angular cross-section, with an indication of an electron-lucent centre. Iterative cross-correlation of more than 200 individual transverse sections has clarified the image and revealed that the FAP fibrils consist of four protofilments arranged

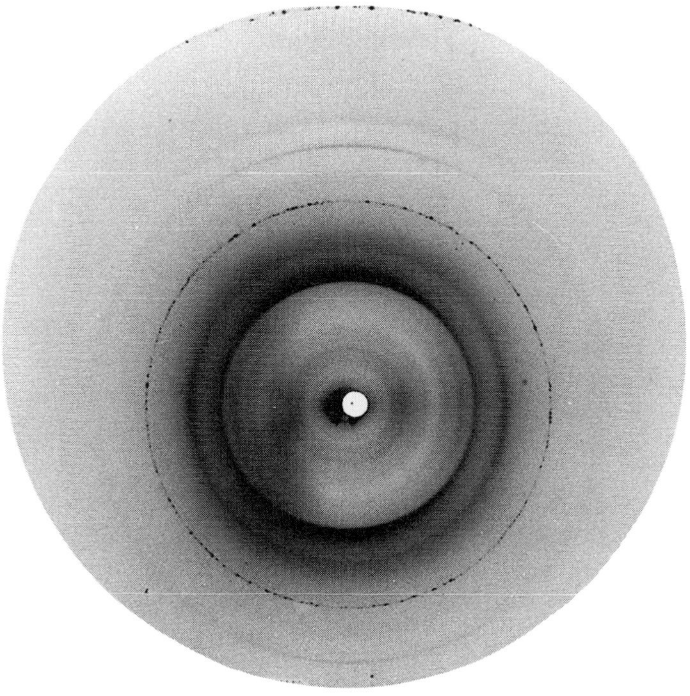

FIG. 1. An X-ray diffraction pattern of the Met30 homozygous FAP amyloid fibrils from vitreous humour. The 'spotty' circle is a powder line from the calibrant (Si: $d = 3.14$ Å).

at the corners of a square about 120 Å on edge, leaving a substantial hollow core along the axis of the fibril (see Fig. 2). The protofilaments are 50–60 Å in diameter, which corresponds closely to the cross-sectional size of the TTR tetramer in the direction parallel to its constituent β-sheets, and perpendicular to the strands in the sheets (Blake et al 1978). This suggests that if FAP amyloid is composed of β-sheets, the observed protofilaments are of the appropriate size to accommodate four β-sheets parallel to their long axes. However, this does not imply that intact TTR tetramers are present in protofilaments. There is considerable evidence that TTR undergoes a structural transition on forming amyloid involving a breakdown of its tetrameric structure to dimers or monomers (Colon & Kelly 1992).

X-ray diffraction

Use of partially orientated samples of homozygous Met30 FAP fibrils from vitreous humour and also heterozygous Met30 FAP fibrils from kidney on the UK national synchrotron radiation source at Daresbury has produced the most detailed X-ray diffraction patterns of amyloid so far obtained from *ex vivo* specimens. These contain diffraction features extending to the edge of the observed patterns, 2.0 Å and 2.2 Å, respectively. A feature of these patterns is that the intense '4.7 Å' meridional reflection, characteristic of the cross-β pattern, is resolved into a close doublet of lines at 4.83 Å and 4.64 Å. We have also observed this doublet in the X-ray patterns of different amyloids. Although this doublet was not resolved in the pattern from the vitreous sample (Fig. 1), its presence can be inferred by noting that the observed harmonic of the 4.83 Å reflection, seen at 2.41 Å, allows its fundamental to be placed accurately at the extreme inner edge of the intense '4.7 Å' reflection, requiring a reflection at about 4.6 Å to explain the observed intensity profile of this dominating reflection.

The observed meridional reflections from these Met30 FAP fibrils are listed in Table 1. Including the close doublet, the meridional reflections can all be indexed within experimental error as Bragg reflections to a repeat of 115 5 Å along the fibril axis. As can be seen from Table 1, the intense 4.83 Å and its second order at 2.41 Å, which characterize the scattering from the β-strands in the cross-β structure, index as the 24th and 48th orders of the 115.5 Å repeat. This shows that whereas the new X-ray pattern is fully consistent with a cross-β type of structure, the β-strands in the FAP fibrils are grouped into units of 24, hydrogen-bonded together into sheets extended along the axis of the fibrils. It does not seem possible to identify this 24-stranded repeating unit present in the fibril with the TTR molecule which contains much smaller β-structures.

If the 24-stranded repeating unit in the fibrils cannot be related to a 'covalent' unit such as the TTR molecule, it probably represents a structural repeating unit of a so far unidentified type. The probable nature of this

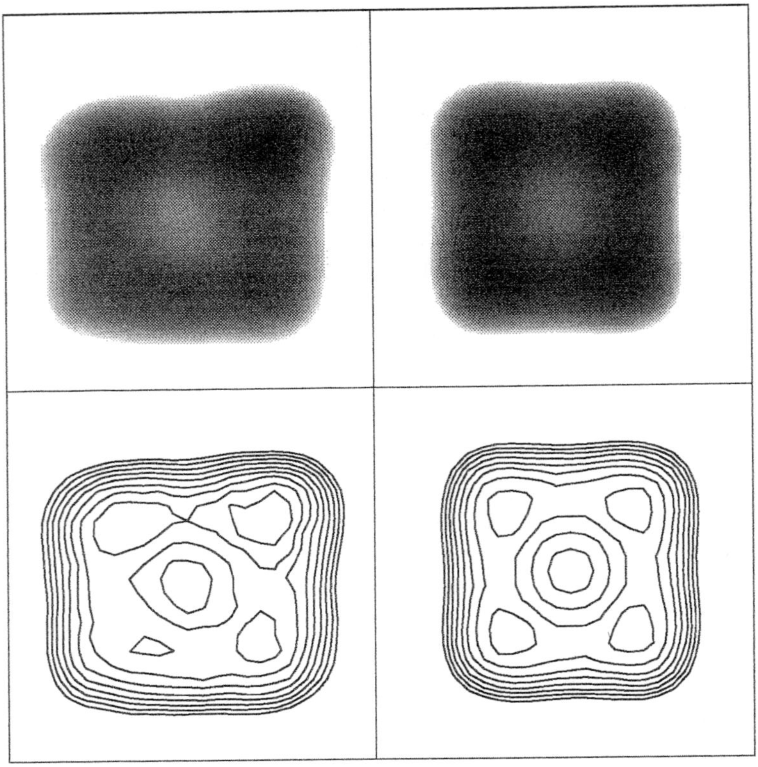

FIG. 2. Cross-sectional electron microscope images of the Met30 FAP amyloid fibril. On the left is the final averaged image (top), and its contoured equivalent (below), and on the right is the result of imposing fourfold symmetry on the final image, in the same format.

TABLE 1 Indices of the meridional reflections

d(obs) (Å)	*Index*	*Calculated repeat (Å)*
4.830	24	115.9
4.625	25	115.6
3.860	30	115.8
3.215	36	115.7
2.880	40	115.2
2.409	48	115.6
2.022	57	115.3

repeating unit is indicated by the observation that the indices of the observed meridional reflections tend to be multiples of three, which is a condition indicative of the presence of a threefold screw axis parallel to the axis of the protofilament. This symmetry operator requires the 24-stranded repeating unit to be composed of three equivalent eight-stranded units, related by a translation of 115.5 Å/3 (or 38.5 Å), and a rotation of 360°/3 (or 120°). A typical eight-stranded β-sheet seen in a globular protein—for example, TTR (Blake et al 1978)—would have a dimension perpendicular to the β-strands of about 38 Å, and a twist of the eighth strand relative to the first of about 120° (see Blake et al 1978). This symmetry operation will therefore generate, from a typically twisted eight-stranded β-sheet, a 24-stranded β-sheet in which the 24th β-strand is twisted by 360° relative to the 0th, around an axis parallel to the fibril axis. This corresponds to a helical arrangement of β-strands in which 24 β-strands form one turn of a helix with a pitch of 115.5 Å, whose axis is parallel to the axis of the protofilament. This 'β-sheet helix' therefore can be identified as the repeating unit implied from the X-ray diffraction pattern of the FAP fibrils. The extension of the X-ray pattern to at least 2.0 Å along the meridian indicates that there is a high degree of crystallinity along the fibril axis, which is only likely to occur if the helical β-sheet structure is extended along the axis of the fibril, or more precisely along the axis of the protofilaments, for long distances relative to the length of the helix. We may therefore regard the protofilaments to be continuously hydrogen-bonded along their total lengths, a factor in explaining the well-known rigidity and stability of the amyloid fibrils.

The equator of the diffraction pattern from the fibrils does not contain Bragg reflections that can be indexed in the same way as the meridional reflections. Instead the diffraction maxima are expected to represent various primary spacings that define the cross-sectional structure of the fibrils. The equatorial reflections from the Met30 FAP fibrils are listed in Table 2. The lowest angle equatorial reflection that is observed is an intense reflection at 64 Å, which corresponds closely with the centre-to-centre spacing of the protofilaments in the fibril as observed in the transverse sections in the electron micrographs (Serpell et al 1995). The so-called 10 Å equatorial reflection of the cross-β structure has been attributed to the characteristic separation of the β-sheets within the fibril. In FAP and other amyloids we have examined, this reflection is often doubled indicating the presence of more than one type of β-sheet separation, and therefore the presence of more than one pair of β-sheets in the protofilament. As argued previously, the diameter of the FAP protofilament is appropriate for four parallel β-sheets which, if arranged symmetrically, would give rise to two different β-sheet spacings: that between sheets 1 and 2, *and* 3 and 4 (say 10.1 Å, see Table 2); and that between sheets 2 and 3 (say 12.6 Å, see Table 2). The reflection at 34 Å could then represent the spacing of β-sheets 1 and 4, and the 20 Å reflection could correspond to the separations of sheets 1

TABLE 2 Spacings of the equatorial reflections

d(obs) (Å)	*Relative intensity*
64	vs
34	s
20.2	vw
12.6	m
10.1	m
7.56	vw
6.05	w
5.32	m
3.94	s

s, strong; m, medium; w, weak; v, very.

and 3, *and* 2 and 4. The equatorial reflections at 6.05 Å and 5.32 Å may be second orders of the main β-sheet spacings. Finally the strong equatorial reflection 3.94 Å will reasonably correspond to the peptide spacing within the regular β-strands arranged perpendicular to the fibril axis.

Molecular model of the amyloid fibril

On the basis of the X-ray and electron microscope data discussed previously, it is possible to build a molecular model that incorporates all the major features that have been indicated. This model is illustrated in Fig. 3. It consists of four β-sheets of indefinite length running parallel to the axis of the protofilament, with their constituent β-strands arranged perpendicular to the axis. Each β-strand is twisted by 15° to its immediate neighbours, a value that is commonly seen in globular proteins, thereby generating a helical twist to the stack of sheets around a common axis coincident to the axis of the protofilament. This helical twist is the most characteristic feature of the present model. If we assume that the four β-sheets of the protofilament occur in two (symmetrical) pairs, each pair enclosing and being stabilized by a hydrophobic core as is normally seen in globular proteins of the 'all-β' type, then the structure that is generated has the character of a double helix. It is in fact a generic structure, albeit one that has not been fully described previously—the β-sheet equivalent of the α-helical coiled coil, which occurs in many natural protein fibres. It is of interest that the β-sheet equivalent is very uncommon, and may only occur in dysfunctional states such as amyloid.

A question of great importance is whether the amyloid structure illustrated in Fig. 3 is representative only of the FAP protofilament, or of amyloid in general. We have used the synchrotron sources at Daresbury and the new

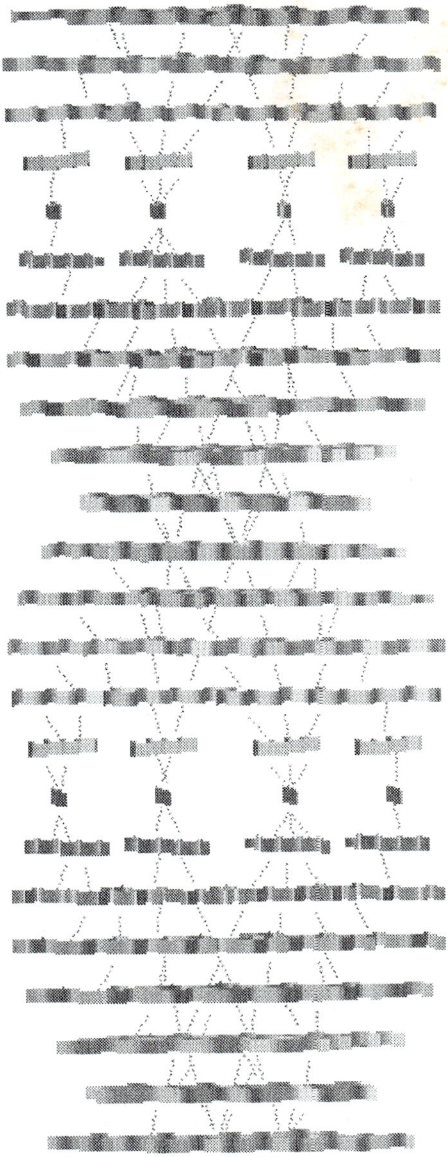

FIG. 3. The molecular model of the protofilament of Met30 FAP, showing one complete helical repeat. The β-strands are represented by the horizontal lines and hydrogen bonds by the broken lines. The helical twist can be perceived by noting the change of the β-strands from being face-on to being end-on, which occurs twice in each helical turn.

European Synchrotron Radiation Source (ESRF) at Grenoble to produce X-ray patterns of other disease-state amyloid fibrils. These include amyloid A, immunoglobulin light chain, apoAI and lysozyme amyloids (kindly provided by Professor Mark Pepys of the Hammersmith Hospital), synthetic fibrils from a fragment of the islet amyloid polypeptide (kindly provided by Dr Ann Clark of the Radcliffe Infirmary), and synthetic fibrils produced from residues 10–19 of TTR. All these amyloids give rise to diffraction patterns that are very similar to those from FAP fibrils, and we can therefore propose that the core structures of these amyloids are related to the model we have outlined here. This does not exclude the possibility, indeed probability, that the detailed structural features of different amyloids may differ widely. For example, amyloid fibrils could be composed of different numbers of protofilaments, or the presence of loops of chains or other structures on the periphery of the β-sheet core could produce protofilaments of different diameters. This to say nothing of the possible presence of glycosaminoglycans or other non-protein components associated with the fibrils. Nevertheless, the presence of a similar β-sheet core, probably in the form of a double helix, is indicated by the X-ray examination.

Acknowledgements

We are grateful for the financial support of the UK Medical Research Council and the European Union's Biomed I Programme.

References

Benson MD, Wallace MR 1989 Amyloidosis. In: Scriver CP, Beaudet AL, Sly WS, Valles D (eds) The metabolic basis of inherited disease. McGraw-Hill, New York, p 2439–2460

Blake C, Geisow M, Rerat B, Rerat C, Swan I 1974 Structure of human plasma prealbumin at 2.5 Å resolution. A preliminary report on the polypeptide chain conformation, quaternary structure and thyroxine binding. J Mol Biol 88:1–12

Blake CCF, Geisow MJ, Oatley SJ, Rerat B, Rerat C 1978 Structure of prealbumin: secondary, tertiary and quaternary interactions determined by Fourier refinement at 1.8 Å. J Mol Biol 121:339–356

Bonar L, Cohen A, Skinner M 1967 Characterization of the amyloid fibril as a cross-β protein. Proc Soc Exp Biol Med 131:1373–1375

Chothia C 1973 Conformations of twisted-β sheets in proteins. J Mol Biol 75:295–302

Colon W, Kelly JW 1992 Partial denaturation of transthyretin is sufficient for amyloid fibril formation *in vitro*. Biochemistry 31:8654–8660

Costa P, Figueira A, Bravo F 1978 Amyloid fibril protein related to prealbumin in familial amyloidotic polyneuropathy. Proc Natl Acad Sci USA 75:4499–4503

Eanes ED, Glenner GG 1968 X-ray diffraction studies on amyloid filaments. J Histochem Cytochem 16:673

Geddes AJ, Parker KD, Atkins EDT, Beighton E 1968 'Cross-β' conformation in proteins. J Mol Biol 32:343–358

Kanda Y, Goodman D, Canfield R, Morgan F 1974 The amino acid sequence of human plasma prealbumin. J Biol Chem 249:6796–6805
Pauling L, Corey R 1951 Configuration of polypeptide chains with favored orientation around single bonds: two new pleated sheets. Proc Natl Acad Sci USA 37:729–735
Pepys MB, Hawkins PN, Booth DR et al 1993 Human lysozyme gene mutations cause hereditary systemic amyloidosis. Nature 362:553–557
Saraiva MJM 1995 Transthyretin mutations in health and disease. Hum Mutat 5: 191–196
Serpell L, Sunde M, Fraser P et al 1995 The examination of the structure of the transthyretin amyloid fibril by image reconstruction from electron micrographs. J Mol Biol 254:113–118
Shirahama T, Cohen AS 1967 High resolution electron microscopic analysis of the amyloid fibril. J Cell Biol 33:679–708
Sipe JD 1992 Amyloidosis. Ann Rev Biochem 61:947–975

DISCUSSION

Kirschner: It is unusual to have so few reflections from a structure such as the one you have described. Do you have any evidence for very small-angle meridional reflections from the proposed large repeat along the fibril axis, for example, at 65 or 115 Å?

Blake: We do have some experimental evidence. Between something over 100 Å and 4.7 Å we don't see any meridional reflections. That is an extraordinary observation when you consider that the TTR molecule is 50 Å in diameter. The explanation could be that in the fibril, TTR is no longer in what you would call a globular state, but instead has become a fibrous protein. I think this is what amyloidosis is, the absorption of a globular protein into a fibrous structure so that the globular characteristics disappear. Otherwise the kind of pattern we are looking at is the sort of pattern one might associate with small peptides; however, we know that here this is not the case, because one can regain the TTR from the amyloid.

Kirschner: Another way to test whether or not the relatively small number of wide-angle reflections that you have used to calculate the large repeat truly belong to this one lattice is to determine whether the half-widths of those reflections are the same. Have you done this?

Blake: We haven't done that specifically, but they appear to be similar. I would point out that they index to the same spacing within three parts in a thousand, which is a very precise agreement.

Kirschner: Is it possible that the few reflections could index to the same period fortuitously?

Blake: They are all rather sharp reflections, looking like Bragg reflections from a highly ordered structure or a highly crystalline material.

Kirschner: Regarding your reflection at 4.7–4.8 Å, which is highly arced: you are proposing that the strands are rigidly perpendicular to the axis of the fibril.

Is it not unusual to have such an arced reflection coming from a structure that is so precisely stacked?

Blake: I don't think so. It simply represents the fact that it is extremely difficult to orient the mass of fibrils to within less than 20°. The striking thing about all electron micrographs of amyloid is that the fibrils don't seem to associate very much with each other. Under these circumstances there is no sort of intrinsic crystallinity within the mass of fibrils, and one simply has to try mechanically to make them more or less parallel to one another—this is difficult to do. The 4.7 Å reflection appears in a wide arc because it is so intensely strong: even where it is much reduced in intensity you can still see it.

Kirschner: One way to approach this would be to use thinner samples. Using a synchrotron beam you might end up seeing sampling along the 4.7 Å arc, indicating that you do have extremely sharp domains along the different fibres, which individually have different orientations.

Blake: We tried using the European synchrotron radiation facility at Grenoble, which has a particularly fine beam. Unfortunately, our sample of FAP was degraded by that time and we got rather poor results.

In terms of further analysis, I think the way forward is to get higher degrees of orientation. This is now the limiting factor: the material is good, but it is difficult to get oriented samples.

Pepys: Your proposal of a final common structure for amyloid fibrils is very attractive. It readily accommodates the TTR structure, but what about the thermodynamic aspects of transforming proteins such as lysozyme or serum amyloid A and its AA fragment, which don't have a well-ordered β-sheet structure in their native state?

Blake: One possibility is that there is an intermediate which is itself structured and about which we know very little. It may be that amyloidotic proteins are converted into this structural intermediate which then is the building block for the amyloid, rather than going directly from the globular form to the amyloid. In cases like tobacco mosaic virus, there is a well defined pathway for doing this in a very rapid way that one would not otherwise imagine. I think it would be worth looking for that intermediate.

Sipe: You showed a diffraction pattern of a peptide from TTR. Is there any particular unique segment of TTR that is fibril-forming?

Blake: In the TTR molecule there are some segments which form amyloid more easily than others, and they happen to correspond to the β-strands. The one that we have the best results for is β-strand A, which consists of residues 10–19.

Sipe: Do the other strands also form amyloid?

Blake: Yes. Others have done experiments with the turns and loops and so on, but these don't appear to form amyloid nearly as readily. One of the most interesting features of the fibril structure is that it can be built from a whole range of different-length polypeptide chains, even from quite small ones. I would guess that the length of a single β-strand would be the lower limit, which is about 9 or 10 residues, but for the upper limit you might just think of polypeptide chains being β-strands linked together covalently and you can have a considerable number of those folded together. So the fibril structure I'm proposing can be accessed from a wide variety of different-length polypeptide chains, which is of course one of the characteristics of amyloid and which is otherwise quite difficult to understand.

Westermark: In most TTR amyloidoses, especially in the senile systemic form where there is only wild-type TTR, but also in the Swedish Met30 variant and the Met111 variant, the TTR molecule is highly spliced. We have had great difficulty in finding the N-terminus in amyloid deposits; we mainly find the C-terminal fragments starting at positions 46, 49 and 52. Would such fragments fit in with your model of fibril formation?

Blake: Possibly. I would emphasize that the model stands independently of whatever mechanism you think is involved for any particular protein. It stands on the basis of the X-ray diffraction patterns, which are basic experimental data. What I've outlined may not be the correct model for TTR, but certainly it stands firmly on good physical foundations. You could probably fit different-length polypeptide chains into the structure, so that if you have TTR with residues 1–49 missing, I don't think that would preclude its incorporation into the fibrils. I started off with TTR because it is convenient to do that, but my model is not dependent on it.

Westermark: Dr Å. Gustavsson in our lab has done a lot of work on synthetic TTR peptides. Recently we have synthesized a segment which is similar to the α-helix and this also forms fibrils.

Blake: If you use structure prediction techniques, you will find that where you get a strong indication of β-sheet you often also get a strong indication of α-helix, and vice versa. So, on the basis of prediction, it is not impossible that α-helices can be converted to β-sheets rather easily, and then be incorporated into the amyloid.

Kelly: Over the past five years we have made 300–400 different peptides that have nothing to do with amyloid disease—that is, the sequences aren't from real proteins—and the vast majority of these peptides self-assemble into something that very closely approaches the amyloid structure. So I agree with your statement that these structures are really thermodynamic minimum. Many peptides have the ability to self-assemble into this type of structure. I believe that there is a critical structure that makes this possible, and you can assess that both from the unfolded state which most peptides exhibit, or from a folded protein like lysozyme, which clearly has to change conformation before it can make fibrils.

Your model can accommodate a variety of different lengths of TTR. Is it possible that instead of a four-stranded subunit, you have a three-strand repeating unit, so you would still have 24 strands but the dimer would be six strands wide instead of eight? This would explain many of the data in the literature, particularly the observation that the N-terminus is often cut off.

Blake: I would have to think about that. This proposal about the nicking of the polypeptide chain has been experimentally determined for a long time, but there doesn't seem to be any definitive evidence that, for example, 49–127 forms amyloid or that in amyloid deposits you can only find that fragment and not the rest of the molecule.

Pepys: Protein sequencing of fibril subunits from our patient with the TTR Val47 mutation (Booth et al 1994) revealed a minor component with the wild-type Gly residue at position 47 as the N-terminus, and most of the material starting at position 49.

Blake: Of course, it is possible that although the chain is nicked, the pieces stay together. I don't think it would affect the model I produced, but it might relate to how one actually incorporates TTR into the fibril.

Pepys: Since we all seem to be attacking your model, I would like to put on record what a spectacular advance it actually is. It is far ahead of everything that has gone before.

Blake: But I do think it is important to question it, because the fact that the fibrils do not form an ordered crystalline array means that we have only the minimum data we need to develop a model like this—one would feel rather more comfortable with further data.

Lundgren: A comment on the N-terminal fragment: in the amyloid from the vitreous body of the eye we find a mixture of nicked and full length peptides and we also often find N-terminal fragments. When we trypsinize these amyloid fibrils, we lose all the full length peptides and end up with the N-terminal and 49–127 fragments. So, at least in the eye material, we think that the cleavage is secondary and not important for fibril formation.

If I understand your model correctly, the four filaments stick together. How do they do that, and how do they build up?

Blake: That's a very interesting question. This raises the possible involvement of proteoglycans in amyloidogenesis. One idea is that they form a sort of structural framework for the filament formation. In addition, I'm not sure whether we have four equivalent protofilaments—that is, a fourfold axis of symmetry—or whether this is a sort of double ribbon. One sees ribbons quite frequently and it may be that these are two ribbons put face to face. There's a hint of asymmetry in the electron micrographs. But that is a problem—and it is a very interesting one, because we never see frayed ends of separate protofilaments. Furthermore, it is very difficult to find electron micrographs of separate protofilaments; they always seem to associate into fibrils of at least two protofilaments, if not more.

Goldgaber: Proteoglycans probably won't explain the fibril-like appearance of synthetic peptides produced *in vitro*.

Blake: No, they are obviously not important to that. We haven't carried out electron microscope studies sufficient to say how many protofilaments in the fibrils form synthetic peptides. It is one of the things I would very much like to see done, because again the question concerns whether they form single protofilaments, or whether they are paired or multiplied. If they are, then it is something other than proteoglycan that is holding them together. And it is quite difficult to envisage what the nature of a connection would be that always operated.

Kelly: It is interesting that some of the fibrils that are formed *in vitro* don't look exactly like the fibrils that you form *in vivo*. In many cases they resemble protofilaments. When we make them in a test tube they often associate laterally into very large entities. It could be that you are correct in suggesting that the proteoglycans help the final assembly and stabilize the fibrils. In addition, often the fibrils we make *in vitro* are unstable. The extracellular matrix components might be critical in stabilizing them and in bringing in the protofilaments.

Blake: So there may be initial forms that then assemble into the final state that we have described.

Merlini: You suggested that amyloid might be a single structural entity with a minimal energy state that various proteins can achieve through different structural reshapings. This common structure offers hope of finding structure-specific drugs which could be active in all kinds of amyloidoses, irrespective of their biochemical composition. One possibility is that potential drugs could be designed to intercalate in the 'helical' structure of amyloid fibrils. Does this possibility fit your model?

Blake: Once you see a ladder structure you immediately think of intercalation of planar molecules as a possible mode of interaction.

Kirschner: With amyloid diffraction patterns that have so few reflections, it is relatively simple to model them. It is crucial, therefore, to come up with ways to test the models. Have you any ideas about testing the model that you propose?

Blake: One important test is to compare electron microscopy and X-ray diffraction data, and we've tried to do this. I showed the optical reconstructions of the fibrils in which there are repeating units of about 40 Å, which would correspond pretty closely with the 115.5 Å divided by three repeat that we saw in the X-ray pattern. That kind of comparison needs to be done, but we do need to increase the quality of the X-ray patterns. I think this is best done by making samples and trying to boost the orientation to produce layer lines and row lines, which give more information. All studies of fibrous proteins have gone through stages where the initial diffraction patterns looked pretty awful, and later on people produced better specimens and better diffraction patterns where you can be doing real crystallography.

Kirschner: It was suggested to me, at a biophysics conference in Jerusalem in 1987, that the cross-β conformation was just a dustbin of protein structure.

This notion goes along with the theme at this symposium that the cross-β conformation is just a minimum-energy state for many of these proteins.

Blake: In relation to that, it is a remarkable thing that in 60 years of X-ray diffraction of fibrous proteins, there have been no natural animal proteins that I'm aware of that have the cross-β structure. If this is true then amyloid is unique in its structure within our bodies.

Kirschner: Amyloid fibrils *do* provide an almost unique example of β-sheets that form an *oligomeric cross-β fibrillar assembly*. However, a number of other naturally occurring proteins also form β-structures which, unlike the amyloid in diseased tissues, have functional roles. For such proteins, the morphologies include fibre, rod, tube, ribbon and plate. β-keratin (Fraser & MacRae 1962), feather keratin (Fraser et al 1971) and silk (Marsh et al 1955a,b) form fibres where the β-strands are parallel to the fibre direction. In contrast, in *Chrysopa* silk the polypeptide chains are oriented perpendicular to the ribbon direction, thus forming a cross-β structure (Geddes et al 1968). The rod-like shafts of the adenovirus fibre (Green et al 1983) and of the tail fibre of bacteriophage T4 (Earnshaw et al 1979) have cross-β arrangements of protein. Cylindrical, ion-channel tubes in membranes, such as formed by α-toxin (Tobkes et al 1985) and porin (Kleffel et al 1985), consist of oligomeric proteins with a β-barrel arrangement in which the chains run normal to the surface of the membrane. As a final example, membrane-like plates in a bacterium cell wall have been identified in which polypeptide chains in the β-conformation run parallel to the surface of the cell wall (Blaurock & Walsby 1976, Blaurock & Wober 1976, Stewart et al 1985).

Kelly: There's a new fold coming out in *Science* in three weeks that's very interesting. It is effectively a left-handed β-helix trimer in the protein UDP-*N*-acetylglucosamine-3-*O*-acyltransferase (Raetz & Roderick 1995).

References

Blaurock AE, Walsby AE 1976 Crystalline structure of the gas vesicle wall from *Anabaena flos-aquae*. J Mol Biol 105:183–199

Blaurock AE, Wober W 1976 Structure of the wall of *Halobacterium halobium* gas vesicles. J Mol Biol 106:871–888

Booth DR, Soutar AK, Hawkins PN, Reilly M, Harding A, Pepys MB 1994 Three new amyloidogenic transthyretin gene mutations: advantages of direct sequencing. In: Kisilevsky R, Benson MD, Frangione B, Gauldie J, Muckle TJ, Young ID (eds) Amyloid and amyloidosis 1993. Parthenon, Park Ridge, NJ, p456–458

Earnshaw WC, Goldberg EB, Crowther RA 1979 The distal half of the tail fibre of bacteriophage T4. Rigidly linked domains and cross-β structure. J Mol Biol 132: 101–131

Fraser RDB, MacRae TP 1962 An investigation of the structure of β-keratin. J Mol Biol 5:457–466

Fraser RDB, MacRae TP, Parry DAD, Suzuki E 1971 The structure of feather keratin. Polymer 12:35–56

Geddes AJ, Parker KD, Atkins EDT, Beighton E 1968 'Cross-β' conformation in proteins. J Mol Biol 32:343–358
Green KM, Wrigley NG, Russell WC, Martin SR, McLachlan AD 1983 Evidence for a repeating cross-β sheet structure in the adenovirus fibre. EMBO J 2:1357–1365
Kleffel B, Garavito RM, Baumeister W, Rosenbusch JP 1985 Secondary stature of a channel-forming protein: porin from *E. coli* outer membranes. EMBO J 4:1589–1592
Marsh RE, Corey RB, Pauling L 1955a An investigation of the structure of silk fibroin. Biochim Biophys Acta 16:1–34
Marsh RE, Corey RB, Pauling L 1955b The structure of Tussah silk fibroin. Acta Cryst 8:710–715
Raetz CRH, Roderick SL 1995 A left-handed parallel β-helix in the structure of UDP-*N*-acetylglucosamine acyltransferase. Science 270:997–1000
Stewart M, Beveridge TJ, Sprott GD 1985 Crystalline order to high resolution in the sheath of *Methanospirillium hungatei*: a cross-β structure. J Mol Biol 183:509–515
Tobkes N, Wallace BA, Bayley H 1985 Secondary structure and assembly mechanism of an oligomeric channel protein. Biochemistry 24:1915–1920

Refined fibril structures: the hydrophobic core in Alzheimer's amyloid β-protein and prion as revealed by X-ray diffraction

Hideyo Inouye and Daniel A. Kirschner*

Department of Biological Sciences, University of Massachusetts at Lowell, Olsen 6, One University Avenue, Lowell, MA 01854, USA

Abstract. From the wide-angle, equatorial X-ray data of a β-amyloid analogue, we previously calculated the electron density of the constituent β-crystallite, which assembles as multimers (four to six crystallites) in building the amyloid fibre. In the scattering region where the spacing $d < \sim 10$ Å, the observed reflections were indexed by an orthogonal lattice with a unit cell having $a = 9.44$ Å, $b = 6.92$ Å and $c = 10.76$ Å. The phases were initially derived from the atomic coordinates of the β-keratin backbone and were optimized by including new peaks (as point atom or sphere) in the subsequent Fourier iteration. The R-factor between the observed and calculated amplitudes was refined to 35%. In further developing our analysis, we have now applied an alternative constraint to the optimization by eliminating the negative electron densities, and found that the R-factor decreased to 19% after three iterations. The refined electron density map fits phenylalanine, indicating that the amyloid core likely comes from the hydrophobic Leu-Val-Phe-Phe residues. We have applied the same type of optimization, using β-silk as an initial phase model, to the hydrophobic H1 domain of the prion protein for which the monoclinic unit cell constants are $a = 9.51$ Å, $b = 7.06$ Å, $c = 15.94$ Å and $\beta = 88.4°$. The R-factor decreased to 11% from 64% after two iterations. The electron density map shows a silk-like quarter-staggered arrangement of β-sheets which, in the intersheet direction, have circular peaks in one β-sheet and elongated peaks in the alternating β-sheet. These peaks were interpreted as arising from the C-terminal alanine-rich domain and N-terminal hydrophobic residues. Skeletal atomic models for these core regions support this interpretation.

1996 The nature and origin of amyloid fibrils. Wiley, Chichester (Ciba Foundation Symposium 199) p 22–39

Amyloid is characterized by Congo red birefringence, an ultrastructure consisting of 60–100 Å diameter fibrils, and a cross-β X-ray diffraction pattern

*Present address: Department of Biology, Higgins Hall, Boston College, Chestnut Hill, MA 02167, USA.

(Glenner 1980). A model for amyloid proposed in 1974 (Cooper 1974) shows a pair of stacks of β-sheets twisted about one another, with the hydrogen bonding along the fibre axis. The cross section is rectangular, and has dimensions of 40 Å × 40 Å (chain and intersheet directions). The stacks in the fibre are separated from one another by 20 Å, resulting in an outermost diameter of 100 Å. We recently proposed a more detailed model based on X-ray analysis of samples of oriented fibres assembled from synthetic peptides having sequences identical to amyloid β-protein (Aβ) of Alzheimer's disease (Inouye et al 1993). The electron density map gave direct evidence that β-crystallites constitute the core structure of amyloid—specifically, four to six β-crystallites assemble into a hollow cylinder. In the current study, we report on our efforts to obtain a refined electron density map that provides additional details about the structure of the β-crystallite. We present a new X-ray refinement strategy for both cylindrically averaged (as a fibre) and spherically averaged (as a powder) scattering objects. Application of this approach to the X-ray patterns from Aβ11–28 and the H1 prion peptide is described.

Methods

Sequences

The Aβ11–28 analogue and H1 peptide correspond, respectively, to residues 11–28 of the Alzheimer's Aβ protein and to the first helical domain of the Syrian hamster prion PrP^{Sc} (Nguyen et al 1995):

11–28: Glu-Val-His-His-Gln-Lys-Leu-Val-Phe-Phe-Ala-Glu-Asp-Val-Gly-Ser-Asn-Lys
a a a a a a a a a a a a a a c c c c

H1: Met-Lys-His-Met-Ala-Gly-Ala-Ala-Ala-Ala-Gly-Ala-Val-Val
a a a a a a a a a a a a a b

Secondary structure predictions based on these primary sequences were carried out as previously described (Inouye & Kirschner 1991) using Garnier's method with a zero decision constant (Garnier et al 1978). The predominant conformation was α-helical (a; see above), with a short stretch of either coil (c) or β-conformation (b) at the C-terminus. Sample preparation for X-ray diffraction was described previously (Inouye et al 1993, Nguyen et al 1995).

Densitometry and measurement of the intensity

The X-ray diffraction patterns were recorded and digitized as described (Inouye et al 1993, Nguyen et al 1995). Two-dimensional intensities were displayed after converting the raw image data to the optical density scale. The intensities of the arced reflections were circularly averaged within a defined angle to reduce random noise. The software for image handling and display were provided and installed by Dr Tom Tibbitts (Boston College, Chestnut Hill, MA; Tibbits & Caspar 1993).

The intensity curve was obtained after subtraction of the background, which was fit by a polynomial. The integral areas and integral widths of the observed peaks were obtained by fitting a Gaussian function to the intensity profile (Inouye et al 1989). The actual fit to the observed peak by the peak function was carried out by optimizing the input data, i.e. the peak heights and half widths, by a least-squares routine. The film coordinates were changed to reciprocal coordinates and the intensity was corrected and normalized.

Strategy to index the reflections

The lattice constants and indices were determined by comparing the observed and calculated spacings for different combinations of indices. The search was constrained by a range of lattice constants and indices. In most cases the unit cell was assumed as either orthogonal or monoclinic and the range of angle was set between 90° and 120°. The lattice constants were subsequently optimized with fixed indices.

Cylindrically and spherically averaged intensity of a crystal with a limited size

We previously used a numerical method to calculate the cylindrically averaged intensity profile (Inouye et al 1993). However, the formulation for the case of a crystallite having a limited number of lattice points was not presented. In the following, the intensity function for this (Fraser et al 1984) will be given. Starting with the Laue function, we write the interference function of the crystallite as

$$I(\mathbf{R}) = \frac{\sin^2 \pi N_a \mathbf{aR}}{\sin^2 \pi \mathbf{aR}} \frac{\sin^2 \pi N_b \mathbf{bR}}{\sin^2 \pi \mathbf{bR}} \frac{\sin^2 \pi N_c \mathbf{cR}}{\sin^2 \pi \mathbf{cR}} \tag{1}$$

where $\mathbf{R}$ is the reciprocal vector, and N_a, N_b, and N_c are the numbers of the unit cell in the **a,b,c** directions. By using the orthogonal unit cell vectors (**a,b,c**), the reciprocal vector is defined as $\mathbf{R} = X\mathbf{a}/a + Y\mathbf{b}/b + Z\mathbf{c}/c$. Replacing $\mathbf{R}$ in equation (1) gives

$$I(X,Y,Z) = \frac{\sin^2 \pi a N_a X}{\sin^2 \pi a X} \frac{\sin^2 \pi b N_b Y}{\sin^2 \pi b Y} \frac{\sin^2 \pi c N_c Z}{\sin^2 \pi c Z} . \tag{2}$$

Since at the origin,

$$\frac{\sin^2 \pi a N_a X}{\sin^2 \pi a X} = N_a{}^2 \, \mathrm{sinc}^2(\pi a N_a X) = N_a{}^2 \exp(-\pi (a N_a)^2 X^2), \tag{3}$$

the Laue function can be given by

$$I(X,Y,Z) = N^2 I(X_0,Y_0,Z_0)\exp\{-\pi[p_x{}^2(X-X_0)^2 + p_y{}^2(Y-Y_0)^2 + p_z{}^2(Z-Z_0)^2]\} \tag{4}$$

where $p_x = aN_a$, $p_y = bN_b$, $p_z = cN_c$ and $N = N_a N_b N_c$. The Bragg reflections are discrete at $X_0 = h/a$, $Y_0 = k/b$ and $Z_0 = \ell/c$ where h,k,ℓ, (Miller indices) are integers. Assuming that a rotation axis is on the Z-axis, the cylindrically averaged intensity for a meridional reflection is

$$I(R,Z) = I(0,0,Z_0)\exp[-\pi p_z{}^2(Z-Z_0)^2]\exp[-\pi R^2(p_x{}^2+p_y{}^2)/2]\, I_0[\pi R^2(p_x{}^2-p_y{}^2)/2] \tag{5}$$

where I_0 is the modified Bessel function of the second kind, given by

$$I_0(x) = \left(\int_0^{2\pi} \exp[x\cos(\phi)]d\phi\right)/2\pi. \tag{6}$$

When the coherent lengths along the x and y axes are the same, i.e., $p_x = p_y = p$, equation (4) is simplified by using the modified Bessel function of the second kind. The cylindrically averaged intensity therefore is given by

$$I_c(R,Z) = I(X_0,Y_0,Z_0)\exp[-\pi p_z{}^2(Z-Z_0)^2]\exp[-\pi p^2(R-R_0)^2]\, i_0(2\pi p^2 R_0 R) \tag{7}$$

where $i_0(x) = \exp(-x)I_0(x)$, and $R_0{}^2 = X_0{}^2 + Y_0{}^2$.

The cylindrically or spherically averaged intensities $I_c(R,Z)$ and $I_s(R)$ can be numerically calculated as a function of the radial coordinates R where $R_{ij} = (X_i^2 + Y_j^2)^{1/2}$ for a cylinder with Z as a cylinder axis, and $R_{ijk} = (X_i^2 + Y_j^2 + Z_k^2)^{1/2}$ for a sphere. The intensities are given by

$$I_c(R,Z) = \sum_i \sum_j I(X_i,Y_j,Z)/R, \quad \text{for } R - \Delta < R_{ij} < R + \Delta \tag{8}$$

$$I_s(R) = \sum_i \sum_j \sum_k I(X_i, Y_j, Z_k)/R^2, \quad \text{for } R - \Delta < R_{ijk} < R + \Delta \qquad (9)$$

where R in the last term refers to the Lorentz type correction factor (Cella et al 1970) which relates the calculated intensity to the observed intensity in the radial direction, and Δ is determined by experimental conditions, and includes the breadth of the incident beam, optical geometry and disorder.

Phase optimization procedure: Fourier synthesis combined with electron density modification

In most fibre diffraction studies one uses the model building approach and bypasses calculating the electron density map. For the fibre X-ray diffraction patterns obtained for the Aβ peptides, however, we found the conventional Fourier synthesis approach to be successful (Inouye et al 1993). Both in fibre and powder diffraction, a difficult problem is to separate from the observed intensity the multiple (superimposed) structure factors that have different indices. By using the predicted ratios among the calculated intensities from the model and dividing the observed intensity in proportion to it, the superimposed reflections can be separated. In conventional crystallography the atom positions and types can then be chosen from the calculated map in the subsequent Fourier iteration. We used a similar approach previously (Inouye et al 1993), but the R-factor did not decrease much. In the new procedure we derived the new map by eliminating negative electron density, where the density is calculated on a relative scale. This solvent flattening type of procedure enhanced the peaks and resulted in a smaller R-factor. This approach has been used by others—e.g. Worthington & Khare (1978) used it to solve the autocorrelation function in membrane diffraction; Stroud & Agard (1979) applied it in interpreting the continuous scattering intensity of nerve myelin; Makowski (1981) applied it to fibre diffraction; and Wang (1985) used the method for single crystal analysis. Our procedure is as follows:

(1) Choose the initial phase model which defines the atomic fraction coordinates (x_j, y_j, z_j) for the jth atom in the unit cell.

(2) Calculate the structure factor $F_{calc}(hk\ell)$ with a given range of h,k,ℓ) and the observed unit cell. The atomic coordinates in the unit cell are derived by symmetry operation. Here, $F_{calc}(hk\ell) = \Sigma_j f_j \exp(i2\pi(hx_j + ky_j + \ell z_j))$ where j refers to the atomic position in the unit cell, and f_j is the atomic factor.

(3) Combine the observed structure amplitude $|F_{obs}(hk\ell)|$ as derived from the observed integral intensity and calculated phase $\phi_{calc}(hk\ell)$. This process is not straightforward because of the multiple indices contributing to the peak in

fibre and powder diffraction. To assign $hk\ell$ indices for the peak, we define the critical value of variation from the observed spacing (see Δ in equations 8 and 9). If the difference between the calculated spacing and the observed one is less than this, the reflection is accepted as a component of the observed peak. Ideally the lower limit of the critical values should be defined by the breadth of the direct beam and the raster size. If the integral width of the direct beam is W_d in film space and the distance between the peak position and the direct beam (L), the two peaks at L and $L+W_d$ can be distinguished. The deviation in Bragg spacing δd is given by

$$\delta d = -W_d(\lambda/4s)(\cos\theta \cos^2 2\theta/\sin^2\theta) \tag{10}$$

where λ is the wavelength, s is the specimen-to-film distance and 2θ is the scattering angle. Here the peak distances L and $L+W_d$ as measured from the origin correspond to the Bragg spacings d and $d+\delta d$, respectively. The extent of deviation increases with an increase of the Bragg spacing. The combined structure factor is given by

$$F(hk\ell) = |F_{obs}(hk\ell)| \exp i\phi_{calc}(hk\ell) \tag{11}$$

where ϕ is the phase angle. The observed structure amplitude is given from the cylindrically averaged intensity $I_c(R,Z)$ or the spherically averaged intensity $I_s(R)$ and the calculated structure amplitude, according to

$$|F_{obs}(hk\ell)|^2 = C(hk\ell)\int I_c(R,Z)dR/LP \text{ or } = C(hk\ell)\int I_s(R)dR/LP \tag{12}$$

where $C(hk\ell)=|F_{calc}(hk\ell)|^2/\Sigma|F_{calc}(hk\ell)|^2$, and LP is the Lorentz-polarization factor. Here, the integration along the radial direction covers the peak centred at $R=R_0$. The indices $(hk\ell)$ for summation should satisfy $|R_{hk}{}^{-1}-R^{-1}|<\delta d$ for cylindrically averaged intensity and $|R_{hk\ell}{}^{-1}-R^{-1}|<\delta d$ for spherically averaged intensity, where R_{hk} and $R_{hk\ell}$ are the radial components of the Bragg reflections in cylindrical and spherical coordinates, respectively. (In our calculation, the deviation was due to the raster size; i.e., 0.1 Å for Aβ, 0.03 Å for H1 lyophilized, and 0.05 Å for H1 dried from acetonitrile.) Note that the observed structure amplitude in this procedure is, therefore, model dependent (Inouye et al 1993).

(4) Calculate the electron density map in a unit cell on a relative scale and fix the negative electron densities as zero. (In our calculation here, the step in the calculation was 0.2 Å.) The zero density here corresponds to the average electron density in the unit cell.

(5) Calculate structure factors. Go back to step (3) above. The iteration is terminated when the R-factor converges.

Results and discussion

X-ray diffraction patterns of Aβ11–28 and H1 domain of PrP prion peptide

X-ray diffraction from Aβ11–28 (Fig. 1A and Table 1) showed a cross-β fibre pattern, in which the rotation axis (as the fibre axis) is along the direction of the H-bond spacing at ~4.7 Å. Due to cylindrical rotation the reflections on the layer lines were indexed two dimensionally as (hkℓ) where h = 0 on the equator, and h = 1 and h = 2 on the first and second layer lines. The widths of the meridional reflections (h00) along the fibre direction were much sharper than those on the layer lines as measured along the radial direction, indicating that the crystallite along the fibre direction was much larger than the one in the other two directions. The crystallite, therefore, has an elongated shape. For H1 (Fig. 1B), the lyophilized sample gave a powder pattern, indicating that the β-crystallites distribute randomly. By contrast, the acetonitrile-treated sample of H1 showed a fibre pattern in which the rotation axis along the equator is in the direction of the β-chain. The widths of the reflections in the intersheet and H-bonding directions were sharp, indicating that the crystallite was a flattened

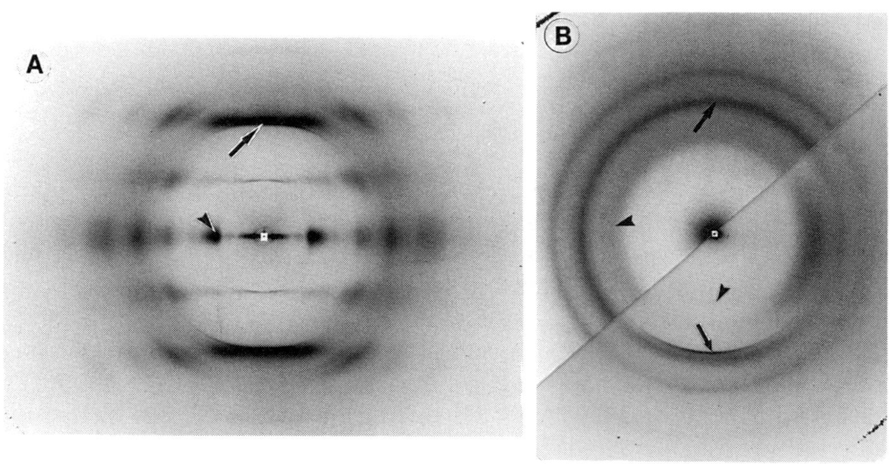

FIG. 1. X-ray diffraction patterns of (A) Aβ11–28 and (B) the H1 domain of PrP^{Sc} (*upper left*, lyophilized; *lower right*, dried from 50% acetonitrile). The H-bonding (arrow) and intersheet (arrowhead) reflections are shown in each pattern. In H1 (lyophilized), it is the (201) reflection that is indicated, while in the other patterns it is the (200) reflection.

TABLE 1 Bragg spacings for Aβ11–28 and H1 PrP peptides

Aβ11–28		*H1 (PrP^{Sc}109–122)*	
		Lyophilized	*Dried from 50% AcN*
$a=9.44$		$a=9.58$	$a=9.51$
$b=6.92$		b –	$b=7.06$
$c=10.76$		$c=11.84$	$c=15.94$
			$\beta=88.4°$
10.76 (Es) (001)	9.15 (1Lm) (100)	5.91 (Cw) (002)	5.67 (Em) (110)
5.45 (Ew) (002)	7.07 (1Lw) (101)	4.44 (Cs) (201)	7.99 (Mw) (002)
4.25 (Em) (012)	5.40 (1Lw) (110)	3.73 (Cm) (202)	4.77 (Ms) (200)
3.51 (Ew) (020)	4.94 (1Lm) (111)	2.98 (Cvw) (004)	4.57 (Mm) (201)
3.32 (Evw) (021)	3.92 (1Lw) (112)		3.94 (Mw) (004)
2.86 (Evw) (022)	4.72 (2Lvs) (200)		3.74 (Mm) (104)
	4.49 (2Lm) (201)		2.97 (Mw) (302)
	3.90 (2Lw) (210)		
	3.66 (2Lm) (211)		
	3.18 (2Lvw) (212)		
	2.77 (2Lvw) (220)		
	3.10 (3Lvw) (300)		

a,b,c, are the β-crystallite unit dimensions, in Å, of the orthogonal or monoclinic lattice. E, equator; M, meridian; C, concentric rings; 1L, 2L, 3L, the first, second and third layer lines; vw, w m, s, vs indicate increasing intensity from very weak→weak→moderate→strong→very strong. AcN, acetonitrile.

sheet. The wide-angle reflections for Aβ11–28 and both types of H1 samples were indexed by an orthogonal or monoclinic lattices (Table 1). The ~4.4 Å reflection in H1 was indexed as (201) where *c* is twice as large as the intersheet separation. Therefore, the unit cell in Aβ is primitive, while in H1 it is face-centered. In the latter, the β-sheets are quarter-staggered in the H-bonding direction (Geddes et al 1968). The former arrangement is similar to that in β-keratin (Fraser & MacRae 1962) and the latter is similar to that in β-silk (Marsh et al 1955a,b).

Iterative Fourier synthesis

Our previous calculation of the β-crystallite electron density for Aβ11–28 was based on the equatorial reflections (Inouye et al 1993). The initial phases were derived from the atomic coordinates of β-keratin (Fraser & MacRae 1962) and the phases were optimized against the observed wide-angle equatorial reflections by choosing peaks to be represented by point atoms or spheres. The R-factor between the observed and calculated amplitudes was refined to 35% from 42% (Inouye et al 1993). In the procedure of Fourier iteration reported here, the phases were refined by the alternative constraint of eliminating negative electron densities (on a relative scale) rather than by picking new atomic positions. Using this strategy, we were able to decrease the R-factor to 21% from 42% after a single iteration, and to 19% after three iterations (Fig. 2 and Table 2). For the diffraction patterns from H1 the initial phases were derived from the atomic coordinates of β-silk (Marsh et al 1955b).

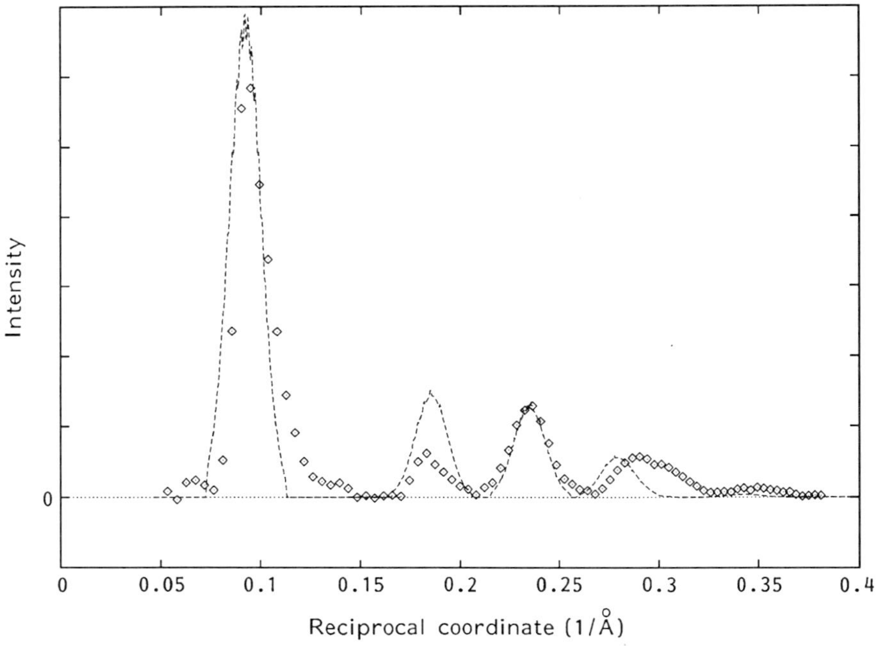

FIG. 2. Equatorial intensity (observed, data points; calculated, dashed line) of Aβ11–28 as a function of reciprocal coordinate (1/Å). The calculated intensity was corrected for the Lorentz and polarization factors in order to fit the observed intensity. The intensity was first calculated every 4.66×10^{-5} Å^{-1}, corresponding to 5 μm at the incident beam position on the film, which was scanned at 50 μm. The specimen-to-film distance was 69.6 mm. The final curve presented here was derived by averaging the calculated intensity data every 50 μm. The areas under the curves were normalized to unity. The fibre tilt and disorientation angles were set to zero. The integral widths of all reflections were set to a constant value (0.02 Å^{-1}) which is the same as that of the 10 Å (001) reflection. Note that the intensity was derived from the calculated structure factors. The electron density map (Fig. 3) was calculated from the observed structure amplitudes and the optimized phases.

TABLE 2 R-factors (%) as a function of number of Fourier iteration

		H1	
Iteration	*Aβ11–28*	*Lyophilized*	*Dried from AcN*
0	41.6	44.5	64.2
1	21.0	25.5	12.5
2	20.0	17.4	11.4
3	19.5	13.4	
4		15.0	
5		15.3	

AcN, acetonitrile.

The R-factor decreased very rapidly and reached 15% and 11% for the lyophilized and acetonitrile treated H1 peptides, respectively (Table 2; see Nguyen et al 1995 for comparison between the observed and calculated intensity).

Skeletal model of Aβ11–28

The calculated electron density map was interactively fit by an atomic model using the XtalView display (McRee 1992). The optimized map (Fig. 3A) showed new peaks located outside the peptide backbone. The peak positions were distant from the backbone and positioned in a diagonal direction from the axis connecting the Cα and Cβ positions. Using XtalView to examine the fit of different sidechains to this peak, we found that phenylalanine fit best. The atomic model of phenylalanine was then refined in XtalView by changing the torsion angle, and the rotation and translation parameters (Fig. 3A). We previously proposed that the β-crystallite portion of the Aβ fibril is likely constituted by hydrophobic residues (Inouye et al 1993). This was based on the observation that the peak positions of the electron density map was consistent with larger or bulkier side chains typical of hydrophobic residues. Here, we report that phenylalanine, in particular, fits the observed peaks. That the hydrophobic phenylalanine is the main component in the β-crystallite explains why a reduced β-sheet content is obtained when the hydrophobic residues Leu-Val-Phe-Phe of the peptide are substituted (Hilbich et al 1992).

Skeletal model of H1 core structure

The electron density projections along the *b*-axis (chain direction) (Fig. 4) showed peaks that were located every ~4.7 Å along the H-bond direction. For

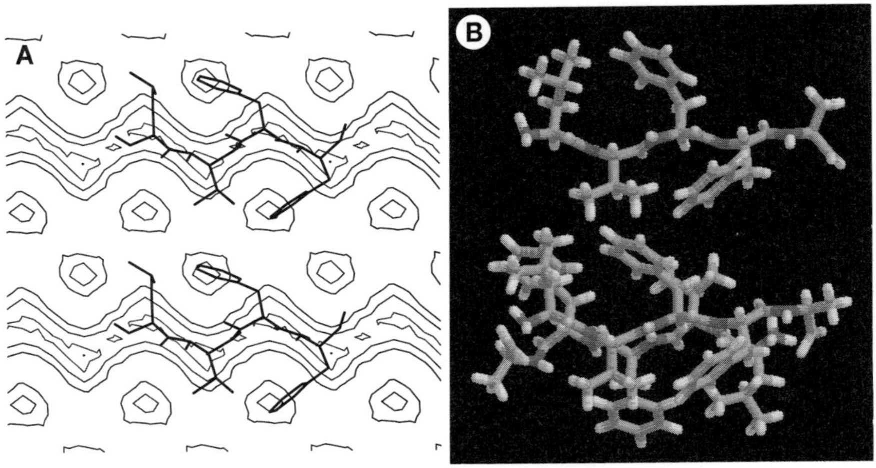

FIG. 3. Electron density map and models of Aβ11–28. (A) The electron density is projected onto the plane defined by the intersheet (vertical) and polypeptide chain (horizontal) directions. The H-bonding direction is normal to the page. The density map was calculated from the observed structure amplitudes and the optimized, calculated phases using XtalView. The peaks in the intersheet space were fit by the side chain of phenylalanine using XtalView's Xfit program. The skeletal model that overlays the density map includes the residues Leu-Val-Phe-Phe in the hydrophobic core. The relative electron densities are between −101 and 104, and the contours are drawn at levels of 0, 40, 80 and 104. (B) Atomic model of the hydrophobic core, which was built using QUANTA. The lower part shows two H-bonded chains that are arranged as antiparallel β-strands.

both types of H1 samples (lyophilized and acetonitrile-treated) the peaks defining each β-sheet were always quarter-staggered along the H-bond direction relative to those on the neighbouring β-sheets. While the electron density peaks in lyophilized H1 were circular in profile similar to the one in the proposed poly-Ala domain with H1 (Nguyen et al 1995), those in H1 treated by acetonitrile were circular in one β-sheet and elongated (in the intersheet direction) in the alternating sheet. The molecular interpretation of this projected density is that in lyophilized H1 the poly-Ala domain forms each entire β-chain, whereas in the acetonitrile-treated H1, there is an intramolecular turn that creates two β-chain domains, one from poly-Ala and one from larger residues. To model this, we used QUANTA (MSI, Inc., Burlington, MA) to build an atomic model, and then fit the electron density map to the model using XtalView. The turn region was assigned to Gly-Ala-Ala and the rest of the residues were built in an anti-parallel β-conformation. The circular peaks were fit by the C-terminal six residues (Ala-Ala-Gly-Ala-Val-Val), and the elongated ones were fit by the N-terminal five residues (Met-Lys-His-Met-

Ala) (Fig. 4, skeletal model). In this arrangement of residues and conformation, the hydrophobic Met, His and Ala residues face the Ala, Gly and Val residues. The intramolecular intersheet interaction is therefore hydrophobic, while the inter-molecular intersheet space, which contains Lys, is hydrophilic.

Conclusion

The transition from α-helix to β-chain appears to be relevant to the neuropathological processes involving Alzheimer's Aβ and PrP. Here we have

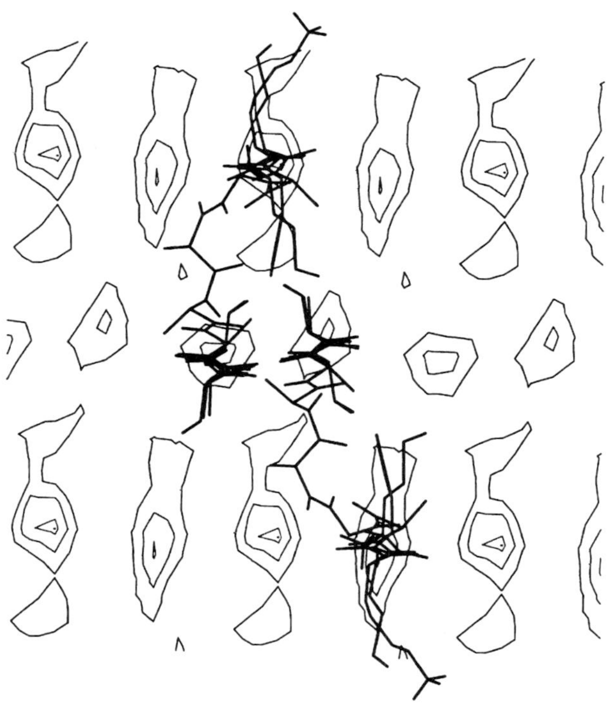

FIG. 4. Electron density map and skeletal model of the acetonitrile-treated H1 peptide of PrP^{Sc}. The density map is projected onto the plane defined by the intersheet (vertical) and H-bonding (horizontal) directions. The polypeptide chain direction is normal to the page, and the screw axis relating the chains is parallel to the H-bonding direction. The electron density was calculated from the observed structure amplitudes and the optimized phases using XtalView. The relative electron densities were between −113 and 141, and the contour level starts at 25 and has an interval of 50. The two types of β-pleated sheets suggested by the localized and less-localized maxima are interpreted here to signify an intramolecular turn in the H1 peptide, with the small side chains of Ala-Ala-Gly-Ala-Val-Val comprising one sheet, and the larger side chains of Met-Lys-His-Met-Ala comprising the other sheet.

shown from electron density maps calculated from X-ray fibre diffraction data that the hydrophobic residues (Leu-Val-Phe-Phe in Aβ and the poly-Ala-rich domain in H1) are in the core regions of the β-crystallites. Such a conformational transition of $\alpha \rightarrow \beta$, therefore, may be driven by hydrophobic interactions between the β-sheets.

Acknowledgements

We thank Kris Grabarek (Oberlin College, Oberlin, OH) for preparing the atomic coordinates of the Aβ core region used in Fig. 3B. The research described here was supported by grants from the National Institutes of Health (NIH-NIA AG08572) and the National Aeronautics and Space Administration (#95-480), and by an Alzheimer's Association Zenith Award (to D. A. K.).

References

Cella RJ, Lee B, Hughes RE 1970 Lorentz and orientation factors in fiber x-ray diffraction analysis. Acta Crystallogr A 26:118–124

Cooper JH 1974 Selective amyloid staining as a function of amyloid composition and structure. Histochemical analysis of the alkaline Congo red, standardized toluidine blue, and iodine methods. Lab Invest 31:232–238

Fraser RDB, MacRae TP 1962 An investigation of the structure of β-keratin. J Mol Biol 5:457–466

Fraser RDB, Suzuki E, MacRae TP 1984 Computer analysis of x-ray diffraction patterns. In: Hall IH (ed) Structure of crystalline polymers. Elsevier Science, London, p 1–37

Garnier J, Osguthorpe DJ, Robson B 1978 Analysis of the accuracy and implications of simple methods for predicting the secondary structure of globular proteins. J Mol Biol 120:97–120

Geddes AJ, Parker KD, Atkins EDT, Beighton E 1968 'Cross-beta' conformation in proteins. J Mol Biol 32:343–358

Glenner GG 1980 Amyloid deposits and amyloidosis. The β-fibrilloses. 1. New Engl J Med 302:1283–1292

Hilbich C, Kisters-Woike B, Reed J, Masters CL, Beyreuther K 1992 Substitutions of hydrophobic amino acids reduce the amyloidogenicity of Alzheimer's disease βA4 peptides. J Mol Biol 228:460–473

Inouye H, Kirschner DA 1991 Folding and function of the myelin proteins. J Neurosci Res 28:1–17

Inouye H, Karthigasan J, Kirschner DA 1989 Membrane structure in isolated and intact myelins. Biophys J 56:129–137

Inouye H, Fraser PE, Kirschner DA 1993 Structure of β-crystallite assemblies formed by Alzheimer β-amyloid protein analogues: analysis by x-ray diffraction. Biophys J 64:502–519

Makowski L 1981 The use of continuous diffraction data as a phase constraint. 1. One-dimensional theory. J Appl Cryst 14:160–168

Marsh RE, Corey RB, Pauling L 1955a An investigation of the structure of silk fibroin. Biochim Biophys Acta 16:1–34

Marsh RE, Corey RB, Pauling L 1955b The structure of Tussah silk fibroin. Acta Crystallogr 8:710–715

McRee DE 1992 A visual protein crystallographic software system for X11/XView. J Mol Graphics 10:44–46
Nguyen JT, Inouye H, Baldwin MA et al 1995 X-ray diffraction of scrapie prion rods and PrP peptides. J Mol Biol 252:412–422
Stroud RM, Agard DA 1979 Structure determination of asymmetric membrane profiles using an iterative Fourier method. Biophys J 25:495–512
Tibbitts TT, Caspar DLD 1993 Deconvolution of disoriented fiber diffraction data using iterative convolution and local regression. Acta Crystallogr A 49:532–545
Wang BC 1985 Resolution of phase ambiguity in macromolecular crystallography. Methods Enzymol 115:90–112
Worthington CR, Khare RS 1978 Structure determination of lipid bilayers. Biophys J 23:407–425

DISCUSSION

Masters: Can you say anything about the kinetics of fibril formation in the model peptide systems that you have worked with?

Kirschner: No, because in our experiments to date, we have only examined fibres that have already formed.

Masters: How do you know that the fibrils are in a stable state by the time you look at them?

Kirschner: Our samples are either in a concentrated gel or in a pellet dried under ambient conditions. The X-ray patterns from fibres in the gel are essentially the same as those in the dry pellets, but much weaker.

Paul Fraser has looked at some of these peptides by FTIR spectroscopy both in solution and as a dry film, and has observed the same type of β-sheet conformation (Fraser et al 1991a). Again, this doesn't address the kinetics, but at least it shows that the conformation in fibres in solution is the same as in the dry state.

J. D. Buxbaum: So many of these peptides seem to show the cross-β structure that you would associate with amyloid disease, yet it has been shown that some of the APP mutations, particularly the Val717 mutations, produce longer amyloid variants that are aggressively pathogenic. However, from what you presented, the 'normal' and longer amyloid variants would all seem to make essentially the same fibrils, so why would some of them be so pathogenic?

Kirschner: These proteins do form similar types of fibrillar structures, which appear to have hydrophobic core domains. What might differ among the various amyloid fibrils are the interactions between their subunits (or β-crystallites, as we call them; Inouye et al 1993). These subunits, which consist of the folded polypeptides, are what assemble into the observable protofilaments and fibrils.

J. D. Buxbaum: What is going to make Aβ1–42 or 1–43 much more pathogenic than Aβ1–40?

Pepys: They are more intensely fibrillogenic: if you put Aβ1–40 into solution, it doesn't make fibrils as rapidly as Aβ1–42 or 1–43.

Kirschner: Aβ1–42 is more hydrophobic, too.

J. D. Buxbaum: So what you are saying is that although all the variants produce the same cross-β structure, the speed or the kinetics of the process of forming the cross-β structure is also important.

Pepys: There is very little Aβ around. It takes more than 50 years for Alzheimer's disease to develop, so kinetics of Aβ aggregation can make a big difference.

Masters: I think biologists are more interested in the toxicity of Aβ amyloid. The solubility and aggregation of the fibrils is one thing, but the actual toxicity of the amyloid is clearly a distinct issue.

Kirschner: One of the problems about some of the toxicity studies is that we really don't know what structural state the peptides are in. They may be fibrils; it could also be the folded subunits (β-crystallites) or short protofilaments which are toxic.

Masters: Biological evidence suggests that the filament is not toxic once it has assembled into a plaque or a long fibril. By the time it gets to this stage it is just sitting doing nothing. This suggests that there is an intermediate stage where something important is happening.

Kirschner: Along those lines, the reverse Aβ peptide (called Aβ40–1) has been shown to be non-toxic (Kowall et al 1991), even though it does have a β-conformation (Fraser et al 1992). The way the peptide is folded or the interaction between the β-subunits could underlie the toxicity.

Kisilevsky: Just a comment about the fibrils being inert: since there is likely to be an equilibrium between monomers (and perhaps even dimers or trimers) and the actual fibril itself, the residual plaque can serve as a huge reservoir providing material to influence the cells around it. I'm not sure that we should immediately conclude that the plaques themselves are innocuous.

Pepys: There is also a strong correlation between the toxicity of different Aβ peptides and their capacity to make fibrils. Nevertheless, there is still a big gap between neurotoxicity by Aβ peptide fibres *in vitro* and what is actually happening in the brain. There is no direct proof that the observed *in vitro* neurotoxicity is the mechanism underlying neuronal loss in Alzheimer's disease.

J. D. Buxbaum: If it is true that the plaques are a reservoir of harmful molecules, then solubilizing the plaques would be horrifically destructive as these molecules would be freed to exert their deleterious effects.

Kirschner: One of the implications of the paradigm of the pentameric arrangement I described or the tetrameric arrangement described by Colin Blake is that different types of interactions between the β-crystallites occur, which lead to formation of the fibril itself. These specific interactions are sites of possible therapeutic interventions. One might also try to interfere with the intersheet interactions within the β-crystallite, to prevent its proper folding and ability to assemble into fibrils.

Kelly: Could you compare your pentameric structure with Colin Blake's structure? Although his was tetrameric, the actual orientation of the strands seemed quite similar.

Kirschner: The orientation has to be the same because of the cross-β diffraction patterns. Thus, in both cases, the polypeptide chains are running perpendicular to the long axis of the fibril.

Kelly: But in your case, do you invoke a twist?

Kirschner: Yes. The individual β-strands are likely to be slightly twisted By contrast, the β-strands in globular proteins are highly twisted (Chothia 1973). In amyloid fibrils, there may also be a twist of the fibril about its long axis, as seen in electron micrographs.

Maury: We have some experience with fibril formation *in vitro* with synthetic gelsolin peptides. Ultrastructurally, amyloid-like fibrils are rapidly formed from short mutant Asn187 and Tyr187 gelsolin peptides corresponding to the mutations found in familial gelsolin amyloidosis syndromes. Some of these wild-type gelsolin peptides also make fibrils. However, these tend to be tiny and either do not take up Congo red or show very weak staining. What are these atypical fibrils?

Kirschner: Has anybody recorded X-ray patterns from such Congo red-negative fibrils to confirm the orientation of the polypeptide chain relative to the long axis of the fibril? One might expect to find evidence for an extended type of β-structure. However, when we examined fibres formed from Aβ19–28, which are Congo red-negative, we recorded, unexpectedly, a cross-β pattern. A similar finding (cross-β X-ray pattern and Congo red-negative) was reported for a 20-mer peptide sequence from the intracellular domain of the Aβ precursor protein (Caputo et al 1992). So there are exceptions that must have to do with the way the Congo red molecules are fitting in and are aligned.

Maury: What about factors such as peptide concentration and incubation time which are known to influence fibril formation?

Kirschner: Those of us who stain synthetic peptide assemblies with Congo red have found that sample thickness is very important. If a sample is too thick you won't get the classic yellow–green birefringence, and if it is too thin you won't see anything. A good example of this in tissue is the so-called 'diffuse' amyloid. This is Congo red negative yet it has been shown to be fibrillar (Davies & Mann 1993). It could just be a question of the concentration or the density of the fibre packing.

Pepys: I agree. The Congo red test is one of relatively low sensitivity

Westermark: The designations 'Congo red positive' or 'Congo red negative' are often used wrongly. One should realize that there is a scale of reaction from very weak positivity (and green birefringence) to the characteristic strong staining.

Blake: Perhaps we should be pressing for an X-ray diffraction analysis criterion for amyloid. After all, it is relatively easy test to do: if you have a protein with a 4.7 Å meridional reflection, it is almost certainly amyloid.

Kirschner: If we agree that amyloid is fibrillar, then this may not be a good sole criterion for amyloid. For example, we have measured the 4.7 Å reflection from the preparations that are clearly amorphous and not fibrillar at the electron microscope level. (By amorphous, I mean no recognizable ordered macromolecular structure.) These samples can give intersheet spacings at around 10 Å. Thus, a criterion for amyloid ought to include both conformational data (from X-ray diffraction, circular dichroism, or infrared spectroscopy) and also morphological data (from electron microscopy). Such a criterion would recognize that the polypeptides fold locally into β-pleated sheets, and that these β-pleated sheets assemble into extended structures (amyloid fibrils).

I would also like to mention that the intensity of the intersheet spacing may range from very weak to very strong compred with the intensity of the 4.7 Å hydrogen bond spacing (see, for example, our collage of Aβ X-ray patterns in Inouye et al 1993).

Blake: I think you can understand that. The β-sheet itself has side chains on either side of it, so in electron density terms it is a very broad sort of feature that doesn't have a particularly sharp character, whereas the 4.7 Å β-spacing should be suitable to be the criterion, because it indicates a series of β-strands, 4.7 Å apart, like a ladder along the length of the fibril, which is its basic characteristic.

Kirschner: The stacking is defined by hydrogen bonding, so it is a very precise distance, whereas the intersheet spacing depends on side-chains and their packing and can range from about 4 to 20 Å (Fraser & MacRae 1973).

Blake: But we're dealing with proteins that have large side chains, so these will be standard.

Kirschner: In prion protein there is a polyalanine-rich area, and you do get much smaller spacing (Nguyen et al 1995).

Kelly: A technical question: am I correct in assuming that most of the data you showed today were obtained with aligned fibrils?

Kirschner: Some were and some weren't. Some of the fibres will align in an external magnetic field. We use a field strength of about 20 000 gauss.

Kelly: How does this work? The dipole in a β-sheet is pretty weak and the electric component to the magnetic field is also pretty weak.

Kirschner: The fibrillar assemblies orient in an external magnetic field as a result of their diamagnetic anisotropy and liquid crystalline domains. In proteins the diamagnetic anisotropy results from oriented peptide bonds as well as oriented magnetic groups (Worcester 1978, Glucksman et al 1986). When planar groups such as the five-atom peptide bond, or five-atom ester bond, or an aromatic (such as the benzene rings in tyrosine, tryptophan or phenylalanine) are placed in a magnetic field, the field induces a magnetic moment. To minimize the energy of the magnetic movement, these groups will tend to orient with their planes parallel to the field. Thus, α-helices and β-sheets tend to orient parallel to the magnetic field. In β-pleated sheet structures, the pleating reduces the relative contribution of the peptide bonds, so that the major contributor would be the aromatic rings. We have observed that the cross-β amyloid fibrils that orient do so parallel to the magnetic field, i.e. with the peptide bonds perpendicular to the field (Fraser et al 1991b). Thus, whether a particular peptide assembly orients in a magnetic field cannot be predicted soley on the basis of its summed diamagnetic anisotropies—the cooperative behaviour of liquid-crystalline domains of the assemblies is also a significant factor (Makowski 1989).

References

Caputo CB, Fraser PE, Sobel IE, Kirschner DA 1992 Amyloid-like properties of a synthetic peptide corresponding to the carboxy-terminus of β-amyloid protein precursor. Arch Biochem Biophys 292:199–205

Chothia C 1973 Conformation of twisted β-pleated sheets in proteins. J Mol Biol 75:295–302

Davies CA, Mann DM 1993 Is the 'preamyloid' of diffuse plaques in Alzheimer's disease really nonfibrillar? Am J Pathol 143:1594–1605

Fraser PE, Nguyen J, Surewicz W, Kirschner DA 1991a pH-dependent structural transitions of Alzheimer amyloid peptides. Biophys J 60:1190–1201

Fraser PE, Duffy LK, O'Malley MB, Nguyen J, Inouye H, Kirschner DA 1991b Morphology and antibody recognition of synthetic β-amyloid peptides. J Neurosci Res 28:474–485

Fraser PE, Nguyen JT, Inouye H et al 1992 Fibril formation by primate, rodent and Dutch-haemorrhagic analogues of Alzheimer amyloid β-protein. Biochemistry 31:10716–10723

Fraser RDB, MacRae TP 1973 The beta conformation. In: Conformations in fibrous proteins and related synthetic polypeptides. Academic Press, New York, p 218–246

Glucksman MJ, Hay RD, Makowski L 1986 X-ray diffraction from magnetically oriented solutions of macromolecular assemblies. Science 231:1273–1276

Inouye H, Fraser PE, Kirschner DA 1993 Structure of β-crystallite assemblies formed by Alzheimer β-amyloid protein analogues: analysis by X-ray diffraction. Biophys J 64:502–519

Kowall NW, Beal MF, Busciglio J, Duffy LK, Yankner BA 1991 An *in vivo* model for the neurodegenerative effects of β-amyloid and protection by substance P. Proc Natl Acad Sci USA 88:7247–7251

Makowski L 1989 Preparation of magnetically ordered specimens for diffraction experiments. In: Sweet RM, Woodhead AD (eds) Synchrotron radiation in structural biology. Plenum, New York, p 341–347

Nguyen JT, Inouye H, Baldwin MA et al 1995 X-ray diffraction of scrapie prion rods and PrP peptides. J Mol Biol 252:412–422

Worcester DL 1978 Structural origins of diamagnetic anisotropy in proteins. Proc Natl Acad Sci USA 75:5475–5477

General discussion I

Fibril structure

Kisilevsky: Colin Blake, the fibrils that you study have often been washed during preparation: how well do you think they reflect the *in situ* state of the aggregated protein that we call amyloid? I'm aware that this is a difficult question.

Blake: It is a difficult question, and I don't think there's any definite answer. However, I would point out that fibrils with different origins, which may or may not have been treated in different ways, seem to give the same kind of X-ray pattern. This implies that their structure is similar, and that it has survived the different purification procedures. It's rather difficult to go further into it than that, because I suspect the question you're really asking is: if one was able to take a sample straight out of the body, would you expect its diffraction patterns to be different from those of the purified samples? I don't know that anybody has done that experiment, but it needs to be done. Could you provide a sample in which one could guarantee that the material was, as it were, untouched by human hand?

Pepys: One could cut a section through a heavily amyloid-laden organ—that's about as close as you could get, but there would be much material present other than amyloid protein.

Blake: Nevertheless, you might detect X-ray patterns from amyloid and separate them from those of lipid and other components.

Benson: A few years ago we did that with frozen tissue from lymph nodes that were practically pure amyloid, and we saw a typical β-pattern.

Damas: We studied FAP fibrils extracted from the kidney (Damas et al 1995). When we did X-ray diffraction experiments on these unpurified fibrils, there were many reflections, some of which were from the protein and others from lipids and P component. We extracted the lipids and P component from the fibrils and we ended up with a different diffraction pattern, which still reflected the β-structure.

Blake: One test of foreign materials is that the lines may have a different half width. That is, they may be sharper or broader than the ones from the protein. We have certainly seen on some of our amyloid patterns sharp lines which are manifestly different—very much sharper, and very variable—these are clearly foreign materials. The most obvious contaminant is lipid, which may be naturally associated with the amyloid in a physical but not in a structural sense, but other materials such as glycosaminoglycans could also contribute. By and large we tend to ignore the foreign lines, but perhaps one should follow this up and see whether they are forming some kinds of arrangements that are in some way in register with the amyloid structure and which therefore might be physically and chemically associated with it. This might help us to understand the involvement of other components in the fibril structure.

Kirschner: With the sizes (cross-sections) of the beams typically used, one is averaging over a large volume of tissue, so several inclusions could be detected.

Blake: Again, you would need to look at the sample by electron microscopy to see what kind of thing is in the X-ray beam.

Costa: Colin Blake, did I understand correctly that your amyloid fibril preparations were from Swedish homozygous patients?

Blake: Yes; Professor Lundgren is the correct person to answer this, because he obtained them.

Lundgren: Most of these samples are from homozygous individuals, and we take them from the vitreous body by making an incision, injecting saline and then withdrawing a sample.

Costa: Have you compared these preparations with fibril preparations from heterozygous patients?

Blake: Yes. There's not a great deal of difference. The fibrils from homozygous patients give rather better patterns, but this may simply be because they were better samples or we had a better X-ray beam. The patterns are manifestly the same; if you take account of the different origins of the fibrils, I think one is looking at the same material. The kidney material had rather more in the way of foreign lines than the vitreous—that is the major difference.

Benson: I'd like to ask a technical question about the preparation of the vitreous amyloid. The vitreous body also has a lot of collagen, and I didn't see any in your samples, so I think you must have done more than just washing out the amyloid. Did you?

Lundgren: These are rather elderly people so there is not much collagen. More than 90% of the protein is transthyretin (TTR) when the material is directly analysed by SDS-PAGE.

Benson: But we see it in the histology of the vitreous body.

Lundgren: There are some individual differences. Usually we have homogeneous gel-like aggregates. But the material may change upon storage in saline and start to form clumps or aggregates, so we usually spin it down.

Kisilevsky: Are these vitreous extracts subsequently washed in water, as with most other amyloid isolation procedures?

Lundgren: We haven't done that, because we have enough material as it is.

Sipe: Would the amyloid P component be part of the fibril?

Lundgren: Yes, it is also there.

Pepys: Did you wash that off?

Lundgren: We can wash it off with citrate.

Pepys: Is that the material Colin Blake used for his diffraction studies?

Blake: No; we simply used the stuff as it came.

Benson: We have extracted the fibrils with citrate, and found both SAP and the P2 protein in the washes. But we were not doing structural studies, we were trying to do biochemistry.

Lundgren: What was the tissue source?

Benson: The same specimen that you referred to. The surgeon takes it out in about 20 cc of saline and then we spin it down.

Blake: Presumably, if they wash off, SAP and P2 are superficial components.

Pepys: SAP is bound to the fibrils in a Ca^{2+}-dependent way and you can wash it off with EDTA or some other Ca^{2+} chelator (Pepys et al 1979). I am surprised that you didn't do that with your preparations that were then subjected to X-ray diffraction. Nevertheless, I don't think that SAP is arranged in an ordered fashion along these fibrils.

Blake: If it is not arranged in an ordered fashion it wouldn't affect the X-ray diffraction data. But on the other hand one would have expected to see it in the electron micrographs—it's relatively large.

Pepys: Yes, you would have seen it in the negatively stained electron micrographs if it was present. Did you wash the sample a few times?

Blake: Yes.

Pepys: If you just wash away the ambient Ca^{2+} down to about 0.5 mM, which only takes a few spins to do, the SAP comes off anyway.

Merlini: Does it come off completely?

Pepys: More remains after washing than if you add EDTA, but if you wash enough in saline it will all come off.

Caughey: What would be the molar ratio to start with?

Pepys: Martha Skinner and I quantified the amount of SAP in amyloid deposits and found it to be up to 15% of the weight of the amyloid fibrils (Skinner et al 1980). But this is a crude estimation. To turn it into a molar ratio is beyond the techniques we have available.

Caughey: Another approach to looking at the structure of *in situ* amyloid plaques might be infrared microscopy. Perhaps you could even take an infrared spectrum from an individual plaque: people have certainly taken infrared spectra from individual red cells.

Kelly: In the *in vitro* amyloid studies we've done, the Met30 fibrils are much more stable than the wild-type fibrils. Those subtle differences may play a significant role in producing a filament stable enough to work with over a long period of time with the P component and other stabilizing factors removed. I think we're going find that there are going to be some variants of a given protein that will be ideally suited to studying and others that won't. For example, if you make wild-type fibrils starting with folded protein and look at them right away by electron microscopy, they look very nice, but if you go back and look at the same material a day later they are no longer fibrils. Whereas the Met30 fibrils prepared in the same way are stable for months.

Pepys: It is jolly lucky, or else we would all be getting wild-type TTR senile amyloid when we are 25 years old instead of 60 years old.

Kelly: Is it possible that there is such a thing as pre-amyloid? That is, aggregated material that is soluble. Because in the peptide work that we've done, by ultra centrifugation we can make material that has a molecular weight of over a million, but it is in solution and it binds to Congo red. If you look at it by FTIR it definitely has a β-conformation. But if you put it in UV, it doesn't scatter light at 330 nm. Could it be that there is actually soluble pre-amyloid?

Kirschner: Perhaps the soluble pre-amyloids are aggregates of β-crystallites that have not yet further organized into fibrillar assemblies. One might also have a micellar type of process. In this scenario, above a certain concentration of polypeptide there is the spontaneous self-assembly of the monomers into micelles, which are soluble aggregates. The micelles would serve as sites for the nucleation of the macromolecular, ordered assemblies (Lomakin et al 1996). If the micelles contain locally organized domains of β-conformation, then this too would be consistent with your observations. Thus, the 'pre-amyloid' might be micelles, with a small degree of secondary structure, or the β-crystallites, with a considerable degree of secondary structure.

Kelly: This all comes back to the toxicity issue: which species is actually toxic? We really don't understand this. Is it the soluble form or is it the fibril?

Kirschner: You can have short fibrils that are still soluble. What are your criteria for 'insoluble'? Is it because it is now visible by electron microscopy, or because if you centrifuge, fibrillar material comes down? I think the criteria are a little fuzzy. The toxicity might have more to do with the folding than with solubility. For example, the proposed structure for Aβ10–35 as a monomer in solution resembles a twisted horseshoe (J. T. Lee & J. E. Maggio, personal communication). This clearly must undergo some re-folding when it assembles with other monomers to form β-crystallites and then the extended fibrillar structure.

Blake: From the work I have done, the only thing that one could say is that the TTR tetramer exists in the form that it does in solution, and that in the long-term in amyloid it forms these stable fibrils. There may be a whole range of intermediates in between those two states, but I don't think the techniques that I've been using are capable of demonstrating what these might be. So we're really looking at long-term stable structures that exist at the two extrema, as it were, of the field of interest.

Kelly: Grant Kraft has used atomic force microscopy to look at fibril formation, effectively as a function of time. He sees a wide range of species that are absorbed out of solution.

Kirschner: Although Grant isn't here to defend his results, one of the questions that came up about this work was that in his specimen preparation there is a wash step. Perhaps what he is looking at is biased to the types of assemblies that are not washed off. What is very interesting is that Grant showed extremely thin fibrils about 8–10 Å wide, which is much smaller than anything any of us has detected using other methods.

Amyloid fibril toxicity

Benson: When we make a term like 'amyloid' all inclusive, we have to incorporate many different ideas. Earlier, Colin Masters introduced the subject of the toxicity of the peptide. The older amyloidologists didn't tend to think in terms of toxicity. The feeling was that it wasn't so much *what* an amyloid deposit was as *where* it was, and as long as they didn't form in the wrong places they could accumulate for a long time and not do anything. In other words, amyloid fibrils cause problems because they're there, whether they crystallize in your kidney or make fibrils in your heart—it is not that they are directly toxic. But then when we include Alzheimer's disease or prion disease in our discussion, we have to start thinking about toxicity. Perhaps we also need to think about toxicity in terms of serum amyloid A (SAA) or immunoglobulin light chain amyloid, and maybe even TTR amyloid.

Kelly: Isn't the peripheral neuropathy in familial amyloidotic polyneuropathy (FAP) caused by the killing of nerve cells, then?

Benson: That is the big question. I'm not a neurologist to answer this, but very often in a rather profound neuropathy one sees few fibrils in the nerves themselves, suggesting that much of the clinical disease may be due to ganglion cell loss in the dorsal root ganglia. However, some of the dramatic improvements in the bowel function of people with liver transplantation cannot be explained by regeneration of nerves. Perhaps there is some toxic element involved that is reversed by liver transplantation.

Pepys: We do see objective improvements in peripheral neuropathy after liver transplantation in FAP. However, it is not clear that this reflects clearance of amyloid or removal of some toxic effect. The suggestion that amyloid fibrils can kill cells by inducing apoptosis is particularly interesting and might explain the notable absence of necrosis and inflammation in most amyloidotic organs. Futhermore, if there were individual differences in the susceptibility of individuals or different organs to this type of toxicity induced by different types of amyloid, it could explain the observed disparities between amount of amyloid and the severity of organ dysfunction. FAP is an extreme example in which there can be terrible neuropathy with very little amyloid, while some patients with other types of acquired or hereditary amyloidosis can have normal liver function with 3 kg of amyloid in their liver.

Kisilevsky: This becomes a question of how one defines 'toxicity'. The very fact that we get changes in physiological function in one organ or another in response to amyloid, means that the amyloid is obviously doing something mechanistically, be it physical or biochemical. To me, that is 'toxicity'. It is very clear that the amyloid, when present, isn't good for you.

Pepys: If you get rid of the amyloid one way or the other then the organ function can recover. The question is: is the amyloid doing harm just by its physical presence and corresponding architectural disruption, or by more subtle and specific interference with normal cellular functions?

Kisilevsky: The possibilities mentioned just represent different mechanisms. Verifying that amyloid is present and it is doing something means that a mechanism must be involved. Amyloid is not just doing something because it's there physically. Its physical presence must operate through some mechanism.

Masters: The critical questions are whether or not there is a pre- or para-amyloid deposition which is causing damage or whether the amyloid itself is only a marker of the disease.

Pepys: The prion diseases differ from other forms of amyloidosis in that there can be severe spongiform encephalopathy with no demonstrable amyloid at all. In contrast, it is clear that in essentially all other situations the amyloid deposits are the actual cause of disease.

Masters: In Alzheimer's disease we suspect that a pre- or para-amyloid state exists in which the Aβ molecule exerts toxicity. The molecular nature of this toxic state, possibly a dimer or tetramer, is an important area for future investigations.

Benson: The suggestion here is that perhaps the amyloid is protective. Once precursor proteins are put into amyloid deposits they are no longer toxic. It is when the substrate is produced so rapidly that you don't have the chance to detoxify it and put it into deposits that you end up with the worst disease.

Merlini: I agree that we still don't know the precise mechanism by which amyloid deposits damage organ function. Studies on renal biopsies have shown that after the resolution of nephrotic syndrome the amount of AA amyloid present is almost the same as during the nephrotic stage (Von Gise et al 1978), or even greater, as in the case of two patients with light chain amyloidosis whose nephrotic syndromes regressed after chemotherapy (Kyle et al 1982). The local cellular reaction probably plays a important role in determining organ damage, which may be more relevant than the structural organization of the protein deposit *per se*. In fact, organ damage can also be induced by amorphous monoclonal light chain deposits, as in light chain deposition disease, and by non-amyloid fibrillary deposits (Verani 1993).

References

Damas A, Sebastião MP, Domingues FS, Costa PP, Saraiva MJ 1995 Structural studies on FAP fibrils: removal of contaminants is essential for the interpretation of X-ray data. Amyloid: Int J Exp Clin Invest 2:173–178

Kyle RA, Wagoner RD, Holley KE 1982 Primary systemic amyloidosis. Resolution of the nephrotic syndrome with mephalan and prednisone. Arch Intern Med 142:1445–1447

Lomakin A, Chung DS, Benedek GB, Kirschner DA, Teplow DB 1996 On the nucleation and growth of amyloid β-protein fibrils: detection of nuclei and quantitation of rate constants. Proc Natl Acad Sci USA 93:1125–1129

Pepys MB, Dyck RF, de Beer FC, Skinner M, Cohen AS 1979 Binding of serum amyloid P component (SAP) by amyloid fibrils. Clin Exp Immunol 38:284–293

Skinner M, Pepys MB, Cohen AS, Heller LM, Lian JB 1980 Studies of amyloid protein AP. In: Glenner GG, Costa PP, de Freitas FF (eds) Amyloid and amyloidosis. Excerpta Medica, Amsterdam, p 384–391

Verani RR 1993 Fibrillary glomerulopathy. Kidney 2:63–66

Von Gise H, Helmchen U, Mikeler E et al 1978 Correlations between the morphological and clinical findings in a patient recovering from secondary generalized amyloidosis with renal involvement. Light- and electron microscopic observations on serial biopsies. Virchows Arch A Pathol Anat Histol 379:119–129

Modulating conformational factors in transthyretin amyloid

M. J. M. Saraiva, M. R. Almeida, I. L. Alves, M. J. Bonifácio, A. M. Damas, J. A. Palha, G. Goldsteins* and E. Lundgren*

*Centro de Estudos de Paramiloidose and Instituto de Ciências Biomédicas, Hospital de Sto. Antonio, 4100 Porto, Portugal and *Department of Applied Cell and Molecular Biology, University of Umeå, Sweden*

Abstract. We have analysed the structure, binding properties, stability and amyloidogenicity of particular transthyretin (TTR) mutations—TTR Met30 and TTR Pro55, both associated with familial amyloid polyneuropathy, and TTR Met119, a non-pathogenic TTR mutation with apparent protective effects on the amyloidogenicity of the Met30 mutation. Our results show that in contrast to the Met30 mutation, the Met119 mutation increases the stability of the tetramer towards dissociation into monomers and confers a higher affinity to thyroxine, which binds on the channel that runs through the tetramer. This variant also shows a greater resistance to amyloid formation *in vitro*, in contrast to the Pro55 variant, which is more susceptible to amyloid formation. Crystallographic studies of the structure of the Pro55 variant are underway and reveal major conformational changes. Interestingly, these changes affect the D strand of TTR, which when deleted or modified *in vitro* leads to accelerated rates of amyloid formation. The conformational changes observed in these 'aggressive' mutations may resemble intermediate forms in the process of amyloidogenesis.

1996 The nature and origin of amyloid fibrils. Wiley, Chichester (Ciba Foundation Symposium 199) p 47–57

Although the fibrils in different amyloid diseases are made up of different proteins, the amyloid formed in each has unifying biophysical characteristics. This could mean that its pathophysiological effects are very similar, but that different disease patterns are due to other unknown intervening factors. The transthyretin (TTR)-related amyloidoses represent a good model for understanding the mechanism of amyloid formation. More than 50 mutations have been described in TTR (Saraiva 1995). Most of these TTR variants are associated with familial amyloidotic polyneuropathies (FAP) and familial amyloidotic cardiomyopathies (FAC), diseases characterized by extracellular deposition of fibrillar material composed of TTR. The most frequent mutation is TTR Met30, associated with FAP, an autosomal dominant disease characterized by lower limb neuropathy and autonomic dysfunction, with generalized amyloidosis predominantly affecting the peripheral nervous system.

Our group has studied the structure, binding properties, stability and amyloidogenicity of particular TTR mutations, including Met30, the clinically severe FAP-related Pro55 and the non-amyloid mutation Met119. The latter variant is most important since it has apparently protective effects on the amyloidogenic properties of Met30. This is suggested by the fact that compound heterozygotic carriers detected in the Portuguese population for Met30 and Met119 have a more benign form of the disease (Alves et al 1993). Additionally, by identifying mutational hot spots, we have expressed recombinant TTR molecules that exhibit accelerated rates of fibril formation.

In this paper we give an account of comparative studies of structure and stability of these mutations with reference to the identification of the conformational steps leading to amyloid formation.

The 'anti-amyloidogenic' nature of the Met119 mutation

In order to compare the amyloidogenic potential of TTR Met119 with normal TTR and /or FAP-associated TTR Met30, we developed a quantitative assay for amyloid formation *in vitro*, using thioflavine T fluorimetry, first validated with native amyloid fibrils extracted post-mortem from the thyroid of an FAP patient. Next, we formed amyloid fibrils from normal TTR by acidification. Amyloid formation from normal TTR was favoured at pH 3.6 with an optimum concentration range of 2–3 mg/ml. TTR Met30 also formed amyloid at the same pH but to a greater extent. When the Met119 variant was tested (Fig. 1) very low amounts of amyloid were detected and only at the more acidic pH of 3.0. These results can be interpreted in the light of the proposal by Colon & Kelly (1992) that normal TTR, upon specific pH conditions, undergoes an equilibrium between a tetramer and a structured amyloidogenic monomer. Mutations in TTR could destabilize the tetramer, allowing the amyloidogenic intermediate to be formed under milder acidic conditions. Taking into account this proposal, the 'anti-amyloidogenic' behaviour found for the Met119 mutation can be explained by stabilization of the tetramer.

This hypothesis was tested by studies of comparative dissociation of TTR Met30 and TTR Met119 in which we analysed serum TTR from heterozygous carriers of these mutations and compound heterozygotes for TTR Met30 and TTR Met119 who have hybrid tetramers with different ratios of the two mutant monomers. The dissociation studies involved isoelectric focusing in semi-denaturing urea. The results obtained are shown in Fig. 2. The tetramers from TTR Met119 heterozygotes are more stable (higher amount of tetramer relative to monomer) than those from the TTR Met30 heterozygotes, which dissociate almost entirely into monomers (the two most cathodal bands). TTR Met30–Met119 from compound heterozygote carriers presents a pattern

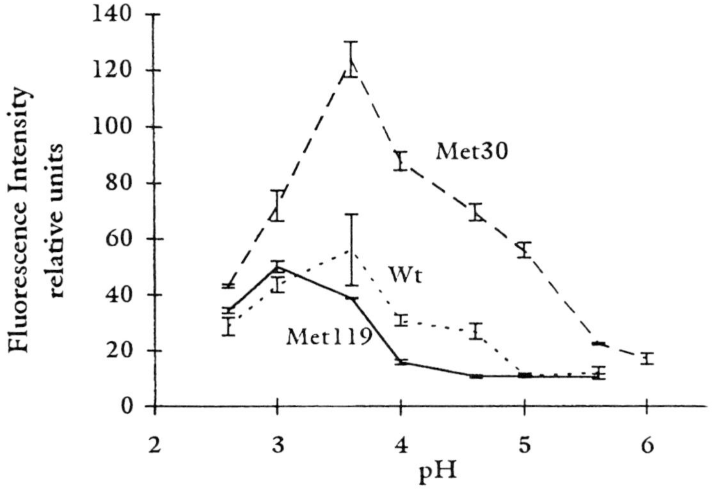

FIG. 1. pH dependence curve of amyloid fibril formation of TTR variants by quantitative thioflavine T-based fluorimetry. Fluorescence was measured at excitation maxima 436 nm and emission maxima 482 nm. Values are means of three assays; error bars give SD. Wt, wild-type.

similar to that from the normal individuals, suggesting that in compound heterozygotes, TTR Met119 stabilizes Met30-containing tetramers.

To further investigate the conformational properties of the Met119 mutant TTR, we undertook ligand binding studies using thyroxine (T_4), a natural ligand of TTR that binds on the interior of a channel that runs through the tetramer. T_4 binding was assayed both in whole serum samples and on isolated TTR from heterozygous Met30 and Met119 carriers and from compound heterozygotic individual carriers of the two mutations. The assays were based on a gel filtration procedure to separate the free from the bound hormone fraction. Table 1 shows the values found for the dissociation constants of the different TTR variants. Whereas Met30 carriers presented low T_4–TTR binding affinity (lower in homozygotes than in heterozygotes), TTR Met119 heterozygotic carriers presented an affinity for T_4 binding approximately 1.5–2 times higher than the affinity of normal TTR and slightly above the affinity of the Met30–Met119 carrier. Thus, the presence of Met119 increases T_4 binding.

To further interpret these data, we crystallized recombinant TTR Met119 and performed X-ray studies at 1.8 Å resolution. The initial interpretation of the data shows that the substitution of Thr119 for Met causes a movement of Leu110, which is in the central region of the channel, anchoring the T_4 complex and leading to the observed increase in binding affinity. In the absence of further structural data on TTR Met119, particularly on the monomer–monomer and dimer–dimer contacts, it remains difficult to explain the

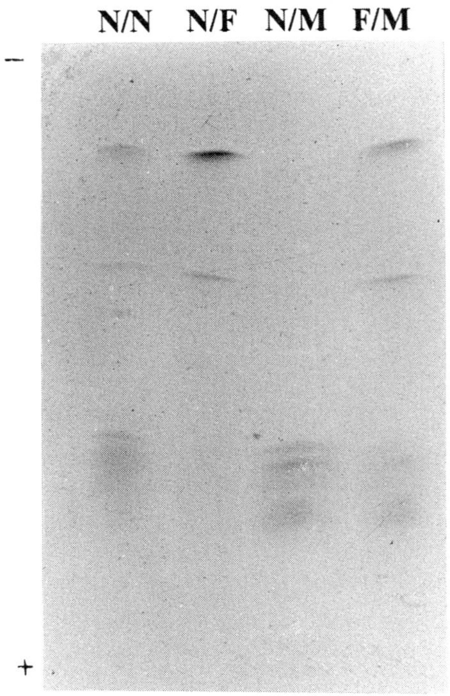

FIG. 2. Isoelectric focusing analysis of serum TTR. Serum samples were analysed in parallel with control sera (NN), from carriers of TTR Met30 (NF), TTR Met119 (NM) and compound Met30–Met119 heterozygotes (FM).

remarkable stability of this variant and how this contributes to its 'anti-amyloidogenic' properties. Such studies are in progress.

The 'pro-amyloidogenic' nature of the Pro55 mutation

In contrast with the Met119 mutation, which appears to protect from the deleterious effects of the Met30 mutation, TTR Pro55 is particularly clinically aggressive (Jacobson et al 1992). Using the amyloid assay described above for the Met119 mutation, we found that TTR Pro55 forms large amounts of amyloid in the pH range 3.6–5, indicating a higher susceptibility to amyloid formation. We performed binding studies with T_4 after certifying that tetrameric species were present. In contrast to the Met119 mutation, the Pro55 mutation presented virtually no binding to thyroxine. In order to further relate this finding with the structure of the mutant, we crystallized recombinant Pro55 and subjected it to X-ray analysis. In addition to presenting a different packing, strand D of each Pro55 monomer undergoes an important structural

TABLE 1 T_4 Binding properties of TTR variants from sera of individuals with different carrier status

Sera	*n*	$K_d \times 10^{-8}$ *M* (±*SD*)	*Relative* K_d
Met30–Met30	1	0.77	0.32
Wild-type–Met30	5	1.58±0.64	0.65
Wild-type–Wild-type	5	2.40±0.32	1
Met30–Met119	5	4.03±0.65	1.68
Wild-type–Met119	5	4.43±1.63	1.85

modification. These preliminary findings open new perspectives for modelling the assembly of TTR molecules into amyloid fibrils and raise the question of whether an intermediate structure occurs when amyloid is formed.

Are there structural intermediates responsible for amyloid formation?

In an independent study, with the aim of approaching the structure of a putative TTR amyloid intermediate, mutations in which the D strand was deleted and/or substituted have been expressed and exhibit greatly accelerated rates of fibril formation, as judged by fluorometric assays. These mutants might contain exposed cryptic epitopes and to test this hypothesis, we have produced and characterized a series of monoclonal antibodies. Under certain conditions the D strand null antibodies did not react with isolated normal TTR or sera from normal individuals, but recognized isolated TTR amyloid variants and sera from carriers of amyloid mutations.

Although further characterization of these antibodies is needed, the fact that they distinguish sera from carriers of amyloidogenic mutations supports the notion that an amyloidogenic intermediate exists and circulates, which under as yet unknown circumstances deposits in tissues as amyloid.

Acknowledgements

This work was supported by grant CT92-1096 from the European Union, Biomed I program.

References

Alves IL, Altland K, Almeida MR, Becher P, Costa PP, Saraiva MJM 1993 Screening of TTR variants in the Portuguese population by HIEF. J Rheumatol 20:185(abstr P2)

Colon W, Kelly J 1992 Partial denaturation of transthyretin is sufficient for amyloid fibril formation *in vitro*. Biochemistry 31:8654–8660

Jacobson DR, McFarlin DE, Kane I, Buxbaum JN 1992 Transthyretin Pro55, a variant associated with early-onset, aggressive, diffuse amyloidosis with cardiac and neurologic involvement. Hum Genet 89:353–356
Saraiva MJM 1995 Transthyretin mutations in health and disease. Hum Mutat 5: 191–196

DISCUSSION

Damas: I would like to describe preliminary X-ray work we have performed on the Pro55 TTR variant. The protein crystallizes in space group C2, with cell constants of $a = 149.99$ Å, $b = 78.74$ Å, $c = 98.95$ Å and $\beta = 100.5°$. X-ray diffraction data were collected to 2.7 Å. The asymmetric unit contains eight monomers which assemble into one tetramer in a general position, and two dimers near the two fold axes. In the case of wild-type TTR, the space group is orthorhombic and there is only one dimer in the asymmetric unit. The crystallographic packing is also different from that of the wild-type protein.

The wild-type protein assembles into crystals with the thyroxine (T_4) binding channels parallel to each other. Interestingly, with Pro55, although the tetrameric structure is present in the crystals, they assemble with their channels perpendicular to each other. Preliminary results concerning the region of substitution indicate that strand D is displaced and, as a result, the interaction between strands A and D is weakened. Furthermore, there is an elongation of the hydrogen bonds between the two dimers that form the tetramer, which suggests a less stable tetrameric structure. We are currently trying to improve the crystal quality and high resolution data will be collected. We think that these results open new perspectives for modelling the assembly of TTR molecules in amyloid fibrils, and support the idea that an intermediate structure might occur when amyloid is formed.

Lundgren: We have deleted or substituted the three amino acids in the D strand, resulting in TTR molecules which spontaneously form precipitates with the tinctorial properties of amyloid. However, the material also forms high molecular weight aggregates, which could be demonstrated on a native PAGE. Compared with the sharp band of the wild-type protein it forms a smear. This might be an intermediate form, before formation of the amyloid proper. We wondered whether the mouse immune system would detect structural features of such a proposed intermediate and therefore we generated monoclonal antibodies. One of these, number 47, could stain the smeary high molecular weight aggregates, but did not detect the wild-type protein. This was also analysed on a gel filtration column, where two peaks appeared with time, while the small peak seems to remain constant in size. We can show on a protein gel that this material is migrating with the same retention time as normal TTR. The large peak is progressively increasing in size. Thus, we might have created an experimental system with which we can study potential pathways for amyloid formation and we have also generated a monoclonal antibody which we propose is detecting an intermediate on the pathway.

Masters: How did you screen your antibodies?

Lundgren: The screening was against the deletion mutant: the injected material was the substitution mutant. We screened for the deletion mutant and excluded those which reacted with wild-type.

Masters: Do the antibodies bind to TTR *in vitro* and inhibit smear formation?

Lundgren: We have not been able to demonstrate that.

Maeda: Maria Saraiva, in your table you showed the T_4 binding properties of the Met30 and Met119 mutant TTRs. In that table, homozygous Met30 TTR has lower affinity for T_4 than heterozygous wild-type–Met30 TTR. However, the familial amyloidotic polyneuropathy (FAP) patients homozygous for the Met30 TTR gene do not show earlier onset than patients heterozygous for the mutant gene. Do you think that there is a relationship between the affinity of TTR for T_4 and its amyloidogenic properties?

Saraiva: One cannot really relate the T_4 binding properties of the molecule with amyloidogenic properties.

Maeda: But homozygous Met30–Met119 TTR has significantly higher affinity for T_4 than homozygous Met30 TTR.

Saraiva: In the compound heterozygous Met30–Met119 individuals, T_4 affinity is increased relative to Met30 heterozygous individuals due to changes in the T_4 binding channel brought about by the Met119 mutation. The anti-amyloidogenic properties of Met119 are related to structural changes that affect other regions of the molecule, most probably involved in monomer–monomer or monomer–dimer contacts, as inferred from the studies on stability and the preliminary X-ray data just presented. Thus, the Met119 mutant is a good example showing that T_4 binding properties are not related to amyloidogenic properties. T_4 binding studies help us to study the conformation of the mutants.

Kelly: Is the D strand in the protein disordered in the crystal structure?

Damas: No, it is not disordered.

Kelly: So you can see the region, but it's just not a strand anymore.

Damas: It's not hydrogen bonded to strand A as in the wild-type protein.

Kelly: I sort of agree with you that this represents a continuum. The surprising result is that the deletions can form amyloid. Did you look at the quaternary structural stability of those deletions? I think that's the critical question, because in fact it may not be the tetramer that's making the fibrils in the deletion cases.

Lundgren: We suspect that they form stable dimers.

Kelly: Stable dimers in solution?

Lundgren: Yes.

Wood: What happens to the 3D structure of TTR at pH 4? Is there any sign of a structure transition that might be necessary for fibre formation?

Blake: We have looked at this and we can't see any difference as we drop the pH from about 6.0 for the native protein down to 3.0.

Kelly: Under what conditions? Is there concentrated ammonium sulfate present?

Blake: Yes.

Kelly: You can't draw analogies from that in solution because ammonium sulfate strongly stabilizes proteins, especially TTR. TTR definitely undergoes conformational changes as the pH changes, unless you discount all we have published over the last five years! It undergoes quite significant conformational changes involving what appears to be the CD loop area.

Goldgaber: Are these changes reversible?

Kelly: They're reversible under the right conditions. Clearly, at high protein concentration it goes to amyloid. At low protein concentration you can have a reversible unfolding. At low temperature you can also do the reversible unfolding and re-folding, but under physiological concentrations and temperature about half the protein goes to amyloid.

Blake: I agree with you that perhaps crystallography is not a very good way of looking at these phenomena. You have to keep the material in the crystalline form if you're going to do this, and so you have to use ammonium sulfate, and that in turn affects the possible conformational dynamics of the molecule.

Kelly: It is important to do these studies in solution at physiological salt concentrations, otherwise quite significant conformational changes and dissociation occur. I think our work is in agreement in that a monomer or a dimer is required for fibril formation.

Blake: It's also interesting that if you look at the distribution of amyloidogenic mutants of TTR, they segregate in the outer parts of molecule, and yet these effects seem to have their major effect at the level of the subunit interface. However, the substitutions themselves seem to avoid the subunit interface. So it is not quite as simple a picture as one might imagine. Pro55 is about as far from the subunit interfaces as you can get in TTR.

Kelly: And the hallmark of that mutant is that it clearly destabilizes the tetramer.

Damas: It is clear that the contacts between the two dimers are elongated in the Pro55 variant, so the tetramer is going to be less stable.

Pepys: Both the Pro55 variant and also the Pro52 variant we have identified (Booth et al 1994) are associated with very early-onset and aggressive clinical amyloidosis. This may be telling us something about the relationship between the degree of destabilization caused by these particular substitutions and propensity to *in vivo* amyloidogenesis.

Costa: Two years ago our clinicians reviewed the case histories of our FAP patients and found 159 patients who presented as sporadic cases: no one was known to have this disease in the family (Coelho et al 1994). In a few dozen of the cases both parents were still alive, and in every case we found that one of them was a carrier of the Met30 TTR variant although none presented any signs of disease. So beyond the amyloidogenicity of the protein itself, many other factors are involved.

Pepys: The penetrance is very much dependent on factors other than the fibril precursor protein itself, and on which we have no handle at all.

Costa: I'm talking about 'clinical' penetrance, because these individuals have the variants circulating at normal levels but don't show any disease.

Maury: Maria Saraiva, I would like to ask you about the quantitative thioflavine-based amyloid fibril assay. I wonder what this assay really measures. Does it give a real estimate of the amyloid fibril concentration or does it reflect the sum of fibrils and various aggregates of peptides in solution?

Saraiva: In this assay we cannot distinguish between aggregating material in solution and fibrillar material, because we don't separate these two materials prior to adding thioflavine. We just measure the total material that binds thioflavine.

Maury: We have used the same method for comparing the fibrillogenicity of various gelsolin peptides and found an accelerated amyloid formation of mutant, disease-related gelsolin peptides as compared with the corresponding wild-type ones (Maury et al 1994).

Lundgren: Our 'soluble' amyloid, i.e. the high molecular weight aggregates, is also thioflavine T positive.

Kisilevsky: Have you any ideas about why certain mutants give you amyloid in particular anatomical places?

Pepys: I think it's wrong to go away with the idea that there is a particularly strong association between many of these mutations and particular anatomical distributions of amyloid. Between families with identical mutations extreme differences exist in anatomical distribution of amyloid, although there are some patterns.

Kisilevsky: As a corollary to that, is it known whether there is a TTR receptor in cells?

Saraiva: There have been reports of TTR being taken by human cell lines in a saturable fashion, namely hepatomas (Divino & Schussler 1990a) and astrocytomas (Divino & Schussler 1990b). For several years there have been unsuccessful attempts to isolate such a human TTR receptor, although a chicken TTR receptor has been characterized (Vieira et al 1995).

J. N. Buxbaum: The paper that talked about receptors actually showed two receptors of different affinities. I don't know if anyone has confirmed that.

Concerning the anatomical distribution of the Pro55 variant, children carrying it get TTR amyloid in the early teenage years and by the time that they die in their early 20s, it is everywhere. This may reflect the protein characteristics of Pro55 TTR more than anything else, and there may be a hierarchy of deposition, but clearly in those patients you could find it every place you look.

Lundgren: It is interesting that the Portuguese patients with the Met30 variant have a different pattern of disease from those in Sweden. In the Swedish homozygous cases the onset is much later and if they get polyneuropathy it comes very late. Usually they start with eye depositions and most of them have eye deposition only. Also, most of them are sporadic cases.

Costa: But in Sweden you have many more asymptomatic carriers than in Portugal. That's why you have so many homozygotic patients. Maybe the cold weather protects them!

Lundgren: I would expect to see a gene dosage effect on the background of the typical Swedish weather.

Maeda: We introduced the human mutant Met30 TTR gene into inbred C57BL/6 mice. We found no significant difference in the serum levels of human TTR among the transgenic mice. However, the age of onset and progression of human TTR-derived amyloid deposition in these mice were variable among them. This indicates clearly that although the protein structure itself is very important to amyloidogenesis, other factors such as the environment affect the age of onset and progression of amyloid deposition.

Pepys: Can you manipulate the age of onset by altering the environment?

Maeda: Yes, if we keep them in SPF (specific pathogen-free) conditions they don't develop amyloid.

Merlini: I would like to address the relationship between protein stability and the tendency to form amyloid. In the case of TTR, does the molecule transported, T_4, stabilize the tetramer and somehow affect the tendency to make amyloid?

Saraiva: To my knowledge, these studies have not been done and I do not have evidence for such a correlation. However, it is known that T_4 stabilizes and increases the half-life of T_4-binding globulin (Grimaldi et al 1982).

Kelly: Under conditions where the wild-type protein can form amyloid without T_4, the addition of T_4 stabilizes the protein to the extent where it can't populate the monomer, and therefore it does not make amyloid. Its stabilization effect is quite marked and is well known in the protein literature. T_4-like molecules might be a therapeutic strategy. T_4 would be a disaster for a number of reasons, but T_4 analogues might be reasonable, especially if they had specificity for TTR over other fibrils.

Palha: But binding of T_4 to TTR should not increase the TTR half-life.

Kelly: Are you talking about biological half-life?

Palha: Yes.

Kelly: Does that necessarily correlate with the stability of the protein?

Palha: I think so. If your concept of stabilization of TTR by T_4 and prevention of amyloid is true, then in hypothyroidism, where T_4 circulating levels are decreased, TTR-related amyloidosis should occur, and it doesn't. With regard to the application of T_4 therapy to TTR-related amyloidosis, one should remember that only about 20% of the circulating TTR molecules carry T_4. Thus large amounts of T_4 or T_4 analogue would be needed to saturate TTR. Finally, it is worth noting that T_4 stabilization of TTR is unlikely to occur in the conditions you mentioned, for the simple reason that T_4 does not bind TTR under the acidic conditions that are used to make amyloid from wild-type TTR. In fact, T_4 binding to TTR occurs at pHs above 7.

Kelly: In biophysical experiments, I'll stake my reputation on the fact that it strongly stabilizes the protein. I don't know what happens in turnover.

References

Booth DR, Soutar AK, Hawkins PN, Reilly M, Harding A, Pepys MB 1994 Three new amyloidogenic transthyretin gene mutations: advantages of direct sequencing. In: Kisilevsky R, Benson MD, Frangione B, Gauldie J, Muckle TJ, Young ID (eds) Amyloid and amyloidosis 1993. Parthenon, Park Ridge, NJ, p 456–458

Coelho T, Sousa A, Lourenço E, Ramaheira J 1994 A study of 159 Portuguese patients with familial amyloidotic polyneuropathy (FAP) whose parents were both unaffected. J Med Genet 31:293–299

Divino CM, Schussler GC 1990a Receptor-mediated uptake and internalization of transthyretin. J Biol Chem 265:1425–1429

Divino CM, Schussler GC 1990b Transthyretin receptors on human astrocytoma cells. J Clin Endocrinol Metab 71:1265–1268

Grimaldi S, Edelhoch H, Robbins J 1982 Effects of thyroxine binding on the stability, conformation and fluorescence properties of thyroxine-binding globulin. Biochemistry 21:145–151

Maury CPJ, Nurmiaholassila EL, Rossi H 1994 Amyloid fibril formation in gelsolin-derived amyloidosis—definition of the amyloidogenic region and evidence of accelerated amyloid formation of mutant Asn-187 and Tyr-187 gelsolin peptides. Lab Invest 70:558–564

Vieira AV, Sander EJ, Schneider WJ 1995 Transport of serum transthyretin into chicken oocytes. A receptor mediated mechanism. J Biol Chem 270:2952–2956

Proteoglycans and amyloid fibrillogenesis

Robert Kisilevsky* and Paul Fraser†

*Department of Pathology, Queen's University and The Syl and Molly Apps Research Center, Kingston General Hospital, Kingston, Ontario, Canada K7L 3N6 and †The Centre for Research in Neurodegenerative Diseases and The Department of Medical Biophysics, University of Toronto, Toronto, Ontario, Canada M5S 1A8

Abstract. A brief discussion of the general structure of proteoglycans is followed by a description of the diverse nature of amyloids. Using the murine form of inflammation-associated (AA) amyloid, we have examined the temporal and anatomical relationship between the heparan sulfate proteoglycan, its mRNA and AA amyloid deposition *in vivo*. The *in vitro* effect of heparan sulfate on the secondary structure of amyloid precursors, and on amyloid peptides, suggests that this interaction is important in amyloidogenesis. The relationship of these two components likely reflects a more general process taking place between basement membrane proteins (which may be synthesized by a variety of cell types within and outside the CNS) and amyloid precursors. A general definition of *in vivo* amyloid deposits emerges from these considerations as do concepts for interfering with amyloidogenesis. Preliminary results showing the effect of small molecule aliphatic sulfonates and sulfates on *in vitro* amyloid β-protein fibrillogenesis and AA amyloidogenesis *in vivo* supports the general process presented and suggests therapeutic strategies for treating amyloid-based diseases.

1996 The nature and origin of amyloid fibrils. Wiley, Chichester (Ciba Foundation Symposium 199) p 58–72

Proteoglycans

Carbohydrates have been known to be part of amyloid deposits for more than a century. In fact, the term amyloid means 'starch-like' and was coined by Rudolf Virchow approximately 140 years ago (Virchow 1854). In attempting to establish that the waxy-appearing deposits characteristic of the then un-named amyloid contained cellulose, he treated cross-sections of such whole tissue with iodine in the presence of sulfuric acid. This reaction gave the typical blue-black positive reaction for starch and cellulose and led him to the term amyloid.

By the 1920s it was apparent that the carbohydrate was a mucopolysaccharide (the older name for what are now known as glycosaminoglycans [GAGs]), thought to be chondroitin sulfate (Boyd 1932). Further characterization of the

X
|
Ala
|
Asp
|
Ser-Xyl-Gal-Gal-GlcA-(GlcNac-GlcA)$_n$
|
Gly
|
Glu
|
Tyr
|
X

FIG. 1. The partial amino acid sequence of the glycosaminoglycan attachment point of perlecan, and the general structure of heparan sulfate with its tetrasaccharide attachment stem.

carbohydrate in amyloid continued through to the 1960s by several groups (Bitter & Muir 1966, Dalferes et al 1967, Pennock 1968). Several GAGs were implicated in amyloid structure, primarily heparan sulfate and chondroitin sulfate. Some work also examined the effect that amyloid had on the tissue culture production of GAGs, where hyaluronan was implicated (Palmoski & Brandt 1975).

With the exception of hyaluronan, GAGs do not occur as free polysaccharide chains in tissues (Kjellen & Lindahl 1991). They are linked to a protein backbone and the entire complex is referred to as a proteoglycan. The general structure of a proteoglycan is illustrated in Fig. 1, where the partial sequence of the GAG attachment site in perlecan, the heparan sulfate proteoglycan found in basement membranes, is shown (Kjellen & Lindahl 1991, Paulsson 1992, Gallagher et al 1992, Noonan & Hassell 1993, Iozzo et al 1994). The GAG proper is a linear polysaccharide. It is attached to the protein core through a serine moiety which is flanked by aspartate and glycine, and through a tetrasaccharide stem composed of xylose, two molecules of galactose, and one of glucuronic acid (Kjellen & Lindahl 1991, Noonan & Hassell 1993, Iozzo et al 1994). Then follows the repeating disaccharide structure characteristic of a GAG which is composed of an alternating hexosamine and a uronic acid. In the case of heparan sulfate (or heparin), this is composed of *N*-acetylglucosamine and glucuronic or iduronic acid. The disaccharide is repeated an indeterminate number of times and may give rise to a polysaccharide chain with molecular mass in the range of 60–70 kDa. The two repeating sugars within the disaccharide are sulfated at particular locations. This is in part determined by whether the glucuronic acid undergoes an epimerization to iduronic acid. Thus, for example, in heparin the disaccharide is fairly uniform with iduronate as the second component, and which ensures a fairly uniform sulfation pattern of heparin along its length. In the case of heparan sulfate, there are stretches of polysaccharide containing iduronic acid as in heparin, and other regions where glucuronic acid predominates. This difference determines areas of high sulfation and low sulfation, respectively.

Potential importance of proteoglycans in amyloidogenesis

Until relatively recently (25 years ago), amyloid was thought to represent a single entity whenever it was identified in tissue. This concept was based on the unique tinctorial, morphological, ultrastructural and protein-organizational characteristics of these fibrillar deposits. The advent of techniques to isolate the fibrils from tissue allowed investigators, for the first time, to characterize the protein(s) responsible for these structures (Pras et al 1968). It was anticipated that a single protein would be identified for such a singular structure. Soon it became apparent that multiple proteins could be responsible for amyloid deposits. Almost twenty have now been characterized (Kazatchkine et al 1993). Each is either associated with a specific disease or a specific pathological process (Table 1).

The potential importance in amyloidogenesis of heparan sulfate and its proteoglycan perlecan emerged from work which attempted to understand why such different amyloidogenic proteins tended to organize themselves into the characteristic deposits. A search for homologous amino acid sequences or consensus sequences among the different amyloidogenic proteins was unfruitful, and alternative explanations were therefore required. One possibility was that there were common components in amyloid deposits which provided an

TABLE 1 A partial listing of amyloid-based diseases with their associated proteins

Disease	*Amyloid protein*
Alzheimer's	Amyloid β-protein
Type II diabetes	IAPP (Amylin)
Dialysis	β_2-microglobulin
Plasma cell dyscrasias	L-chain or H-chain
Inflammation	SAA
CJD/GSS/Kuru/Scrapie	Prion
FAP	Mutant TTR or apoAI
Senile cardiac	Normal TTR

CJD, Creutzfeldt–Jakob disease; FAP, familial amyloidotic polyneuropathy; GSS, Gerstmann–Sträussler–Scheinker syndrome; IAPP, islet amyloid polypeptide; SAA, serum amyloid A; TTR, transthyretin.

environment or scaffold for each of these different proteins to aggregate in a particular way, namely as an amyloid.

To determine the potential importance of the carbohydrate moiety we did a series of experiments to establish the temporal relationship of protein fibril and carbohydrate appearance during the course of amyloid deposition (Snow & Kisilevsky 1985). The model used was that of inflammation-associated (AA) amyloid deposition in the mouse. The skeleton of the pathogenetic process of AA amyloidogensis is fairly well understood (Kisilevsky & Young 1994).

AA amyloidogenesis

In humans, AA amyloid is seen associated with inflammatory conditions regardless of the cause, be it infections, tumours or familial inflammatory disorders such as the serositis and pleuritis seen in familial Mediterranean fever.

In animals, the pathogenetic process can be broken down into two groups of events. The first is rapid and includes the activation of inflammatory cells which release cytokines such as interleukin 1, interleukin 6 and tumour necrosis factor. These operate on the liver, in the presence of steroids, to induce hepatic acute-phase protein synthesis (Kushner & Rzewnicki 1994). Among these are two proteins of the serum amyloid A (SAA) family, SAA_1 and SAA_2, which are produced in enormous quantities during the early phases of inflammation. In the mouse, the SAA_2 isoform serves as the precursor to the fibril protein which is deposited as amyloid (Hoffman et al 1984). In humans, both isoforms may be found, but SAA_1 predominates (Liepnieks et al 1995). However, the precursor on its own, even in large quantities, though necessary is not sufficient to cause amyloid. The levels of the two SAA isoforms regularly increase 500–1000-fold above normal levels (from 1–5 μg/ml to 500–1000 μg/ml) with every inflammatory reaction. If this were all that was necessary, virtually everyone would develop the AA form of amyloid because the plasma levels of the precursor increase with every viral infection, trauma, myocardial infarction as well as the chronic inflammatory diseases that are usually associated with amyloid, such as rheumatoid arthritis or cystic fibrosis (Skinner et al 1988, Chan et al 1992).

In animal models it became apparent that a slower process is also taking place (Kisilevsky & Boudreau 1983). This process provides a factor, originally called amyloid enhancing factor (AEF) but which we now recognize as a nidus, around which fibrillogenesis is likely to occur. In the presence of this nidus, and with a sufficient concentration of SAA, fibrillogenesis takes place extremely rapidly, giving rise to large histologically demonstrable deposits of AA amyloid in 36 h (Kisilevsky & Boudreau 1983). There are therefore two ways in which AA amyloid can be induced. One is to use standard inflammatory induction protocols and wait for AEF to be generated endogenously. In such models in highly susceptible mouse strains AA amyloid first appears in the spleen in approximately two weeks (Kisilevsky & Boudreau 1983). The second is to prepare an AEF extract and administer it to recipient mice together with the inflammatory stimulus. Such mice develop splenic amyloid in 36–48 h (Kisilevsky & Boudreau 1983). Once amyloid deposition begins, the kinetics of deposition is the same in both cases (Kisilevsky & Boudreau 1983).

It is therefore possible to devise both rapid and slow models of AA amyloid deposition. With these two models it became possible to investigate when in the course of amyloid induction the carbohydrate component appeared. Its appearance before or together with the fibrils would indicate that the carbohydrate was worthy of further study as a factor in the genesis of the amyloid deposit; its appearance after the fibrils would have eliminated it from a potential causative role.

Heparan sulfate proteoglycan and amyloidogenesis

Using such models it was possible for us to demonstrate that regardless of the inflammatory stimulus used, the induction protocol chosen and speed of induction, or the tissues examined, it was impossible to separate the appearance of the carbohydrate from the appearance of the amyloid fibrils (Snow & Kisilevsky 1985). It therefore became of interest to identify the nature of the carbohydrate. This was shown to be heparan sulfate, which increased in the spleen in direct proportion to the amount of amyloid (Snow et al 1987). No other GAG appeared to be taking part in this process. The heparan sulfate coincided anatomically with the amyloid deposits, as did the heparan sulfate proteoglycan. Further studies with gold-labelled antibodies to the protein core showed that the intact proteoglycan was part of the amyloid fibril itself, and that the GAGs were being deposited in a periodic fashion along the fibril (Snow & Kisilevsky 1988, Snow et al 1991).

In the mouse, the acute phase forms of SAA occur in two molecular species, SAA_1 and SAA_2. Sequence analysis has shown that SAA_2 is the precursor to murine AA amyloid deposits. If the interaction between heparan sulfate and SAA_2 was important in altering the conformation of this precursor so that it took on more β-sheet structure (the characteristic of amyloid) this should be demonstrable by circular dichroism. The spectrum of SAA_1 and SAA_2 were therefore examined in the presence of different GAGs (McCubbin et al 1988). It was shown convincingly that molecules such as chondroitin sulfate could reduce the α-helical structure of both isoforms but did not increase the β-sheet or β-turn structures. In the case of SAA_1, neither heparin nor heparan sulfate had any significant effect on secondary structure. However, in the case of SAA_2, heparan sulfate removed all the random coil structure and converted it into β-sheet β-turn conformation. This was the first demonstration that the interaction of two components normally found in amyloid could lead to a change in protein secondary structure which is characteristic of amyloid.

Furthermore, it was only the combination of the amyloidogenic form of SAA and heparan sulfate that resulted in this change. These findings were then substantiated by others (McCubbin et al 1988, de Beer et al 1993). It was subsequently shown by *in vivo* studies that the mRNA for perlecan, the heparan sulfate proteoglycan of interest, was increasing in the spleen at least coincident with and possibly preceding the amyloid deposit (Ailles et al 1993).

Other basement membrane proteins and amyloidogenesis

Many of the findings with perlecan, a basement membrane protein, have since been shown to be true for several other basement membrane proteins, such as laminin, collagen IV, fibronectin and entactin. These components are also deposited coincidentally with AA amyloid (Lyon et al 1991) and, in the case of the laminin B2 chain (J. Stewart & I. D. Young, personal communication) and the α_1-collagen IV chain (Woodrow et al 1994), their mRNAs increase in a similar manner to that of perlecan. Furthermore, binding interactions can be shown to take place between uncomplexed basement membrane proteins and SAA (Ancsin & Kisilevsky 1994). These results suggest that there is an alteration in basement membrane protein metabolism which occurs very early in the course of amyloidogenesis. This is in keeping with previous morphological studies showing early amyloid deposits taking place in relation to basement membranes (Linke et al 1989, Yamaguchi et al 1992). Moreover, these basement membrane proteins may be important players in the pathogenetic events leading to amyloid deposition generally. Findings similar to those with AA amyloid have been made with the amyloid β-protein (Aβ) found in Alzheimer's disease. Laminin, collagen IV and fibronectin have been identified in senile plaque amyloid (Perlmutter & Chui 1990, Howard & Pilkington 1990). Laminin mRNA levels are markedly increased in the brains of Alzheimer's patients but not in age-matched controls (Murtomaki et al 1992). High affinity binding can be demonstrated between perlecan or laminin and the β-amyloid protein precursor (APP) (Narindrasorasak et al 1991, 1992, 1995). Heparan sulfate influences the secondary conformation of Aβ, increasing its β-sheet structure considerably and influencing the linear growth and lateral aggregation of Aβ fibrils (Fraser et al 1992, 1994).

GAG binding sites and amyloid proteins

These results with heparan sulfate and the AA and Aβ forms of amyloid suggested that there were binding sites on amyloid precursors for this GAG. On the basis of consensus heparan sulfate binding sequences discovered in several apolipoproteins (Cardin & Weintraub 1989), these were predicted to be present in murine acute phase SAA between residues 82–87 and (using the APP695 numbering scheme) residues 98–104, 324–331, 608–613 in APP

(Kisilevsky 1989). In the latter case, both the 98–104 and the 608–613 were substantiated by others and our own unpublished work (Fraser et al 1992, Snow et al 1995). The immunohistochemical demonstration of perlecan in at least five different amyloids (inflammation, type II diabetes, Alzheimer's, Gerstmann–Sträussler–Scheinker syndrome and familial amyloidotic polyneuropathy), indicates that this process is likely to be a general one rather than one restricted to AA and Aβ amyloids. It suggests further that amyloid should be thought of as being composed of two groups of components, a disease specific protein and a set of common components most of which are constituents of basement membrane structure (serum amyloid P, perlecan, laminin, collagen IV, entactin and apolipoprotein E).

Potential therapeutic approaches to amyloidogenesis

If the binding interactions between the amyloidogenic proteins and heparan sulfate are important in the process of amyloidogenesis, as demonstrated in the AA and Aβ types of amyloid, then small molecules that mimic structural elements of the opposite faces of the binding site should be able to interfere with amyloid deposition both *in vivo* and *in vitro*.

TABLE 2 Correlation of *in vivo* and *in vitro* effects of compounds provided by Neurochem Inc.

Neurochem Inc.compounds[a]	*CD [mdeg]*[b]	*Percentage β-sheet*	*Splenic area with amyloid as a percentage of non-treated control*[c]
Control	−0.808	100.0	100
WAS-2	−0.654	80.9	55
WAS-3	−0.660	81.7	35
WAS-4	−0.754	93.3	90
WAS-5	−0.595	69.9	8
WAS-6	−0.514	52.4	11
WAS-7	−0.558	63.6	54

[a]WAS 2–7 are, respectively: 1,2-propane disulfonate; 1,4-butane disulfonate; 1,2-ethane disulfate; 1,3-propane diol disulfate; and 1,4-butane diol disulfate.
[b]Circular dichroism (CD) [mdeg] taken at 218 nm. Aβ β-sheet content was measured after its incubation with heparin in the absence and subsequent addition of the WAS compounds.
[c]The percentage of murine splenic area occupied by amyloid was measured six days after amyloid induction. Treated animals received the WAS compounds in their drinking water (at a concentration of 50 mM) one day after induction and were sacrificed five days later. Amyloid was measured by image analysis after tissue staining with Congo red (Kisilevsky et al 1995).

Such experiments have been shown to be successful (Kisilevsky et al 1995). Small molecules which mimic elements of the structure of heparan sulfate can interfere with both the *in vivo* induction and persistence of AA amyloid deposits and, furthermore, can interfere with the heparan sulfate induction of Aβ β-sheet formation and Aβ fibrillogenesis *in vitro*. There is a satisfying correlation between the effects of these compounds *in vivo* with AA amyloid, and their *in vitro* effect in reducing Aβ β-sheet structure (Table 2). These results provide additional support for the general amyloidogeneic process presented and also suggest general strategies for the medical treatment of amyloid-based diseases (Kisilevsky 1996).

Acknowledgements

This work represents the combined efforts of many students, collaborators, and post-doctoral fellows in addition to the authors. These include Drs B. D. Greenberg, M. Guo, S. Inoue, C. Kay, D. A. Kirschner, L. Lemieux, A. Lyon, W. McCubbin, S. Narindrasorasak, A. Snow, W. Szarek, D. Weaver and I. Young. Past and present students include L. Ailles, J. Ancsin, J. Stewart, S. Thomas and S. Woodrow.

This work has been supported by the Medical Research Council of Canada, the USA National Institutes of Health, The Alzheimer's Society of Canada, The Alzheimer's Society of Ontario, The Kidney Foundation of Canada, The Canadian Arthritis Society, The Upjohn Co. and Neurochem, Inc.

References

Ailles L, Kisilevsky R, Young ID 1993 Induction of perlecan gene expression precedes amyloid formation during experimental murine AA amyloidogenesis. Lab Invest 69:443–448

Ancsin JB, Kisilevsky R 1994 Characterization of SAA: laminin binding. In: Kisilevsky R, Benson MD, Frangione B, Gauldie J, Muckle TJ, Young ID (eds) Amyloid and amyloidosis 1993. Parthenon, Park Ridge, NJ, p 105–107

Bitter T, Muir H 1966 Mucopolysaccharides of whole human spleens in generalized amyloidosis. J Clin Invest 45:963–975

Boyd WA 1932 Textbook of pathology: an introduction to medicine, 2nd edn. Lea & Febiger Philadelphia, PA, p 107

Cardin AD, Weintraub HJR 1989 Molecular modeling of protein–glycosaminoglycan interactions. Arteriosclerosis 9:21–32

Chan KW, Lo WK, Cheng IKP 1992 Nephrotic syndrome associated with angiofollicular lymph node hyperplasia, and subsequent amyloidosis. Pathology 24:229–230

Dalferes ER, Radhakrishnamurthy B, Berenson GS 1967 Acid mucopolysaccharides of amyloid tissue. Arch Biochem Biophys 118:284–291

de Beer MC, de Beer FC, McCubbin WD, Kay CM, Kindy MS 1993 Structural prerequisites for serum amyloid A fibril formation. J Biol Chem 268:20606–20612

Fraser PE, Nguyen JT, Chin DT, Kirschner DA 1992 Effects of sulfate ions on Alzheimer-β/A4 peptide assemblies: implications for amyloid fibril–proteoglycan interactions. J Neurochem 59:1531–1540

Fraser PE, Kirschner DA, Nguyen JT, Abraham CR, McLachlan DR 1994 Binding of sulfated-proteins and alpha-1-antichymotrypsin to Alzheimer Aβ: different actions of amyloid associated proteins. In: Kisilevsky R, Benson MD, Frangione B, Gauldie J, Muckle TJ, Young ID (eds) Amyloid and amyloidosis 1993. Parthenon, Park Ridge, NJ, p 341–343

Gallagher JT, Turnbull JE, Lyon M 1992 Patterns of sulfation in heparan sulfate: polymorphism based on a common structural theme. Int J Biochem 24:553–560

Hoffman JS, Ericsson LH, Eriksen N, Walsh KA, Benditt EP 1984 Murine tissue amyloid protein AA: NH_2-terminal sequence identity with only one of two serum amyloid protein (ApoSAA) gene products. J Exp Med 159:641–646

Howard J, Pilkington GJ 1990 Antibodies to fibronectin bind to plaques and other structures in Alzheimer's disease and control brain. Neurosci Lett 118:71–76

Iozzo RV, Cohen IR, Grassel S, Murdoch AD 1994 The biology of perlecan: the multifaceted heparan sulfate proteoglycan of basement membranes and pericellular matrices. Biochem J 302:625–639

Kazatchkine MD, Husby G, Araki S et al 1993 Nomenclature of amyloid and amyloidosis. Bull WHO 71:105–108

Kisilevsky R 1989 Theme and variations on a string of amyloid. Neurobiol Aging 10:499–500

Kisilevsky R 1996 Anti-amyloid drugs: potential in the treatment of diseases associated with aging. Drugs & Aging 8:75–83

Kisilevsky R, Boudreau L 1983 The kinetics of amyloid deposition. I: The effect of amyloid enhancing factor and splenectomy. Lab Invest 48:53–59

Kisilevsky R, Young ID 1994 Pathogenesis of amyloidosis. In: Husby G (ed) Clinical rheumatology, vol 8, no 3: Reactive amyloidosis and the acute phase response. Bailliere Tindall, London, p 613–626

Kisilevsky R, Lemieux LJ, Fraser PE, Kong XQ, Hultin PG, Szarek WA 1995 Arresting amyloidosis *in vivo* using small-molecule anionic sulfonates or sulfates: implications for Alzheimer's disease. Nat Med 1:143–148

Kjellen L, Lindahl U 1991 Proteoglycans: structures and interactions. Annu Rev Biochem 60:443–475

Kushner I, Rzewnicki DL 1994 The acute phase response: general aspects. In: Husby G (ed) Clinical rheumatology, vol 8, no 3: Reactive amyloidosis and the acute phase response. Bailliere Tindall, London, p 513–530

Liepnieks JJ, Kluve-Beckerman B, Benson MD 1995 Characterization of amyloid A protein in human secondary amyloidosis: the predominant deposition of serum amyloid A1. Biochim Biophys Acta 1270:81–86

Linke RP, Huhn D, Casanova S, Donini U 1989 Immunoelectron microscopic identification of human AA-type amyloid: exploration of various monoclonal AA-antibodies, methods of fixation, embedding and of other parameters for the protein-A gold method. Lab Invest 61:691–697

Lyon AW, Narindrasorasak S, Young ID et al 1991 Codeposition of basement membrane components during the induction of murine splenic AA amyloid. Lab Invest 64:785–790

McCubbin WD, Kay CM, Narindrasorasak S, Kisilevsky R 1988 Circular dichroism and fluorescence studies on two murine serum amyloid A proteins. Biochem J 256:775–783

Murtomaki S, Risteli J, Risteli L, Koivisto UM, Johansson S, Liesi P 1992 Laminin and its neurite outgrowth-promoting domain in the brain in Alzheimer's disease and Down's syndrome patients. J Neurosci Res 32:261–273

Narindrasorasak S, Lowery D, Gonzalez-DeWhitt P, Poorman RA, Greenberg B, Kisilevsky R 1991 High affinity interactions between the Alzheimer's β-amyloid precursor proteins and the basement membrane form of heparan sulfate proteoglycan. J Biol Chem 266:12878–12883

Narindrasorasak S, Lowery DE, Altman RA, Gonzalez-DeWhitt PA, Greenberg BD, Kisilevsky R 1992 Characterization of high affinity binding between laminin and the Alzheimer's disease amyloid precursor proteins. Lab Invest 67:643–652

Narindrasorasak S, Altman RA, Gonzalez-DeWhitt P, Greenberg BD, Kisilevsky R 1995 An interaction between basement membrane and Alzheimer amyloid precursor proteins suggests a role in the pathogenesis of Alzheimer's disease. Lab Invest 72:272–282

Noonan DM, Hassell JR 1993 Perlecan, the large low-density proteoglycan of basement membranes—structure and variant forms. Kidney Int 43:53–60

Palmoski MJ, Brandt KD 1975 Stimulation of glycosaminoglycan biosynthesis by amyloid fibrils. Biochem J 148:145–147

Paulsson M 1992 Basement membrane proteins—structure, assembly, and cellular interactions. Crit Rev Biochem Mol Biol 27:93–127

Pennock CA 1968 Association of acid mucopolysaccharides with isolated amyloid fibrils. Nature 217:753–754

Perlmutter LS, Chui HC 1990 Microangiopathy, the vascular basement membrane and Alzheimer's disease: a review. Brain Res Bull 24:677–686

Pras M, Schubert M, Zucker-Franklin D, Rimon A, Franklin EC 1968 The characterization of soluble amyloid prepared in water. J Clin Invest 47:924–933

Skinner M, Pinnette A, Travis WD, Shwachman H, Cohen AS 1988 Isolation and sequence analysis of amyloid protein AA from a patient with cystic fibrosis. J Lab Clin Med 112:413–417

Snow AD, Kisilevsky R 1985 Temporal relationship between glycosaminoglycan accumulation and amyloid deposition during experimental amyloidosis: a histochemical study. Lab Invest 53:37–44

Snow AD, Kisilevsky R 1988 A close ultrastructural relationship between sulfated proteoglycans and AA amyloid fibrils. Lab Invest 57:687–698

Snow AD, Kisilevsky R, Stephens C, Anastassiades T 1987 Characterization of tissue and plasma glycosaminoglycans during experimental AA amyloidosis and acute inflammation. Quantitative and qualitative analysis. Lab Invest 56:665–675

Snow AD, Bramson R, Mar H, Wight TN, Kisilevsky R 1991 A temporal and ultrastructural relationship between heparan sulfate proteoglycans and AA amyloid in experimental amyloidosis. J Histochem Cytochem 39:1321–1330

Snow AD, Kinsella MG, Parks E et al 1995 Differential binding of vascular cell-derived proteoglycans (perlecan, biglycan, decorin, and versican) to the β-amyloid protein of Alzheimer's disease. Arch Biochem Biophys 320:84–95

Virchow R 1854 Zur Cellulosefrage. Virchows Arch Pathol Anat Physiol 6:416–426

Woodrow SI, Gore J, Kisilevsky R, Young ID 1994 Type IV collagen gene expression in experimental splenic AA amyloidosis. In: Kisilevsky R, Benson MD, Frangione B, Gauldie J, Muckle TJ, Young ID (eds) Amyloid and amyloidosis 1993. Parthenon, Park Ridge, NJ, p 195–197

Yamaguchi H, Yamazaki T, Lemere CA, Frosch MP, Selkoe DJ 1992 Beta-amyloid is focally deposited within the outer basement membrane in the amyloid angiopathy of Alzheimer's disease—an immunoelectron microscopic study. Am J Pathol 141: 249–259

DISCUSSION

Kirschner: Are you aware of our finding that sulfate ions at 5–50 mM, but not phosphate or selenate ions, induce substantial lateral and linear aggregation of Aβ fibrils (Fraser et al 1992)? How does this work relate to what you find here?

Kisilevsky: Yes, I was aware of the work you and Paul Fraser have done with free sulfate. We're not using free sulfate here. If you look at whether the agents are effective or not at inhibiting the process of fibrillogenesis, *in vivo* or *in vitro*, there is a structural relationship between the spacing of the sulfonates or sulfates. By using free sulphate, I suspect you are probably doing much the same thing as if you were putting in heparin or heparan sulfate. The organization and the spatial orientation of the sulfates in the latter two compounds is quite different from the ones we have been using as inhibitors. I suspect that the spatial orientation or stereochemistry of the sulfates is going to turn out to be critical in understanding their role in the process of fibrillogenesis.

Kirschner: As you know, Congo red contains two sulfonate groups, which differ from the sulfate esters found in glycosaminoglycan chains, but are still capable of electrostatic interactions. How does this relate to your example?

Kisilevsky: That's a good question—I don't know the answer. The sulfonates on Congo red are really quite far apart relative to the molecules that we've been using. In the cell culture systems that Byron Caughey has been using (and probably others), we do not know whether the Congo red is acting as it is or is being metabolized to an active agent. One may end up with a Congo red derivative that is really quite different from Congo red itself. Most of the studies involving Congo red have actually used it to inhibit the cellular 'toxicity' of amyloid. I suspect the cells may be doing something to that Congo red.

Sipe: I was wondering about the order of events in which your test compound inhibits amyloid formation. Have you administered the compound to mice with established amyloid or do you administer it simultaneously with amyloid enhancing factor (AEF) and an inflammatory stimulus?

Kisilevsky: These experiments have been done in many different ways. Some of our collaborators have actually used the compound before the amyloid induction protocol, and it is effective in this way. We can give it within 24 h of the induction protocol and it is effective. We have also given it a week later, after amyloid has been established. In this latter case one can show that the amyloid actually starts to disappear in those animals. The rate of disappearance is equivalent to that of an amyloid-induced animal that has received only one inflammatory stimulus. In this latter case amyloid increases for 10–14 days and then starts to disappear (Kisilevsky et al 1995). If you give the agents a week after you have induced amyloid, the amyloid starts to disappear quite readily. So it has its effect both early on and later.

Sipe: And what is the nature of the nidus in AEF?

Kisilevsky: The precise nature is not known. There are many different proteins that might have this function. Per Westermark has shown quite nicely that if you take islet amyloid polypeptide (IAPP) or Aβ and allow them to form a fibril, and then use those fibrils as an AEF, they actually work. The same proteins in a non-fibril form are not effective. It appears that certain conformational elements are necessary and once those elements are present it can provoke the endogenous amyloid protein to take the fibril conformation. The prion protein is an excellent example of this.

Pepys: You showed the mRNA for the heparan sulfate proteoglycan (HSPG) being turned on only when you gave AEF and silver nitrate. That's not compatible with AEF just being a nidus.

Kisilevsky: It is true that AEF and silver nitrate lead to an increase of HSPG mRNA. Neither AEF nor silver nitrate alone give this response. This is still compatible with AEF being a nidus, but HSPG mRNA synthesis occurs immediately downstream mechanistically. I think the silver nitrate is necessary to provoke inflammation and thereby provide a precursor pool, generating the serum amyloid A (SAA). It is clear that without the SAA you will not get any amyloid: we showed this many years ago (Kisilevsky et al 1979).

Frangione: Do you have intact SAA in your AEF?

Kisilevsky: No. You certainly have AA peptides, but if you purify the AA protein from the AEF you can show the purified protein has no such property. The reason is as follows. Crude AEF, when denatured for example with guanine or urea and if followed by dialysis, loses its AEF property. There is something about the conformation of AEF that is necessary for its activity. What I'm saying about AEF actually is recapitulating a lot of what has been said about the prion protein.

Frangione: It seems more likely that you do have intact SAA in AEF as well as intact serum amyloid P component (SAP) and histones (F. Gervais, personal communication).

Kisilevsky: That depends upon when you isolate AEF. If you isolate AEF very early after you provoke amyloid, then you will get out intact SAA; later, you get AA fragments.

Frangione: AEF drastically shortens the usual time (15–21 d) needed for inducing fibril formation in the mouse and AA deposition appears within 48–72 h.

Kisilevsky: What strain is this?

Frangione: C57BL/6.

Kisilevsky: Those mice are relatively resistant to forming amyloid. Our data were obtained with CBA/J animals. In CBA/J animals the SAA is there early, but as the amyloid ages, AA peptides predominate. As far as the SAP is concerned, I agree with you, it is there too, but once you denature and purify the SAP it doesn't have any activity either. I believe the critical experiments were conducted by Per Westermark with the pure IAPP and Aβ peptides. These showed conclusively that the conformation was the critical factor in AEF activity.

Frangione: It is possible that the silver nitrate activation also increases enzymic activity, causing degradation of SAA. The AA thus formed may be the nidus.

Kisilevsky: In that case purified AA should have AEF activity, and it doesn't. This was published many years ago (Axelrad et al 1982).

Frangione: But isn't it true that in normal mice, part of the SAA is already degraded in the liver, and they have AA fragments in the circulation?

Kisilevsky: Yes, they have AA fragments in the circulation.

Frangione: The possibility that a circulating AA can induce amyloid formation after its concentration is altered should be considered.

Kisilevsky: That the AA fragment is in the circulation says little about its conformation. It is the conformation that is important for the nidus, as shown by Per Westermark. His work shows that if you take IAPP and it is not in a fibrillar form, it doesn't have the 'AEF' property. It is not enough just to show that the protein is present in the circulation.

Sipe: The CE/J mouse strain, which has a unique isoform of SAA that is a hybrid between SAA_1 and SAA_2, is not susceptible to the AA type of amyloidosis and yet it does have AEF (Kandel et al 1994). What is this agent?

Pepys: Normal mice have AEF. The homegenate of any nucleated cell population has AEF activity (Baltz et al 1986).

Goldgaber: When you use the word nidus, are you implying that amyloid formation is an extracellular process?

Kisilevsky: Yes, that's what I think.

Goldgaber: What are the experimental data to support that? The fact that you showed an increase in mRNA for HSPG suggests that intracellular events are extremely important in amyloid formation.

Kisilevsky: Showing that an mRNA is there for a particular protein doesn't tell you anything at all where that protein can operate. For example, we know that albumin mRNA is present in the liver, but albumin functions primarily in the circulation. The fact that HSPG mRNA is present in spleen cells, and we can actually identify where in the spleen this is, doesn't say anything at all about where (intracellularly or extracellularly) the protein product is operating.

Goldgaber: Have you any experimental data showing that AEF works as a nidus in the extracellular space?

Kisilevsky: None, other than the fact that AA amyloid occurs in the extracellular space within hours after AEF has been given to an inflamed mouse. *In vitro* experiments with AEF and SAA have not been feasible for a variety of reasons.

J. N. Buxbaum: Can I follow up on the basement membrane components: do you think that these are excess components that are made independently of normal basement membrane function, or do you think the basement membrane components are available to participate in amyloidogenesis?

Kisilevsky: Given that the mRNAs for the basement membrane proteins are increasing in parallel with the HSPG mRNA, I think *de novo* synthesis is probably an important factor. The basement membrane proteins already there have organized themselves in such a way (i.e. an intact basement membrane) that they will not interact with the amyloid precursors. We have been able to show this both with SAA and Aβ. That's why I think that nascent basement membrane proteins or an unravelling of existing basement membrane structure is critical. Interestingly, if you stain these amyloid deposits immunohistochemically, you can show that although all the components necessary for basement membrane formation are present, there is no structurally organized basement membrane there. The building blocks are present, but they are not organized properly when part of an amyloid deposit. The components that would normally organize themselves into a basement membrane have been interfered with in some way. Basement membrane components that should interact do not do so in the presence of amyloid precursors. We have been able to show this *in vitro* (Narindrasorasak et al 1995).

J. N. Buxbaum: Supporting this would be the fact that you rarely find amyloid in contact with the basement membrane, but certainly in the immunoglobulin light chain system the non-amyloid deposits are always in contact with the basement membrane and the amyloid deposits are not.

Kisilevsky: I think we have to be careful before we draw mechanistic conclusions from human material that's been examined where the pathogenetic process has been going on for weeks or months. The fact that well established amyloid deposits may not be in apposition to a pre-existing basement membrane is not surprising. These deposits are being looked at late in the disease. We can show the same thing is true in a mouse late in its disease. In those cases where we can monitor the process from its inception, the deposits are all associated with an anatomic area where basement membranes are certainly made and turned over.

Westermark: Have you tried your anti-amyloid small molecules on other amyloid models, for example the transthyretin (TTR) mouse model?

Kisilevsky: We haven't tried the anti-amyloid agents in other *in vivo* models, although we have looked at their effects on other amyloid proteins *in vitro*. They're effective with other amyloid proteins, including TTR.

Caughey: We have used related compounds such as Congo red and sulfated glycans in the scrapie tissue culture system, and have shown very potent inhibition of the protease-resistant prion protein formation by these compounds (Caughey & Race 1992, Caughey & Raymond 1993).

Westermark: What is their mechanism of action?

Kisilevsky: On the basis of binding data, we are speculating that they are interfering with the interaction of HSPG and the amyloid protein. For example, Paul Fraser is currently examining the binding parameters of Aβ with heparin, in the presence and absence of these compounds.

Caughey: We've shown that these compounds inhibit the interaction between prion protein and heparin. Their potency correlates with their potency as inhibitors of prion protein formation in cell culture as well as their ability to prevent scrapie in animals.

References

Axelrad MA, Kisilevsky R, Willmer J, Chen SJ, Skinner M 1982 Further characterization of amyloid enhancing factor. Lab Invest 47:139–146

Baltz ML, Caspi D, Hind CRK, Feinstein A, Pepys MB 1986 Isolation and characterisation of amyloid enhancing factor. In: Glenner GG, Osserman EF, Benditt EP, Calkins E, Cohen AS, Zucker-Franklin S (eds) Amyloidosis. Plenum, New York, p 115–121

Caughey B, Race RE 1992 Potent inhibition of scrapie-associated PrP accumulation by Congo red. J Neurochem 59:768–771

Caughey B, Raymond GJ 1993 Sulphated polyanion inhibition of scrapie-associated PrP accumulation in cultured cells. J Virol 67:643–650

Fraser PE, Nguyen JT, Chin DT, Kirschner DA 1992 Effects of sulfate ions on Alzheimer-β/A4 peptide assemblies: implications for amyloid fibril–proteoglycan interactions. J Neurochem 59:1531–1540

Kandel R, Gonnerman WA, Sipe JD, Greene L, Cathcart ES 1994 AEF produced by amyloid-resistant CE/J mice. In: Kisilevsky R, Benson MD, Frangione B, Gauldie J, Muckle TJ, Young ID (eds) Amyloid and amyloidosis 1993. Parthenon, Park Ridge, NJ, p 122–124

Kisilevsky R, Benson MD, Axelrad MA, Boudreau L 1979 Effects of a liver protein synthesis inhibitor on plasma SAA levels in a model of accelerated amyloid deposition. Lab Invest 41:206–210

Kisilevsky R, Lemieux LJ, Fraser PE, Kong XQ, Hultin PG, Szarek WA 1995 Arresting amyloidosis *in vivo* using small-molecule anionic sulfonates or sulfates: implications for Alzheimer's disease. Nat Med 1:143–148

Narindrasorasak S, Altman RA, Gonzalez-DeWhitt P, Greenberg BD, Kisilevsky R 1995 An interaction between basement membrane and Alzheimer amyloid precursor proteins suggests a role in the pathogenesis of Alzheimer's disease. Lab Invest 72:272–282

Molecular mechanisms of fibrillogenesis and the protective role of amyloid P component: two possible avenues for therapy

M. B. Pepys*, G. A. Tennent*, D. R. Booth*, V. Bellotti*, L. B. Lovat*, S. Y. Tan*, M. R. Persey*, W. L. Hutchinson*, S. E. Booth*, S. Madhoo*, A. K. Soutar†, P. N. Hawkins*, R. Van Zyl-Smit‡, J. M. Campistol°, P. E. Fraser¶, S. E. Radford§, C. V. Robinson§, M. Sunde§, L. C. Serpell§ and C. C. F. Blake§

**Immunological Medicine Unit and †MRC Lipoprotein Team, Clinical Sciences Centre, Royal Postgraduate Medical School, Hammersmith Hospital, Du Cane Road, London W12 0NN, UK, ‡Renal Unit, Groote Schuur Hospital, Observatory 7925, Cape Town, South Africa, °Renal Transplant Unit, Hospital Clinic, Villarroel 170, 08036 Barcelona, Spain, ¶Centre for Research in Neurodegenerative Diseases & Department of Medical Biophysics, University of Toronto, 6 Queen's Park Crescent West, Toronto, Ontario, Canada M5S 1AB and §Laboratory of Molecular Biophysics and Oxford Centre for Molecular Sciences, South Parks Road, University of Oxford, Oxford OX1 3QU, UK*

Abstract. Amyloid deposits regress when the supply of fibril precursor proteins is sufficiently reduced, indicating that amyloid fibrils are degradable *in vivo*. Serum amyloid P component (SAP), a universal constituent of amyloid deposits, efficiently protects amyloid fibrils from proteolysis *in vitro*, and may contribute to persistence of amyloid *in vivo*. Drugs that prevent binding of SAP to amyloid fibrils *in vivo* should therefore promote regression of amyloid and we are actively seeking such agents. A complementary strategy is identification of critical molecular processes in fibrillogenesis as targets for pharmacological intervention. All amyloidogenic variants of apolipoprotein AI contain an additional positive charge in the N-terminal fibrillogenic region of the protein. This is unlikely to be a coincidence and should be informative about amyloidogenesis by this protein. The two amyloidogenic variants of human lysozyme, caused by the first natural mutations found in its gene, provide a particularly powerful model system because both the crystal structure and folding pathways of wild-type lysozyme are so well characterized. The amyloidogenic variant lysozymes have similar 3D crystal structures to the wild type, but are notably less thermostable. They unfold on heating, lose enzymic activity, and aggregate to form amyloid fibrils *in vitro*.

1996 The nature and origin of amyloid fibrils. Wiley, Chichester (Ciba Foundation Symposium 199) p 73–89

Amyloidosis is a pathological condition in which normally soluble autologous proteins are deposited in tissues as abnormal insoluble fibrils with characteristic ultrastructural morphology and the unique tinctorial property of binding Congo red and then giving apple-green birefringence in polarized light (Pepys 1994). The predominant feature of their protein secondary structure is antiparallel β-sheets arranged with their long axes perpendicular to the fibril long axis (Glenner 1980). The fibrils in the different forms of amyloidosis are derived from different and completely unrelated proteins but the fibril morphology and X-ray diffraction patterns are remarkably similar, indicating that during fibrillogenesis the precursors adopt a common structural arrangement (Blake et al 1996, this volume). Further evidence of shared properties is that *in vivo* all amyloid deposits contain serum amyloid P component (SAP), a normal non-fibrillar plasma glycoprotein of the pentraxin family that undergoes Ca^{2+}-dependent binding to all types of amyloid fibril (Pepys 1994).

Amyloid deposits are composed mainly of the amyloid fibrils themselves and, in the systemic amyloidoses, organ dysfunction and disease are definitely caused by the deposits themselves. In Alzheimer's disease the absolute amount of amyloid in the intracerebral and cerebrovascular deposits is usually rather small, but nevertheless there is strong evidence, especially from genetic forms of Alzheimer's disease, of a correlation between amyloid and dementia (Hardy 1992, Cummings & Cotman 1995). In contrast, in the spongiform encephalopathies associated with prions there is sometimes a dissociation between neuropathology and the overt presence of amyloid (Pepys 1994).

The introduction of *in vivo* scintigraphy with radiolabelled human SAP has enabled the natural history of systemic amyloidosis to be monitored for the first time during life (Hawkins et al 1988, 1990a,b, Hawkins 1994). It has demonstrated that the usual inexorable progression of clinical amyloidosis is mostly a reflection of the progressive and frequently incurable nature of the primary disorders that are complicated by amyloidosis. When the underlying disease can be eliminated or controlled, reducing availability of the precursor proteins that form the amyloid fibrils, deposition may stop and in many patients amyloid regresses, sometimes rapidly and extensively. This is generally associated with clinical benefit unless target organ damage is already irreversible. These observations greatly encourage active approaches to treatment of all types of amyloidosis. Unfortunately, in many situations it is not possible to reduce the supply of fibril precursors and alternative anti-amyloid strategies are therefore required.

The classical approach of the pharmaceutical industry to such problems is to identify a cellular or molecular target and then to screen compound libraries for active materials that can be starting points for drug development. However, knowledge of the molecular structure of the target of drug action should facilitate progress from an initial 'hit' and may enable rational drug design. We have been pursuing two parallel approaches to novel therapies for amyloidosis. Firstly, we have identified SAP as a possible contributor to the persistence of amyloid deposits *in vivo*, and therefore as a target for therapy. Secondly, we are using the natural mutations that cause hereditary amyloidosis to elucidate the molecular pathways of fibrillogenesis in the hope of recognizing steps susceptible to pharmacological intervention.

Hereditary apolipoprotein AI amyloidosis

Hereditary amyloidosis can be caused by point mutations in the genes encoding a number of different proteins, including transthyretin, gelsolin, cystatin C, apolipoprotein AI (apoAI), fibrinogen and lysozyme (Pepys 1994). These mutations are responsible for single residue substitutions in the mature sequence and, although these apparently do not affect the physiological functions of the molecules involved, they are sufficient to render these normally soluble proteins amyloidogenic. They have their effect by destabilizing the native structure, and/or by promoting normal or abnormal cleavage to yield amyloidogenic fragments. However, there is no consistent pattern in the nature of the amino acid substitutions in any of these proteins, except apoAI. Each of the three known amyloidogenic point mutations in apoAI encode substitution of neutral residues by the cationic residue arginine: Gly26Arg, Trp50Arg and Leu60Arg, and each one results in acquisition of a single extra positive charge by the mature molecule (Booth et al 1995).

We have lately investigated two newly discovered kindreds with autosomal dominant non-neuropathic hereditary systemic amyloidosis in whom we have identified apoAI as the amyloid fibril protein. One is a very large Spanish family with a unique clinical presentation in which the affected members in three generations have developed massive and ultimately fatal hepatic amyloidosis in adult life (Booth et al 1996). There is little or no overt sign of other organ involvement although deposits are very widespread and extensive at autopsy. The amyloid fibril protein was shown to be apoAI by immunohistochemical staining of amyloidotic tissue obtained at post mortem. The index case was found to be a heterozygote for a mutation in exon 4 in the apoAI gene in which 35 nucleotides had been deleted from the wild-type sequence and five nucleotides inserted, maintaining the reading frame. The mutation was readily demonstrable by gel analysis of the exon 4 PCR product, and this test was used to screen all members of the family from whom samples could be obtained. The observed DNA changes encoded deletion of residues 60–71 of the wild-type amino acid sequence and their replacement by two new residues, valine and threonine. The protein subunits of amyloid fibrils isolated from spleen were precisely characterized by electrospray mass spectrometry and corresponded exactly to N-terminal fragments comprising residues 1–83 and 1–92 of apoAI including the variant sequence predicted by the mutant allele. There was no evidence for any wild-type apoAI sequence in the fibrils. This is the first example of an amyloidogenic deletion mutation to be described.

The second kindred is of English/Scottish origin and now lives in South Africa. The clinical presentation is with adult-onset, slowly progressive but ultimately fatal amyloid nephropathy. Other visceral involvement is present but is generally silent. The amyloid fibril protein has been identified as apoAI by immunohistochemistry on biopsy material as no autopsy tissue is available. The fibril subunits have therefore not yet been characterized in protein studies, but sequencing of the apoAI gene revealed a hitherto undescribed in-frame deletion mutation, encoding loss of residues Glu70–Trp72 in mature apoAI with replacement of position 70 by Asp. This is present in all affected family members but not in any of their normal relatives.

Both the Spanish and the South African deletion mutations result in acquisition by the variant apoAI molecules of one additional positive charge compared with the mature wild-type protein. This finding, in conjunction with the three amyloidogenic point mutations that have the same charge effect, strongly implies that the position and the nature of the charge change play a critical role in promoting amyloid fibril formation. Some possible mechanisms, that are not mutually exclusive, include destabilization of the native structure leading to fibrillogenic aggregation, facilitation of proteolytic cleavage to yield a fibrillogenic fragment, and enhancement of interaction with the polyanionic glycosaminoglycans that are universally associated with amyloid deposits and are tightly bound to the fibrils (Snow et al 1987, Nelson et al 1991a). Interestingly, it has recently been demonstrated that the N-terminal fragment of putatively normal wild-type apoAI commonly forms amyloid fibrils both in aged dogs (Johnson et al 1992) and in man (Westermark et al 1995, 1996, this volume), and that intact wild type apoAI can be induced to form amyloid fibrils *in vitro* (Wisniewski et al 1995). The amyloidogenic effect of the mutations may therefore represent an enhancement and/or acceleration of the processes responsible for these 'normal' phenomena of ageing. We are currently expressing apoAI and its amyloidogenic variants *in vitro* in order to study their aggregation, folding and cleavage behaviour and to compare them with the wild-type and variant proteins isolated from the plasma of affected heterozygotes.

Hereditary lysozyme amyloidosis

The discovery of hereditary non-neuropathic systemic amyloidosis caused by the first known natural mutations in the human lysozyme gene opened up a powerful new model system (Pepys et al 1993). The two variants were Ile56Thr and Asp67His. Subsequently we have identified a third affected family carrying the His67 mutation in which the proband required orthotopic liver transplantation following rupture of the amyloidotic liver, and he has subsequently undergone removal of a heavily amyloid-laden spleen. Abundant *ex vivo* lysozyme His67 amyloid fibrils are therefore available. However in order to study the molecular mechanisms of amyloid fibrillogenesis it was necessary to produce the variant and wild-type proteins *in vitro* by recombinant technology. This was achieved in the baculovirus system and the purified products were crystallized and their 3D structures solved to atomic resolution by X-ray crystallography.

The structure of recombinant wild-type lysozyme was identical to that previously reported for natural lysozyme. The Thr56 variant crystallized under different conditions from wild-type lysozyme but in the same crystal form, and its structure was very similar indeed to that of the wild-type. It did not contain the potentially stabilizing new hydrogen bond that we had predicted might be possible with Thr in place of Ile56 (Pepys et al 1993). In contrast, the His67 variant, which crystallized under different conditions and in a different crystal form, confirmed our prediction (Pepys et al 1993) that this substitution would have significant structural effects. His67 cannot make the three hydrogen bonds made by the wild-type residue Asp67 that are essential to stabilize this domain of the molecule, and the two adjacent loops are separated by about 10 Å more than in the wild-type structure.

These exciting results suggested that both of the amyloidogenic variants would be less stable than wild-type lysozyme, and this was independently found to be the case. When the proteins are heated, the two variants progressively lose enzymic activity while the wild-type is unaffected, and at 65 °C they are completely inactivated when the wild-type is still almost intact. Loss of activity in the variants is associated with aggregation, not seen with the wild-type, to yield Congophilic, green birefringent material, electron micrographs of which reveal typical amyloid fibrils.

Heat-induced aggregation and amyloid fibrillogenesis involve unfolding of the lysozyme variants as compared to the wild-type, as shown by intrinsic tryptophan fluorescence and mass spectrometric amide protection studies. Analysis of the circular dichroism spectra, showing loss of tertiary structure before loss of secondary structure, suggests that the fibrillogenesis pathway may proceed via a molten globule intermediate. It is certainly clear from Fourier transform infrared spectroscopy that the native His67 variant contains predominantly α-helical secondary structure, as known from the crystal structure, and that on heat aggregation it changes to adopt a predominantly β-sheet conformation with a spectrum closely resembling that of *ex vivo* His67 amyloid fibrils. However, this pathological conformational change is entirely reversible *in vitro*. When *ex vivo* His67 amyloid fibrils, which lack any lysozyme enzyme activity, are completely solubilized and denatured in guanidine hydrochloride and then renatured by careful dialysis under appropriate conditions they yield fully active enzyme which is identified by electrospray mass spectrometry as homogeneous, intact, His67 lysozyme.

The remarkable finding of a reversible interconversion between a native, normally folded, precursor protein and amyloid fibrils has not been reported for any other amyloid protein. Lysozyme may represent a special case but nevertheless it illuminates the folding and aggregation mechanisms involved in formation of typical amyloid fibrils from a soluble globular protein and may thus assist rational development of fibrillogenesis inhibitors with therapeutic potential in other types of amyloidosis.

SAP protects amyloid fibrils against proteolysis

The demonstration by radiolabelled SAP scintigraphy that amyloid deposits in amyloidoses caused by amyloid A protein (AA) (Hawkins et al 1993a), immunoglobulin light chains (AL) (Hawkins et al 1993b), β_2-microglobulin (Nelson et al 1991b) and transthyretin (TTR) (Holmgren et al 1993) can often regress significantly when the supply of fibril precursor proteins is adequately reduced, indicates that the deposits are in a dynamic state. An attractive approach to treatment in situations in which precursor supply cannot be controlled would therefore be to enhance regression. Unfortunately nothing is known about the mechanisms responsible for clearance of amyloid from the tissues. However it must involve proteolysis and presumably is mediated by the activity of macrophages and/or the parenchymal cells of the affected tissues. Many years ago I proposed that SAP, which coats the amyloid fibrils in all known amyloid deposits, might protect the fibrils from degradation by masking their abnormal structure with its own normal conformation (Hind et al 1984, Pepys 1986). In addition the avid binding of SAP to amyloid fibrils should stabilize them regardless of the mechanisms by which they may be degraded *in vivo*. More recently, we have confirmed that SAP isolated from tissue amyloid deposits is indeed absolutely unaltered with respect to circulating SAP (Pepys et al 1994), and we have identified hepatocytes as the only cells in the body that mediate significant catabolism of SAP (Hutchinson et al 1994). Finally, the high resolution crystal structure of SAP (Emsley et al 1994) demonstrates the molecular basis for the extreme proteinase resistance of SAP itself (Kinoshita et al 1992). These observations refocused our attention on the concept of amyloid fibril protection by SAP, and we have now confirmed it experimentally (Tennent et al 1995).

Firstly, we found that SAP undergoes Ca^{2+}-dependent binding to amyloid fibrils formed *in vitro* from pure synthetic Alzheimer's disease amyloid β-peptide (Aβ), in the absence of any glycan, and the binding constant is the same as for *ex vivo* amyloid fibrils. Secondly, having bound to these fibrils or to *ex vivo* Aβ, AA, AL or apoAI amyloid fibrils, SAP then dramatically protects them from proteolysis by a variety of bacterial, digestive and lysosomal enzymes. Thirdly, SAP is protective only when actually bound to and coating the fibrils. SAP is not an enzyme inhibitor and if it is present in the digestion mixtures but is prevented from binding to the fibrils by the 4,6-cyclic pyruvate acetal of galactose (methyl 4,6-*O*-[(R)-1-carboxylethylidene]-β-D-galactopyranoside; M*O*βDG), its low molecular weight sugar ligand, then no protection is observed. If SAP within amyloid deposits mediates similar protection of amyloid fibrils *in vivo* then it may make a significant contribution to their persistence, accumulation and pathogenicity.

Our therapeutic strategy is thus to identify pharmaceutically acceptable molecules that inhibit and reverse binding of SAP to amyloid fibrils *in vivo*, in the hope that if this can be done without undue toxicity then regression of amyloid should be enhanced. A screening and evaluation programme in collaboration with Hoffmann-La Roche, Basle, is currently in progress. Availability of active compounds would enable us to test the hypothesis very rigorously in the experimental mouse model of AA amyloidosis. Another powerful test will be SAP knockout mice, in which the SAP gene has been deleted by homologous recombination, provided they can survive without SAP. We have created four separate strains and are presently investigating them (M. Botto, M. C. M. Bickerstaff, A. E. Bygraves, M. J. Walport & M. B. Pepys, unpublished work 1995). These approaches should define the role of SAP in amyloidogenesis and its potential as a target for drug therapy.

Conclusions

Increasingly precise information about molecular mechanisms of amyloid fibrillogenesis, derived from experiments of nature (the hereditary amyloidoses), and about the properties of SAP, derived from experiments in the laboratory, provides a powerful background for novel approaches to therapy of amyloidosis.

Acknowledgements

This work was supported in part by programme, project and fellowship grants from the Medical Research Council and the Arthritis and Rheumatism Council for Research.

References

Blake CCF, Serpell LC, Sunde M, Sandgren O, Lundgren E 1996 A molecular model of the amyloid fibril. In: The nature and origin of amyloid fibrils. Wiley, Chichester (Ciba Found Symp 199) p 6–21

Booth DR, Tan SY, Booth SE et al 1995 A new apolipoprotein AI variant, Trp50Arg, causes hereditary amyloidosis. Quart J Med 88:695–702

Booth DR, Tan SY, Booth SE et al 1996 Hereditary hepatic and systemic amyloidosis caused by a new deletion/insertion mutation in the apolipoprotein AI gene. J Clin Invest 67, in press

Cummings BJ, Cotman CW 1995 Image analysis of β-amyloid load in Alzheimer's disease and relation to dementia severity. Lancet 346:1524–1528

Emsley J, White HE, O'Hara BP et al 1994 Structure of pentameric human serum amyloid P component. Nature 367:338–345

Glenner GG 1980 Amyloid deposits and amyloidosis. The β-fibrilloses. 2. N Engl J Med 302:1333–1343

Hardy J 1992 Framing β-amyloid. Nat Genet 1:233–234

Hawkins PN 1994 Studies with radiolabelled serum amyloid P component provide evidence for turnover and regression of amyloid deposits *in vivo*. Clin Sci 87:289–295

Hawkins PN, Myers MJ, Lavender JP, Pepys MB 1988 Diagnostic radionuclide imaging of amyloid: biological targeting by circulating human serum amyloid P component. Lancet I:1413–1418

Hawkins PN, Lavender JP, Pepys MB 1990a Evaluation of systemic amyloidosis by scintigraphy with ^{123}I-labeled serum amyloid P component. N Engl J Med 323:508–513

Hawkins PN, Wootton R, Pepys MB 1990b Metabolic studies of radioiodinated serum amyloid P component in normal subjects and patients with systemic amyloidosis. J Clin Invest 86:1862–1869

Hawkins PN, Richardson S, Vigushin DM et al 1993a Serum amyloid P component scintigraphy and turnover studies for diagnosis and quantitative monitoring of AA amyloidosis in juvenile rheumatoid arthritis. Arthritis & Rheum 36:842–851

Hawkins PN, Richardson S, MacSweeney JE et al 1993b Scintigraphic quantification and serial monitoring of human visceral amyloid deposits provide evidence for turnover and regression. Quart J Med 86:365–374

Hind CRK, Collins PM, Caspi D, Baltz ML, Pepys MB 1984 Specific chemical dissociation of fibrillar and non-fibrillar components of amyloid deposits. Lancet II:376–378

Holmgren G, Ericzon B-G, Groth C-G et al 1993 Clinical improvement and amyloid regression after liver transplantation in hereditary transthyretin amyloidosis. Lancet 341:1113–1116

Hutchinson WL, Noble GE, Hawkins PN, Pepys MB 1994 The pentraxins, C-reactive protein and serum amyloid P component, are cleared and catabolized by hepatocytes *in vivo*. J Clin Invest 94:1390–1396

Johnson KH, Sletten K, Hayden DW, O'Brien TD, Roertgen KE, Westermark P 1992 Pulmonary vascular amyloidosis in aged dogs. A new form of spontaneously occurring amyloidosis derived from apolipoprotein AI. Am J Pathol 141:1013–1019

Kinoshita CM, Gewurz AT, Siegel JN et al 1992 A protease-sensitive site in the proposed Ca^{2+}-binding region of human serum amyloid P component and other pentraxins. Protein Sci 1:700–709

Nelson SR, Lyon M, Gallagher JT, Johnson EA, Pepys MB 1991a Isolation and characterisation of the integral glycosaminoglycan constituents of human amyloid A and monoclonal light-chain amyloid fibrils. Biochem J 275:67–73

Nelson SR, Hawkins PN, Richardson S et al 1991b Imaging of haemodialysis-associated amyloidosis with ^{123}I-serum amyloid P component. Lancet 338:335–339

Pepys MB 1986 Amyloid P component: structure and properties. In: Marrink J, van Rijswijk MH (eds) Amyloidosis. Martinus Nijhoff, Dordrecht, p 43–50

Pepys MB 1994 Amyloidosis. In: Frank MM, Austen KF, Claman HN, Unanue ER (eds) Samter's immunologic diseases, 5th edn. Little, Brown & Co., Boston, MA, p 637–655

Pepys MB, Hawkins PN, Booth DR et al 1993 Human lysozyme gene mutations cause hereditary systemic amyloidosis. Nature 362:553–557

Pepys MB, Rademacher TW, Amatayakul-Chantler S et al 1994 Human serum amyloid P component is an invariant constituent of amyloid deposits and has a uniquely homogeneous glycostructure. Proc Natl Acad Sci USA 91:5602–5606
Snow AD, Willmer J, Kisilevsky R 1987 Sulfated glycosaminoglycans: a common constituent of all amyloids? Lab Invest 56:120–123
Tennent GA, Lovat LB, Pepys MB 1995 Serum amyloid P component prevents proteolysis of the amyloid fibrils of Alzheimer's disease and systemic amyloidosis. Proc Natl Acad Sci USA 92:4299–4303
Westermark P, Mucchiano G, Marthin T, Johnson KH, Sletten K 1995 Apolipoprotein AI-derived amyloid in human aortic atheroslcerotic plaques. Am J Pathol 147:1186–1192
Westermark P, Sletten K, Johnson KH 1996 Ageing and amyloid fibrillogenesis: lessons from apolipoprotein AI, transthyretin and islet amyloid polypeptide. In: The nature and origin of amyloid fibrils. Wiley, Chichester (Ciba Found Symp 199) p 205–222
Wisniewski T, Golabek AA, Kida E, Wisniewski KE, Frangione B 1995 Conformational mimicry in Alzheimer's disease: role of apolipoproteins in amyloidogenesis. Am J Pathol 147:238–244

DISCUSSION

Maeda: What do you think the function of SAP is?

Pepys: It must have a very important function because it's so stably conserved and because there are no polymorphisms. It is the main DNA and chromatin binding protein in plasma (Pepys & Butler 1987). It selectively dissociates H1 histone from native long chromatin and thereby solubilizes the chromatin (Butler et al 1990). Consequently, one very important function could be that it participates in the handling of chromatin released when cells die. If chromatin were not efficiently cleared from the extracellular environment it could become auto-immunogenic and/or be a source of inappropriate genetic material. SAP is also a lectin (Hind et al 1984) and binds to certain bacteria, including *Streptococcus pyogenes* (Hind et al 1985), which is one of the most potent human pathogens. Consequently, it might be involved in innate immunity. I would guess that a molecule as ancient as this has probably got a number of functions. The short answer is, however, that we don't know exactly what these are, and that's why—just as you are—we are making the SAP knockout mice.

Maeda: If it does have such an important function, SAP deficiency might be lethal to the SAP knockout mice.

Pepys: If we don't get knockout mice, then we'll have to hope that they die sufficiently late in embryogenesis for us to discern the role of SAP. I suspect that they will be born, but then something will happen: for instance, they might succumb to infection or get lupus.

Goldgaber: Bob Kisilevsky, in your talk you presented a very interesting story but you didn't mention SAP, and Mark Pepys has also presented a beautiful story without mentioning heparan sulfate proteoglycan (HSPG). Could you present a story in which both molecules play a critical role?

Kisilevsky: You have given me an opportunity to describe some work I have been doing with Dr Sadayuki Inoue (McGill University). His background is in extracellular matrix and basement membrane components and studying their high resolution appearance by electron microscopy. Because he knew that I was working with basement membrane proteins, he asked me to give him some amyloidotic tissue, to see whether he could find structures with an appearance similar to that of these molecules when purified. From previous work he already knew the characteristics of SAP, HSPG and CSPG (chondroitin sulfate proteoglycan). The material he examined was spleen with amyloid of about a week or so. On the surface of the amyloid fibrils at very high resolution one can see what he calls 'double track' structures. The spacing between the two tracks is 4.5–5 nm. Dr Inoue feels that this is absolutely characteristic of HSPG. This can be seen even without antibody staining on the surface of the fibril. In deeper cuts along the longitudinal axis of the fibril, again one can recognize a double-track structure. The spacing here is only about 3 nm, which is characteristic of CSPG. A distribution curve of the spacing in these two types of 'double tracks' shows that the two classes don't overlap. At the periphery, where amyloid is just aggregating, one can see pentameric structures. These 'pentosomes' represent the subunit of SAP. When the core of the fibrils is examined, the pentosome is at its centre. In areas at the edge of where the amyloid seems to be aggregating, the pentosome is associating with the CSPG, and it converts eventually into a typical amyloid fibril. The question is: where is the AA in this fibril? He has tagged affinity purified antibodies to the AA with 5 nm and 1 nm gold particles. These labelled antibodies associate with fine strands 1–2 nm in width on the surface of the amyloid fibril. In the absence of antibodies we can make out the fine fibril that is apparently the AA fibril. When these are put together in a composite arrangement, Dr Inoue thinks the SAP is actually critical to fibril assembly and occurs in the core of the amyloid fibril, on top of which there are CSPG and HSPG, the latter associated with the filaments of AA. These findings suggest that SAP has a role to play that is perhaps different than we've imagined, and potentially much more important than we thought. It may be critical in setting up the core around which the amyloid fibril is actually put together.

J. N. Buxbaum: Intuitively and experimentally we all know that it is easy to get SAP out of amyloidotic tissues with the early salt washes, suggesting that the association between SAP and the fibril is relatively loose. Your results suggest a more intimate and perhaps tighter association. Unless the interaction is a 'hit and run' process, which is not suggested by your findings, it is hard to reconcile the ease of extraction with a stable natural function, unless you are just washing the cores out of a central hollow tube.

Kisilevsky: The material just described was examined *in situ*. Amyloid fibrils may look quite different after extraction from tissue. When you think of the washing techniques that we use to prepare semipurified fibrils, this is not as surprising as it may seem. CSPG and HSPG both have lots of glycosaminoglycans, which would soak up water intensely. In the absence of saline these would lift off the fibril surface.

Pepys: But all the SAP is out long before you do that. SAP comes out in the first two washes with citrate or EDTA.

Kisilevsky: I would agree that the SAP may be gone in the first few washes.

Goldgaber: Are you suggesting that when you extract the amyloid from the tissue you will wash away SAP, and then what you are left with is re-formed amyloid which was not there to begin with?

Kisilevsky: Yes. The amyloid may have been there but in a different form. This is a possibility we should keep in mind.

Pepys: We will soon know whether SAP really is important for amyloidogenesis, because we will have SAP knockout mice as a unique experimental model. My guess is that they will get amyloid but that this amyloid won't persist. We all know that typical amyloid fibrils can form *in vitro* from pure protein precursors in the absence of SAP. However, these fibrils are readily degraded by proteolysis. SAP protects these and *ex vivo* fibrils from proteolysis *in vitro* and may therefore also do so *in vivo* (Tennent et al 1995).

J. N. Buxbaum: There are other data relevant to this, from the system that is least-well represented at this meeting—the immunoglobulin light chains. Some light chains make fibrils, and other light chains deposit but fail to make fibrils. The latter always sit on the basement membrane and never have SAP, whereas those that make fibrils always have SAP. Thus the crucial issue with respect to SAP binding may not be deposition *per se*, but the final form of the deposit (fibrillar or non-fibrillar) and, as suggested by Mark Pepys, its long term stability.

Westermark: Do the transgenic mice that over-express human SAP get amyloidosis more easily?

J. N. Buxbaum: Murakami et al (1992) and Tashiro et al (1991), using two different approaches, answered that question in mice transgenic for human Met30 TTR. When they increased endogeneous murine SAP production by treating the animals with lipopolysaccharide for a period sufficient to produce AA amyloid in the transgenics, they did not find any increase in the degree of human TTR deposition, as defined histologically. Similarly, when they made double transgenics (for both human SAP and TTR Met30) the animals did not appear to have a more rapid rate or greater extent of amyloid accumulations than in the TTR Met30 single transgenics.

Pepys: This hasn't been tested for AA amyloid. However, it is not a very rigorous experiment, because in mice their own SAP is a dramatic acute phase reactant: they can produce huge amounts of it. If it turns out that SAP knockout mice don't get amyloidosis, a much more instructive experiment would be then to cross them with SAP transgenic mice and restore amyloidosis in that way.

Kisilevsky: The hamster amyloid model at least partly answers that question. The female hamster protein, which is the equivalent of SAP, seems to predispose those animals to amyloidosis.

Pepys: I don't think it is clear as that, because other factors could be involved, even though we first reported many years ago the correlation, in different strains of mice and with different stimuli, between the capacity to make SAP and the ease of getting amyloid (Baltz et al 1980). The female hamsters are a dramatic example of the association as they get amyloidosis very easily and spontaneously whereas male hamsters get it with much more difficulty (Snel et al 1989, Coe & Ross 1990). This correlates beautifully with the amount of hamster SAP they have, but it still does not establish a causative relationship. We hope the SAP knockout mice will prove this point.

Sipe: The SAP concentrations in the female hamsters are dramatically higher than those found in other animals. Although the model of spontaneous AA amyloidosis in ageing female golden Syrian hamsters may not be 'clean' in the sense that it cannot be synchronized in the way that the accelerated murine model using amyloid enhancing factor can, it does offer one unique advantage. This is that amyloidogenic events can be analysed in the absence of confounding factors due to the massive inflammatory stimulation required by other experimental models. In particular, the pathogenic role of SAP can be analysed. In the absence of inflammation, after one month of age, SAP concentration can be as high as 2–3 mg/ml in the female, compared with 40–50 μg/ml for human and 50–100 μg/ml for mouse. SAP concentration in male hamsters is comparable to humans and mice. The incidence of spontaneous amyloidosis in female hamsters at 6 months is 25%; in male hamsters it is virtually nil. It should be emphasized that the amount of inflammation evident in female hamsters who have developed amyloidosis spontaneously is miniscule compared with hamsters or mice who have received daily injections of casein or lipopolysaccharide for 7–28 d or more.

Westermark: I have a question regarding the *in vitro* studies with binding of SAP to the fibrils formed *in vitro.* Do fibrils formed from segments of precursor proteins behave in the same way as fibrils containing the complete protein? For example, have you used Aβ1–40 and have you also tested fragments thereof?

Pepys: Yes, we have used Aβ1–40, 1–42 and 1–28 (although the latter doesn't make fibrils or spin down very nicely). These experiments were all done some time ago with centrifugation assays, but we're now working with the biosensor method. This is a better system in that you can immobilize the fibrils, quantify how much is there, put SAP on and see how many molecules are bound. We don't know about very short length fragments, but we have looked at some of your TTR peptides and at your islet amyloid polypeptide, and SAP binds to the fibrils formed from them, although possibly in smaller amounts than to fibrils formed from larger proteins.

Westermark: Does this mean that you don't think that SAP binds to a special motif on the amyloid fibrils?

Pepys: On the contrary, I think there is a special motif. There is something structurally in common between all the different types of amyloid fibrils, and SAP detects it.

Westermark: And that is not a shared sequence?

Pepys: No, it is a 3D motif. My hypothesis, already many years old, is that it's a β-bend where the sheets turn around and fold back on themselves (Pepys 1986). There's an exposed carbonyl group there which selectively coordinates Ca^{2+} over other cations. I suspect this is the ligand to which SAP binds. Interestingly, we have some new data which support this concept.

J. N. Buxbaum: A clinical question: in your boy with the His67 lysozyme mutation and liver transplant, the proband in the third lysozyme amyloid family, how much lysozyme was made in the liver? Since there are other sources of lysozyme, presumably he is still making the mutant.

Pepys: Lysozyme is the major secreted protein of macrophages, so the liver transplant is not likely to protect him. Some is also made by the hepatocytes. I don't think anybody has ever quantified the relative amounts. This might give us an opportunity to look at that. In theory, he may well re-develop amyloid in the liver later on.

Kirschner: What do the electron micrographs of your SAP Aβ preparations show?

Pepys: We haven't done any electron microscope studies of those.

Kirschner: What do you predict?

Pepys: In electron micrographs of fibrils that have been extracted *ex vivo* without any attempt to wash the SAP off, one sees pentamers and decamers of SAP in a range of orientations along the fibril. However, this is very difficult to interpret because if you have pure SAP, in the absence of other proteins but in the presence of Ca^{2+} that is required for ligand binding, the SAP autoaggregates with high efficiency. You can then see many spectacular structures in the electron micrographs (Painter et al 1982). In our experiments looking at pure SAP binding to pure Aβ fibrils, the self-aggregation of SAP is prevented by the presence of 40 mg/ml bovine serum albumin which reduces the free ionizable Ca^{2+} concentration (Baltz et al 1982). This material is therefore not suitable for electron microscope studies.

Kirschner: In electron micrographs of lysozyme amyloid, the fibres appear very different from fibres you get in Alzheimer's disease. For instance, these look much more like thick ribbons or plates. Do you have any idea about the orientation of the polypeptides? How would you build a fibre from lysozyme?

Blake: With great difficulty, because the molecule starts off being largely α-helical—even worse than that, it has four disulfide bridges linking the polypeptide chain. Consequently, any model is going to be speculative in the extreme. All one can say at the moment is that we have X-ray diffraction patterns of the fibrils and they appear to conform to the normal characteristics.

Kirschner: But presumably the lysozyme is denatured?

Blake: Yes.

Kirschner: Given that, it seems to question whether X-ray crystallography on crystals of amyloid would be relevant to understanding the fibril structure.

Blake: That's probably true.

Pepys: We have lately made a unique observation in the lysozyme amyloid system. The isolated *ex vivo* fibrils have no lysozyme enzymic activity, but they can be dissolved and dissociated in guanidine. The free subunits, corresponding to intact variant lysozyme molecules, can then be carefully renatured to yield fully active native lysozyme. If the intrachain disulfide bridges are broken by inclusion of mercaptoethanol during dissociation of the fibrils, no active product can be obtained. This lysozyme variant is thus able, remarkably, to undergo an enormous secondary structural rearrangement from a native state with little β-structure into a predominantly β-sheet fibril and back again.

Blake: I think it's beyond our capabilities at the moment to model that.

Masters: A brief question on the occurrence of SAP on tangles. Surely it is in the wrong cellular compartment—how does SAP gain access to intracellular tangles, or do you only see it only on extracellular tangles?

Pepys: I haven't done this work myself. Others have claimed that they can immunostain, with appropriate specificity controls, SAP on quite a high proportion of tangles (Kalaria & Grahovac 1990, Kalaria & Perry 1993, Kalaria et al 1991a,b, Kimura et al 1994, Duong et al 1993, Perlmutter et al 1995). I presume that these are tangles that are exposed because either they are extracellular or they are in cell bodies which are defunct and are permeable to protein molecules.

Caughey: You mentioned nucleic acid binding properties of SAP. Is there any relationship between its amyloid binding properties and its nucleic acid binding properties?

Pepys: SAP binds to a number of polyanions (Pepys et al 1977), but it binds particularly avidly to DNA (Pepys & Butler 1987). In binding chromatin, SAP is binding to the DNA not to the histones. In fact it selectively displaces H1 histone, thereby unwrapping the nucleosome core structure so that the long chromatin unravels and becomes soluble (Butler et al 1990). Normally, 0.5 M salt is required to displace H1, but SAP knocks it off completely under physiological conditions, so it is a very high avidity binding.

Caughey: Do nucleic acids interfere somehow with binding to amyloid or vice versa?

Pepys: The cyclic 4,6-pyruvate acetal of galactose, M*O*βDG (Hind et al 1984), is the best characterized specific Ca^{2+}-dependent ligand for SAP. At millimolar concentrations it completely inhibits binding of SAP to amyloid fibrils. M*O*βDG at high concentration will inhibit also SAP binding to DNA, which suggests it is going through the same site. On the other hand, at appropriately low concentrations of M*O*βDG, you can actually see enhancement of SAP binding to DNA, which is something we found rather favourable, because the downside of our drug strategy is that we're going to block the normal ligand binding function of SAP and that might have some toxicity. So it is rather encouraging to us that something could inhibit SAP binding to amyloid and yet enhance its binding to the DNA, which might be a physiologically relevant function. But it does address the fact that the binding probably involves the same sort of binding site.

Wood: Both M*O*βDG and DNA prevent precipitation of SAP by Ca^{2+} ions. They inhibit an intermolecular interaction of SAP molecules involving the Ca^{2+} sites. The phosphodiester backbone of DNA could interact directly with the Ca^{2+} sites on SAP in a similar way to the carboxylate group of M*O*βDG and in principle could compete with amyloid binding.

Goldgaber: How does M*O*βDG work? Why do you need five molecules of M*O*βDG for one molecule of SAP to see an effect?

Pepys: SAP is a ligand binding molecule that recognizes the structure of amyloid. The same part that recognizes the amyloid presumably recognizes the M*O*βDG, so M*O*βDG is acting as a competitive inhibitor of SAP binding to amyloid fibrils. However, it's not a very good inhibitor of SAP binding and that's why so much MOβDG is needed. The molecules from our drug screening program have much higher affinity and should therefore be more appropriate to use *in vivo*.

Goldgaber: Does the SAP monomer bind to amyloid fibrils or does it have to be the pentamer?

Pepys: Monomers of SAP can only be obtained under extreme denaturing conditions. I'm not aware of any evidence for renatured monomers of SAP that display any functional or binding activity, and there are clearly many important, stabilizing inter-protomer contacts in the pentamer crystal structure (Emsley et al 1994).

Goldgaber: Were the binding sites for SAP determined using a monomer?

Pepys: No, it was on a pentamer (Emsley et al 1994).

Kelly: Mark Pepys, you mentioned that the intermediate that leads to lysozyme fibrils is a molten globule. This, and the fact that you have three disulfides, really limits the type of β-structure you can get. Typically you don't see disulfide bonds between strands that are next-door neighbours. This is destabilizing. Using those two pieces of evidence, can you make a model where you have one strand or a β-hairpin which polymerizes? Is the fibril unusually large?

Pepys: It's not unusually large.

Blake: For the lysozyme sequences available you can see where the links are made. The disulfide bridge can go between two β-strands of different sheets—that is favourable. Whether you could build something like that, I don't know.

References

Baltz ML, Gomer K, Davies AJS, Evans DJ, Klaus GGB, Pepys MB 1980 Differences in the acute phase responses of serum amyloid P component (SAP) and C3 to injections of casein or bovine serum albumin in amyloid susceptible and resistant mouse strains. Clin Exp Immunol 39:335–360

Baltz ML, De Beer FC, Feinstein A, Pepys MB 1982 Calcium-dependent aggregation of human serum amyloid P component. Biochim Biophys Acta 701:229–236

Butler PJG, Tennent GA, Pepys MB 1990 Pentraxin–chromatin interactions. Serum amyloid P component specifically displaces H1-type histones and solubilizes native long chromatin. J Exp Med 172:13–18

Coe JE, Ross MJ 1990 Amyloidosis and female protein in the Syrian hamster. J Exp Med 171:1257–1267

Duong T, Doucette T, Zidenberg NA, Jacobs RW, Schiebel AB 1993 Microtubule-associated proteins tau and amyloid P component in Alzheimer's disease. Brain Res 603:74–86

Emsley J, White HE, O'Hara BP et al 1994 Structure of pentameric human serum amyloid P component. Nature 367:338–345

Hind CRK, Collins PM, Renn D et al 1984 Binding specificity of serum amyloid P component for the pyruval acetal of galactose. J Exp Med 159:1058–1069

Hind CRK, Collins PM, Baltz ML, Pepys MB 1985 Human serum amyloid P component, a circulating lectin with specificity for the cyclic 4,6-pyruvate acetal of galactose. Biochem J 225:107–111

Kalaria RN, Grahovac I 1990 Serum amyloid P immunoreactivity in hippocampal tangles, plaques and vessels: implications for leakage across the blood–brain barrier in Alzheimer's disease. Brain Res 516:349–353

Kalaria RN, Perry G 1993 Amyloid P component and other acute phase proteins associated with cerebral Aβ-deposits in Alzheimer's disease. Brain Res 631:151–155

Kalaria RN, Galloway PG, Perry G 1991a Widespread serum amyloid P immunoreactivity in cortical amyloid deposits and the neurofibrillary pathology of Alzheimer's disease and other degenerative disorders. Neuropathol Appl Neurobiol 17:189–201

Kalaria RN, Golde TE, Cohen ML, Younkin SG 1991b Serum amyloid P component in Alzheimer's disease: implications for dysfunction of the blood–brain barrier. Ann NY Acad Sci 640:145–148

Kimura M, Arai H, Takahashi T, Iwamoto N 1994 Amyloid P-component-like immunoreactivity in β/A4-immunoreactive deposits in Alzheimer-type dementia brains. J Neurol 241:170–174

Murakami T, Yi S, Maeda S et al 1992 Effect of serum amyloid P component level on transthyretin-derived amyloid deposition in a transgenic mouse model of familial amyloidotic polyneuropathy. Am J Pathol 141:451–456

Painter RH, de Escallon I, Massey A, Pinteric L, Stern SB 1982 The structure and binding characteristics of serum amyloid protein (9.55 α1-glycoprotein). Ann NY Acad Sci 389:199–213

Pepys MB 1986 Amyloid P component: structure and properties. In: Marrink J, van Rijswijk MH (eds) Amyloidosis. Martinus Nijhoff, Dordrecht, p 43–50

Pepys MB, Butler PJG 1987 Serum amyloid P component is the major calcium-dependent specific DNA binding protein of the serum. Biochem Biophys Res Commun 148:308–313

Pepys MB, Dash AC, Ashley J 1977 Isolation of C-reactive protein by affinity chromatography. Clin Exp Immunol 30:32–37

Perlmutter LS, Barron E, Myers M, Saperia D, Chui HC 1995 Localization of amyloid P component in human brain: vascular staining patterns and association with Alzheimer's disease lesions. J Comp Neurol 352:92–105

Snel F, Niewold TA, Baltz ML et al 1989 Experimental amyloidosis in the hamster: correlation between hamster female protein levels and amyloid deposition. Clin Exp Immunol 76:296–300

Tashiro F, Yi S, Eakasugi S, Maeda S, Shimada K, Yamamura K 1991 Role of serum amyloid P component for systemic amyloidosis in transgenic mice carrying human transthyretin gene. Gerontology 37:56S–62S

Tennent GA, Lovat LB, Pepys MB 1995 Serum amyloid P component prevents proteolysis of the amyloid fibrils of Alzheimer's disease and systemic amyloidosis. Proc Natl Acad Sci USA 92:4299–4303

General discussion II

Human calcitonin fibrillogenesis

Arvinte: I am going to present results from our studies on calcitonin fibrillation. I will focus on aspects of the mechanism of formation of human calcitonin fibrils that may be relevant to the understanding of the mechanism of amyloid fibrillogenesis in general.

Human calcitonin (hCT) is a 32 amino acid peptide hormone which belongs to the human amyloid protein family (Husby 1992). It adopts an α-helical conformation in the presence of structure-inducing agents such as ethanol (Arvinte & Drake 1993). In aqueous solution, hCT has a strong tendency to aggregate and form fibrils. As illustrated in Fig. 1 (*Arvinte*), the kinetics of hCT fibrillation can be followed by turbidity measurements (Arvinte et al 1993). The length of time the solution is clear before the onset of turbidity (i.e. the lag time of the onset of fibrillation, or the fibrillation time, t_f) is dependent on a variety of parameters, including temperature, pH, ionic strength and hCT concentration. As an example, the dependence of the fibrillation time on the initial hCT concentration in solution is shown in Fig. 2 (*Arvinte*). In a double logarithmic plot (inset, Fig. 2 [*Arvinte*]) this dependence yields a linear relationship independent of temperature, pH, ionic strength and other additives. A similar linearity in the *ln*/*ln* representation has been described for the fibrillation of sickle cell haemoglobin (Hofrichter et al 1974). In this case, the linearity was explained by a double nucleation mechanism (see inset, Fig. 2 and Figs 3, 4 [*Arvinte*]) (Hofrichter et al 1974, Ferrone et al 1980, 1985, Samuel et al 1990). According to the scheme presented in Fig. 3 (*Arvinte*), the first step—the homogeneous nucleation step—consists of the formation of a critical nucleus. For this, hCT molecules collide to form transient complexes, and with time there is an increased probability that aggregates are formed containing a larger number of molecules. When a complex contains a critical number of molecules (i.e. a critical nucleus) it can become a stable aggregate with negligible dissociation back to monomers (Fig. 3 [*Arvinte*]). The stability of the critical nucleus is related to an equilibrium associated with conformational changes in the constituent hCT molecules. Until the critical nucleus is reached, the transitory association of molecules is homogeneous (i.e. there is no preferential direction towards aggregation).

In the critical nucleus, the molecules have adopted ordered conformations. Recent nuclear magnetic resonance (NMR) studies of hCT fibrillation have revealed that during the initial aggregation stage (i.e. when critical nuclei are

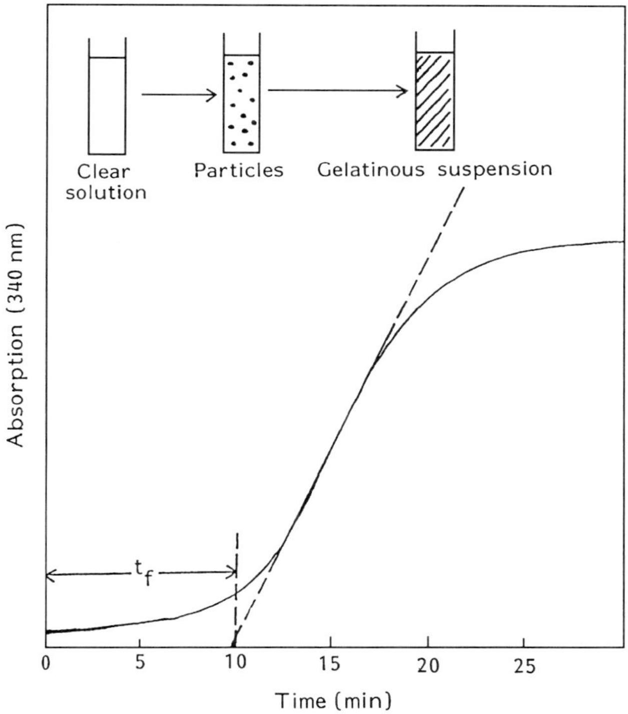

FIG. 1. (*Arvinte*) Changes in absorption during the fibrillation of a human calcitonin solution.

formed) hCT adopts an α-helical conformation (Kanaori & Nosaka 1995). Changes in the surface of the critical nucleus take place so that there are a restricted number of sites where new molecules can bind to the nucleus. The aggregate will now grow not homogeneously but heterogeneously, bidirectionally, to yield a protofibril. Protofibrils interact laterally and form fibrils, cables and bundles (Bauer et al 1995). The growth of the protofibrils and the subsequent building of complex fibrillar structures represents the heterogeneous fibrillation step, the second step in the double nucleation model (Fig. 3 [*Arvinte*]). As documented in Figs 3 and 4 (*Arvinte*), the double nucleation model predicts that the slope of the plot of the logarithm of the fibrillation time vs. the logarithm of the protein concentration (Figs 3, 4 [*Arvinte*]) will be equal to the number of molecules in the critical nucleus (Hofrichter et al 1974). For hCT, *ln*/*ln* plots constantly give a slope around 4, indicating that the critical nucleus consists of four hCT molecules (Fig. 4 [*Arvinte*]). Electron microscopic analysis of different hCT fibrillar structures yields further evidence that the critical nucleus for hCT consists of four molecules. As revealed in Fig. 5 (*Arvinte*), a plot of the fibril pitch vs. fibril diameter gives an intercept that

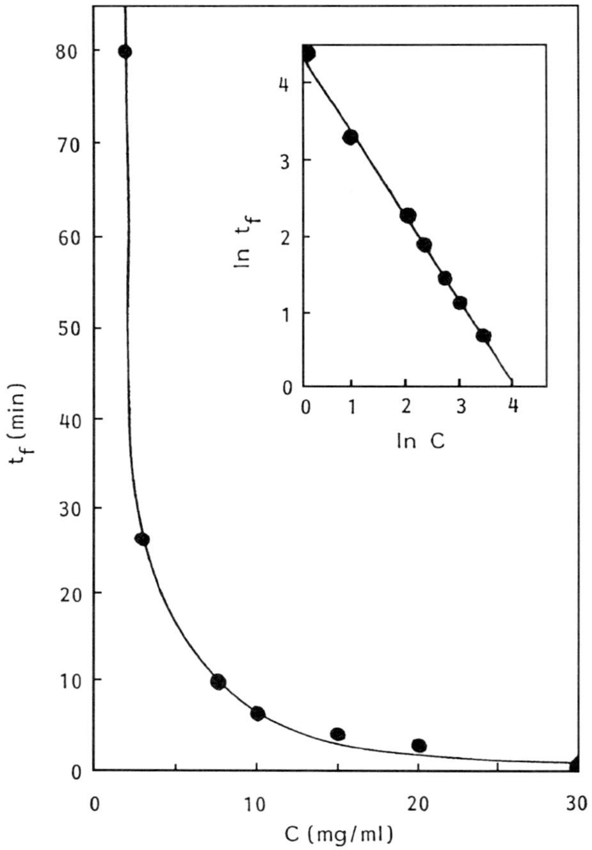

FIG. 2. (*Arvinte*) Dependence of the human calcitonin (hCT) fibrillation time on the initial concentration (C) of hCT in solution. Aqueous solutions of hCT were mixed with phosphate buffer to a final solution composition of 5 mM phosphate buffer, pH 7.4, 145 mM NaCl. From kinetic measurements of the changes of absorption over time (see Fig. 1) the fibrillation times, t_f, were measured. Experiments were performed at 22 °C. The inset shows a double logarithmic plot of initial concentration against t_f.

indicates a diameter of 4 nm (Bauer et al 1995). This value can be interpreted as the diameter of the smallest fibril (the protofibril). This interpretation is in agreement with the smallest fibril (protofibril) observed by electron microscopy which has a diameter of about 4 nm (Bauer et al 1995). As outlined below, a diameter of 4 nm is obtained from a molecular model of four hCT molecules in the critical nucleus (Fig. 6 [*Arvinte*]). A cross-section containing more than five hCT molecules will generate a protofibril diameter larger than 4 nm.

Two important aspects in elucidating the mechanism(s) of protein fibrillation are the determination of the secondary structure of the protein and the geometrical arrangement of the protein subunits within the fibrils. NMR

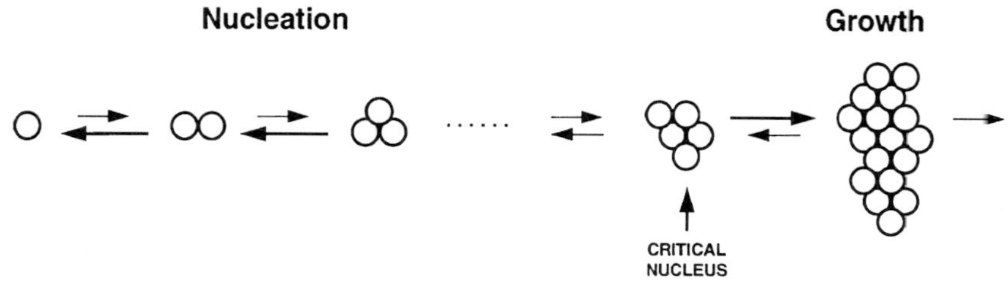

$\ln t_f = n \ln C_o + b$ **The Fibrillation Equation***

n = number of monomers in the critical nucleus
b = constant
C_o = initial peptide concentration
t_f = fibrillation time

* Hofrichter, Ross, Eaton, (1974) Proc. Natl. Acad. Sci. USA 71, 4864

FIG. 3. (*Arvinte*) Double-nucleation fibrillation model.

studies have shown that hCT adopts an α-helical conformation in the initial fibrillation state and that hCT amphiphilicity appears to be important for the hCT association (Kanaori & Nosaka 1995). Circular dichroism (CD) and Fourier-transform infrared spectroscopy (FTIR) experiments have shown that

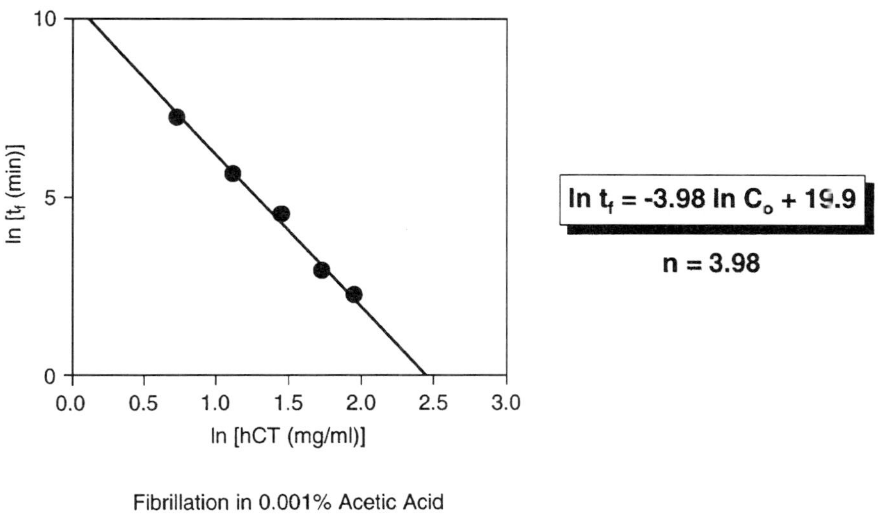

FIG. 4. (*Arvinte*) Double logarithmic plot of the dependence of the fibrillation time, t_f, on the hCT concentration in solution, C_o. The fibrillation equation (Fig. 3) predicts four hCT monomers in the critical nucleus (n = 4).

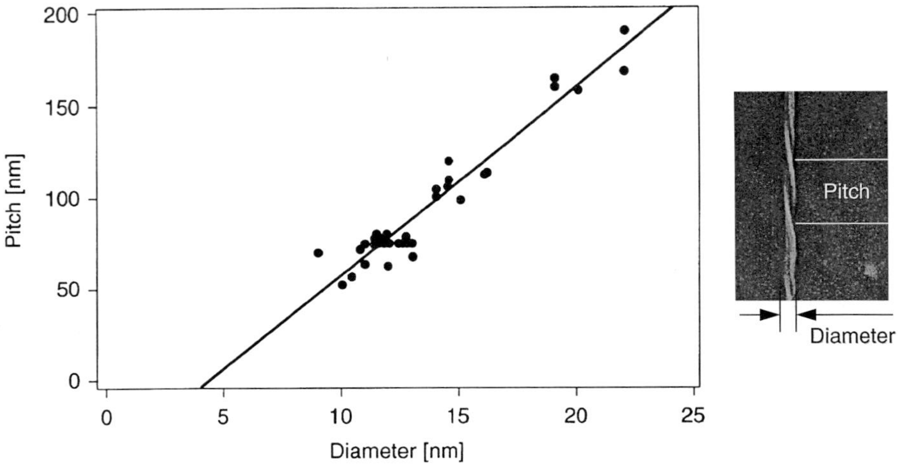

FIG. 5. (*Arvinte*) Plot of the pitch (crossover spacing) of fibrils versus their diameter. On the right is shown an example of the pitch and the diameter measured from an electron micrograph of a human calcitonin fibril.

in the fully fibrillated state the hCT molecules adopt both an amphipathic α-helical conformation and a β-sheet conformation (Arvinte et al 1993, Bauer et al 1994).

Different molecular models for the association of hCT molecules within the critical nucleus and in fibrils have been investigated. It was assumed that the experimentally observed α-helical and β-sheet conformations are present in every hCT molecule within the fibril: amphipathic α-helix between Met8 and Phe22, and the β-sheet structure between Thr25 and Pro32 (the R-sheet consists of hydrophobic amino acids). Any molecular model for the critical nucleus has to be in agreement with the following experimental data: (1) after the critical nucleus is formed the fibrillation is fast (Fig. 1 [*Arvinte*]); (2) the number of hCT molecules in the critical nucleus is around four (Fig. 4 [*Arvinte*]); (3) the hCT molecule in the critical nucleus and in the fibrils adopts an amphipathic α-helical conformation with the hydrophilic face of the α-helix oriented towards the aqueous environment and the hydrophobic side to the fibril interior; (4) hCT molecules within fibrils have a β-sheet conformation component with the β-sheets embedded in a hydrophobic environment; and (5) the diameter of the protofibril is about 4 nm. Any model should include an explanation for the formation of the critical nucleus. The critical nucleus has to be thermodynamically stable and should act as a template for fibril growth.

The optimal molecular model for the critical nucleus found to fulfil these criteria is presented in Fig. 6 (*Arvinte*) (different molecular models for the critical nucleus have been evaluated: T. Arvinte, K. Borlin & H. R. Karfunkel,

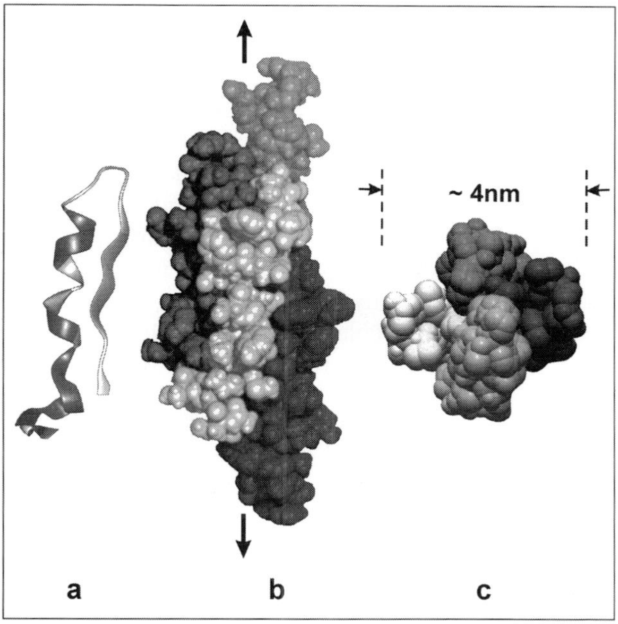

FIG. 6. (*Arvinte*) Proposed model for human calcitonin (hCT) critical nucleus and for the protofibril growth. The critical nucleus is formed from four hCT molecules which adopt α-helical and β-sheet conformations. (a) Ribbon diagram representation of the secondary structure adopted by an hCT molecule in the critical nucleus. (b) Side view of the critical nucleus. (c) Top view of the critical nucleus. The critical nucleus acts as a seed for the growth of the protofibril: arrows in (b) indicate the directions of growth.

unpublished results). The critical nucleus is a tight bundle of four hCT molecules. In this model the hCT molecule in the nucleus adopts the α-helical and the β-sheet conformations (Fig. 6a [*Arvinte*]). The four α-helices of the four hCT molecules in the critical nucleus have axes oriented along the fibril axis (Fig. 6b [*Arvinte*]); since the helices are amphipathic they form a hydrophilic surface around the nucleus. The four hCT molecules in the critical nucleus should be oriented in alternating directions. This arrangement generates no electrical dipole component from the four dipoles of the α-helices (Cohen & Parry 1990) and forms two identical ends for the critical nucleus. In the hydrophobic interior of the nucleus anti-parallel and intermolecular β-sheets are predicted to exist. Each hCT molecule in the critical nucleus is shifted relative to its neighbours by a quarter of its α-helical length (Fig. 6b [*Arvinte*]). This arrangement (a shift between hCT molecules of quarter of the hCT α-helical length and a tight bundle of four hCT molecules in alternating directions) will generate a protofibril in which all hCT molecules are in the same equilibrium state, having the same neighbouring conditions. The α-helix in the hCT molecule is right-handed. The best geometrical fit of four right-handed α-helices in a critical nucleus will be a left-handed bundle (Fig. 6b [*Arvinte*]). Thus, the protofibril will be a left-handed helical array of hCT molecules. This left-handed character of protofibrils is likely to be the basis for the macroscopic left-handed fibrils and bundles observed by electron microscopy (e.g. the fibril in Fig. 5 [*Arvinte*]; Arvinte et al 1993, Bauer et al 1995). The critical nucleus has two identical ends which are hydrophobic and act as templates for the protofibril growth (arrows in Fig. 6b,c [*Arvinte*]). The molecules which bind to the hydrophobic ends are stabilized by their interactions with the hCT molecules of the critical nucleus and with each other. The helical bundle arrangement of the hCT molecules in the critical nucleus determines the uniform growth of the protofibril. In contrast, a flat bundle arrangement of four hCT molecules in the critical nucleus (with the same secondary structure as in Fig. 6a [*Arvinte*]) will not permit a uniform growth of the protofibril.

An alternative structure in agreement with the 4 nm diameter of the protofibril is a screw-ladder model where the α-helices are oriented perpendicular to the direction of the fibril growth. This model is unlikely because it is not able to accommodate the amphipathic character of the helix; nor does it give rise to a critical nucleus since its growth would be uniform from the very beginning. In contrast, in the critical nucleus model proposed in Fig. 6 (*Arvinte*), the first three or four molecules should associate weakly; after the critical nucleus is formed the growth of the protofibril is fast and the association of hCT molecules is tighter. These two types of hCT interactions, a weak one before the critical nucleus is formed and a stronger one during the fibril growth, explain the observed lag time in fibrillation (Fig. 1 [*Arvinte*]) and the double nucleation mechanism (Fig. 3 [*Arvinte*]).

The models investigated for the critical nucleus were based on the molecular dimensions of hCT molecules and on interactive molecular modelling. I should stress that the suggested structure for the hCT critical nucleus and hCT fibrils, although in agreement with experimental data, have no direct structural experimental support.

In summary, the nucleation-dependent aggregation mechanism proposed and developed by Hofrichter and co-workers for the fibrillation of sickle cell haemoglobin (Hofrichter et al 1974, Ferrone et al 1980, 1985) explain the kinetics of hCT aggregation. The double-nucleation mechanism has also been used to explain the fibrillation of several variants of 13 amyloid proteins (Jarrett et al 1993) and of prion proteins (Jarrett & Lansbury 1993). These results suggest that the double-nucleation fibrillation may be a general aggregation mechanism for *in vitro* and *in vivo* amyloid formation.

Kirschner: If one were to do an X-ray diffraction experiment with an oriented pellet of these fibrils, you clearly would not get a cross-β-type pattern, because your β-strands are parallel to the axis of the fibre. You would also expect to observe an α-helical pattern superimposed on the β-pattern. This would be a straightforward test of your model.

Arvinte: These are experiments which we plan to do. It is interesting to note that the 4 nm diameter of the protofibril observed by electron microscopy is so small that it is difficult to find other possibilities for the molecular arrangement of hCT in the fibrils which incorporate the α-helix and β-sheet structural components.

Kirschner: Have you done neutron or X-ray scattering experiments?

Arvinte: No. We would like to perform such experiments

J. N. Buxbaum: Do you envision this happening *in vivo* driven simply by mass action? As the amount of calcitonin accumulates, do you just get to a critical concentration and then the fibrils begin to form?

Arvinte: There are indications that calcitonin may be secreted in aggregated/fibrillated form in non-pathological conditions. Immunoreactive studies have shown that after a spicy meal, high molecular mass forms of endogenous hCT are present in the circulation of healthy humans (Wimalawansa 1990). Studies of tumours of medullary carcinoma of the thyroid have shown the presence of intracellular and also extracellular hCT (and procalcitonin) amyloid fibrils (Berger et al 1988). I suspect that the growth of the fibrils *in vivo* (for example, inside the secretory granules) is hindered in space so we do not see all the complex structures seen *in vitro*.

J. N. Buxbaum: But you think that it's driven by mass action?

Arvinte: Yes. I expect that the hCT local concentration is the driving factor for fibrillation. We studied the fibrillation of human calcitonin under a large variety of conditions: pH, temperature, ion concentration and in the presence of additives such as sugars and cellulose derivatives. In all our experiments we observed the linearity in the double logarithmic plot between the fibrillation time and the hCT concentration in solution. This linearity, predicted by the double nucleation mechanism, suggests that the same mass-driven mechanism is likely to occur *in vivo*.

Proteolysis of amyloidogenic proteins

Kisilevsky: Earlier, we discussed whether various peptides can form amyloid *in vivo*. I think we have to be very careful in interpreting what peptides can and can't do, *vis-à-vis* amyloid formation, based on which peptides are present in an amyloid deposit that has been in a patient for months to years. Clearly, we know that these peptides have been derived by proteolysis from something much larger. However, we lack good animal models with which to study most amyloidoses, and consequently we don't know when this proteolytic attack on the parent protein takes place. Until we have models where we can determine exactly where the proteolytic attack occurs we should exercise caution in deciding when this proteolytic cleavage takes place. From the data we have currently, the attack could be either pre- or post-fibrillogenic.

Benson: Even though we have only three mutations in fibrinogen α-chains that cause amyloid, we are on fairly firm ground when we assume that proteolysis must be occurring before the fibril is formed, no matter how late we may isolate the amyloid. The part of the fibrinogen α-chain that forms this kidney-directed amyloid is called the 'protease-sensitive' part of the molecule: it's very difficult to isolate it. I suspect that a protein this big has to be proteolysed somewhat before that part can then incorporate into some sort of fibril.

Kisilevsky: Even in this example, do we have any information about the way in which the fibrinogen chain actually forms a fibril? If we don't, we can't be sure whether or not this mutation is simply allowing the protein to make a fibril which then has an exposed region and can still be subjected to proteolysis.

J. N. Buxbaum: We don't have a model: we have one observation made many years ago. In a patient with light chain amyloid we demonstrated a fragment inside the synthesizing cell which was secreted as a polymer. Ten years later, when the patient died, we got the amyloid tissue and the fibril subunit was exactly the same size as the one we found inside the cells at the time of synthesis.

Pepys: But that's really not so remarkable. In β_2-microglobulin, the molecule of 11 815 Da is the same molecule that forms the amyloid, without the need for proteolysis. With lysozyme, the whole variant lysozyme, with no trace of wild-type protein, is found in the amyloid without proteolysis.

Benson: My understanding is that β_2-microglobulin is proteolysed and that a significant amount of fibril protein has Lys57 clipped out.

Sipe: Bob Kisilevsky, why do you think this issue is so important?

Kisilevsky: One of the things I find difficult to understand is that in one patient, at a particular site, you may have a series of peptides that are present within the amyloid deposit, and within that same patient at another site, the predominant fragment is different. One would have to postulate either (1) that proteolysis is going on all the time and that the different peptides are being sequestered at different anatomic sites, or (2) that the same process of fibrillogenesis is taking place everywhere, but that the complement of enzymes in different anatomic sites is likely to be different. Consequently, once the fibrils have been laid down they are subject to different proteolytic attacks, resulting in different final peptide products. I find the second process much more satisfying mechanistically than to have to postulate that there are a whole range of peptides, each of which can be incorporated into an amyloid deposit and which all do exactly the same thing, namely, make amyloid fibrils.

Sipe: We've heard that many different peptide fragments of transthyretin (TTR) can form amyloid fibrils.

Kisilevsky: I agree that we can do this *in vitro*, but I don't think we have any evidence that this can take place *in vivo*.

Merlini: Another possibility might be that different organs have different complements of enzymes and that local processing could play a role in the onset and growth of amyloid deposits. This could account at least in part for organ specificity.

Kisilevsky: In the absence of data we can come up with all kinds of possibilities. The point I am making is that most of us are thinking along one particular line: the predominant view is that proteolysis is taking place as a pre-fibrillogenic event, and then deposition of amyloid occurs later. I don't think the data are there to support this.

Sipe: In which forms of amyloid that we've discussed would you say that this is the case?

Kisilevsky: It's been the case historically with AA and AL amyloids. Furthermore, virtually any time we find amyloid present as a fragment of a larger molecule, that's the view we tend to take.

Pepys: I agree with you. The only problem is that this was George Glenner's view—his early experiments with Bence–Jones proteins led him to it—and George has historically been proved right in almost everything he said! Even if the data aren't there yet, the chances are that George will turn out to have been right on this one as well.

Westermark: There are distinctive histological patterns of AA amyloidosis and each pattern correlates closely to specific species of AA protein. For example, there are long protein AA species in the vascular deposition pattern (Westermark et al 1989). Shirahama & Cohen (1980) published a paper concerning the redistribution of AA amyloidosis. They induced AA amyloidosis, which appeared in the spleen. When they stopped this induction, they claimed that the amyloid was redistributed from the spleen to the kidney, as far as I remember. Has anyone repeated this experiment? Is it an example of cleavage before fibril formation?

Kisilevsky: The inference is that the amyloid seen early in one location is the precursor to the amyloid seen later in another location. A temporal difference between the appearance of amyloid in those two sites doesn't make one the precursor to the other.

Westermark: Perhaps not, but the finding that the amyloid disappeared from the spleen and instead was deposited in the kidneys was intriguing. A simultaneous finding of a circulating N-terminal fragment of SAA would have of course been stronger circumstantial evidence of redistribution.

Masters: It doesn't have to be one or the other, it could also be both.

Prusiner: The reason people think the other way—and I think the evidence is pretty good for it—is that in several cases there's no good evidence that these proteins polymerize into any kind of ordered structures which could then be clipped.

Kisilevsky: And yet, as we were discussing earlier, the actual site of cleavage with the various secretases can be quite variable. How come?

Prusiner: That is because it's a pathological process. Often we expect these pathological processes to be as highly controlled as normal physiological processes, but this simply isn't the case. These problems aren't meant to be dealt with on an ongoing basis—these are diseases that often kill the organism.

Goldgaber: Biological infidelity is the rule rather than the exception. Even in the most 'sacred' act, the replication of DNA, there are mismatches. Infidelity exists in every biological system, and the implementation of every biological function is imprecise. In the case of enzymes that are supposed to cut other molecules at a specific site, the precision of the cut depends on the conditions. Not every molecule is cut at exactly the same site. Molecules that are cut at another site are always generated, even under optimum conditions.

Benson: We have occasionally made cleavages with trypsin or chymotrypsin that weren't supposed to happen. Enzymes are like people—kind of imperfect.

Kelly: In the case of TTR mutations there is quite a bit of variability: in some patients you see nearly all full length and others you see a lot of proteolysis. A proteolysis event could be critical for nucleation, but may be undetectable because it is occurring at such a low level. If the fibrils are predominantly full length protein, it still could be that the proteolytic cut is important for getting the nucleation process going. When you cut a protein, in most cases it destabilizes it, and it does change the conformation, which seems to be the link between these different proteins.

J. N. Buxbaum: I would like to ask a general question that is related to this issue. Many people in this room have isolated core peptides of amyloidogenic precursors that form fibrils and bind Congo red *in vitro*. Do these core peptides have a role to play *in vivo* in the process of fibrillogenesis, or are they just a kind of surrogate that we can manipulate in a test tube?

Prusiner: They must be significant—they can be isolated from amyloidotic tissue and they are seen in patient after patient with the same disease.

J. N. Buxbaum: That is certainly true for the intact amyloidogenic proteins, but what you don't isolate are the core peptides, i.e. the minimal peptides that in the test tube will give us this phenomenon (Table 1 [*Buxbaum*]). The question is: does fibrillogenesis function around these cores *in vivo*, or are we just looking at artifices that may not have a great deal to do with what's going on *in vivo* and other more complicated events are in place?

Conceptually, the importance of the 'core' seems intuitive. For instance, normal species variation in the amino acid 23–30 segment of islet amyloid polypeptide correlates with a tendency of the species to develop islet amyloid (Westermark et al 1990). The multiple amyloidogenic amino acid substitutions in TTR seem to defy systematization, being either conservative or not; involving residues in β-strands, α-helix, random coil or junctions between defined segments (Saraiva 1995). The longest mutation-spared region comprises residues 115–121 of the H-strand, a region reported to have core properties under relatively physiological conditions (Gustavsson et al 1991). I

TABLE 1 (*Buxbaum*) Fibrillogenic peptides

Amyloidogenic protein	*Core peptide sequences*	*Residues*	*Reference*
Gelsolin	S F N N G D C F I L D	182–192	Maury et al 1989
Transthyretin	C P L M V K V L D A V Y T I A A L L S P Y S	10–20 105–115	Gustavsson et al 1991
Islet amyloid polypeptide	S N N F G A I L S P	20–29	Westermark et al 1990
Serum amyloid A	S F F S F L G E A F D	2–12	Westermark et al 1992
Amyloid β-protein	Q K L V F F A E D V G S N K	14–28	Gorevic et al 1987
Scrapie prion protein	A G A A A A G A D C V N I T I K Q H T V T T D I K I M E R V V E Q M C T T Q Y	113–120 178–191 202–218	Gassett et al 1992

TABLE 2 (*Buxbaum*) Amyloid fibril precursors

Protein	*Subunit size (Da)*
Immunoglobulin light chains	500–30 000
Serum amyloid A	4500–7500
β_2-microglobulin	12 000–25 000
Cystatin	12 000–13 000
Amyloid β-protein	4000
Transthyretin	10 000–14 000
Apolipoprotein AI	9000
Gelsolin	9500
Islet amyloid polypeptide	3900
Procalcitonin	3400
Scrapie prion protein	27 000
Atrial natriuretic factor	3500
Lysozyme	14 000
α-fibrinogen	7000–10 000
Apolipoprotein AII (mouse)	8700
Insulin (Degu)	6000

would like to propose that the cores are significant *in vivo*, and are kept from extensively aggregating during denaturation by their protein context. What does context mean? While precursor size (Table 2 [*Buxbaum*]) ranges from approximately 3500 Da to 250 kDa, fibril subunit size tends to be under 20 kDa and in most cases under 10 kDa. Thus there seems to be a bulk or mass constraint. Almost all the proteins—the scrapie form of prion protein (PrP^{Sc}) being the major exception—have substantial β-sheet configuration in the native state, hence native conformation also plays a role (Gassett et al 1992). Given the data suggesting that 'off-pathway' folding may generate the fibril precursor, I propose that changes in the intramolecular context produced by mutations, proteolysis or glycosylation, affect the rate and/or extent of off-pathway folding (Kelly & Lansbury 1994). Protein concentration and interactions with other molecules may also play a role. This process is more likely to occur in proteins of particular native structures, perhaps in molecules containing more than one peptide with 'core' properties (as has been demonstrated for TTR and PrP; Gustavsson et al 1991, Gassett et al 1992), whereas other structures may be resistant to polymerization or predisposed to less ordered patterns of aggregation under the same (*in vitro* or *in vivo*) conditions.

If this hypothesis is correct, then mutations which disrupt the core should prevent or diminish fibrillogenesis *in vitro* and *in vivo*. Such seems to be the case when a Thr119 mutation occurs in Met30 TTR (Colon et al 1996, this volume). The hypothesis predicts that Thr119 would reduce the *in vitro* fibrillogenic potential of any TTR mutation.

Prusiner: Clearly, the situation *in vivo* is more complicated than in the test-tube. *In vitro* experiments give some very interesting biophysical handles on what's happening, but do not represent precisely what is going on in the animal.

References

Arvinte T, Drake AF 1993 Comparative study of human and salmon calcitonin secondary structure in solution with low dielectric constants. J Biol Chem 268:6415–6422

Arvinte T, Cudd A, Drake AF 1993 The structure and mechanism of formation of human calcitonin fibrils. J Biol Chem 268:6415–6422

Bauer HH, Müller M, Goette J, Merkle HP, Fringeli UP 1994 Interfacial adsorption and aggregation association changes in secondary structure of human calcitonin monitored by ATR-FTIR spectroscopy. Biochemistry 33:12276–12282

Bauer HH, Aebi U, Häner M et al 1995 Architecture and polymorphism of fibrillar supramolecular assemblies produced by *in vitro* aggregation of human calcitonin. J Struct Biol 115:1–5

Berger G, Berger N, Guillaud M-H, Trouillas J, Vauzelle J-L 1988 Calcitonin-like immunoreactivity of amyloid fibrils in medullary-thyroid carcinomas: an immuno-electron microscope study. Virchows Archiv A Pathol Anal Histopathol 412:543–551

Cohen C, Parry DAD 1990 α-helical coiled coils and bundles: how to design an α-helical protein. Proteins Struct Funct Genet 7:1–15

Colon W, Lai Z, McCutchen SL, Miroy GJ, Strang C, Kelly JW 1996 FAP mutations destablilize transthyretin facilitating conformational changes required for amyloid formation. In: The nature and origin of amyloid fibrils (Ciba Found Symp 199), Wiley, Chichester, p 228–242

Ferrone FA, Hofrichter J, Sunschine HR, Eaton WA 1980 Kinetic studies on photolysis-induced gelation of sickle cell hemoglobin suggests a new mechanism. Biophys J 32:361–381

Ferrone FA, Hofrichter J, Eaton WA 1985 Kinetics of sickle cell haemoglobin polymerization. 2. A double nucleation mechanism. J Mol Biol 183:611–631

Gassett M, Bladwin MA, Lloyd DH et al 1992 Predicted α-helical regions of the prion protein when synthesized as peptides form amyloid. Proc Natl Acad Sci USA 89:940–944

Gorevic PD, Castaño EM, Sarma R, Frangione B 1987 Ten to fourteen residue peptides of Alzheimer's disease fibril formation and its characteristic X-ray diffraction pattern. Biochem Biophys Res Commun 147:854–862

Gustavsson Å, Engström U, Westermark P 1991 Normal transthyretin and synthetic transthyretin fragments form amyloid-like fibrils *in vitro*. Biochem Biophys Res Commun 175:1159–1164

Hofrichter J, Ross PD, Eaton WA 1974 Structure of hemoglobin S fibers—optical determination of molecular orientation in sickled erythrocytes. Proc Natl Acad Sci USA 71:4864–4868

Husby G 1992 Nomenclature and classification of amyloid and amyloidoses. J Intern Med 323:511–512

Jarrett JT, Lansbury PT Jr 1993 Seeding 'one dimensional crystallization' of amyloid: a pathogenic mechanism in Alzheimer's disease and scrapie? Cell 73:1055–1058

Jarrett JT, Berger EP, Lansbury PT Jr 1993 The carboxy terminus of the β-amyloid protein is critical for the seeding of amyloid formation. Implications for the pathogenesis of Alzheimer's. Biochemistry 32:4693–4697

Kanaori K, Nosaka AY 1995 Study of human calcitonin fibrillation by proton nuclear magnetic resonance spectroscopy. Biochemistry 34:12138–12143

Kelly JW, Lansbury PT Jr 1994 A chemical approach to elucidate the mechanism of transthyretin and β protein amyloid fibril formation. Amyloid: Int J Exp Clin Invest 1:186–205

Maury CPJ, Nurmiaho-Lassila EL, Rossi H 1994 Amyloid fibril formation in gelsolin-derived amyloidosis. Lab Invest 70:558–564

Samuel RE, Salmon ED, Briehl RW 1990 Nucleation and growth of fibers and gel formation in sickle cell hemoglobin. Nature 345:833–835

Saraiva MJM 1995 Transthyretin mutations in health and disease. Hum Mutat 5: 191–196

Shirahama T, Cohen AS 1980 Redistribution of amyloid deposits. Am J Pathol 99:539–550

Westermark GT, Sletten K, Westermark P 1989 Massive vascular AA-amyloidosis: a histologically and biochemically distinctive subtype of reactive systemic amyloidosis. Scand J Immunol 30:605–613

Westermark P, Engström U, Johnson KH, Westermark GT, Betsholtz C 1990 Islet amyloid polypeptide: pinpointing amino acid residues linked to amyloid fibril formation. Proc Natl Acad Sci USA 87:5036–5040

Westermark GT, Engström U, Westermark P 1992 The N-terminal segment of protein AA determines its fibrillogenic property. Biochem Biophys Res Commun 182:27–33

Wimalawansa SJ 1990 Effects of *in vivo* stimulation on molecular forms of circulatory calcitonin and calcitonin gene-related peptide in man. Mol Cell Endocrinol 71:13–19

Metabolism of amyloid proteins

M. D. Benson*†, B. Kluve-Beckerman*, J. J. Liepnieks*†, J. R. Murrell*, D. Hanes* and T. Uemichi*

*Indiana University School of Medicine, Department of Medicine, Division of Rheumatology, c/o Veterans Affairs Medical Center (583/111Rh) and †Richard L. Roudebush–Veterans Affairs Medical Center, Department of Medicine, Section of Rheumatology, 1481 West 10th Street, Indianapolis, IN 46202-2884, USA

Abstract. Metabolic processing of amyloid precursor proteins is an important factor in the genesis of practically all forms of amyloidosis. Of the three major forms of systemic amyloidosis, reactive amyloid (amyloid A protein; AA) formation shows the most consistent role of partial proteolysis of serum amyloid A (SAA) to AA proteins which form fibrils. Immunoglobulin amyloidosis is also usually associated with C-terminal degradation of the fibril precursor light chain protein. Although it is commonly thought that transthyretin amyloidosis is associated with fibril formation from the tetrameric circulating plasma transthyretin, chemical analyses of transthyretin fibril deposits show significant fragmentation of the fibril protein constituents. In addition, it has been documented that proteolytic fragments are the fibril subunit proteins in gelsolin, cystatin C, Alzheimer's β-amyloid precursor protein and apolipoprotein AI (apoAI) amyloidoses. Notable exceptions to the role of proteolysis in amyloid fibril formation would appear to be the lysozyme and β_2-microglobulin amyloidoses. Few studies have examined the metabolism of amyloid-forming proteins. Perhaps the best data are on apoAI, which show decreased plasma residence time for the amyloidogenic Gly26Arg apoAI (1.8 d vs. normal 4.5 d). Similarly, preliminary data show increased clearance of Val30Met transthyretin when compared with the wild-type protein (18 h vs. 26 h). Also, biosynthetically ^{35}S-labelled SAA proteins reconstituted with HDL show increased plasma clearance of murine SAA_2, the amyloid fibril subunit protein, when compared with murine SAA_1. Few data are available on metabolism of amyloid immunoglobulin light chain proteins, but it has been shown that radiolabelled Bence–Jones proteins are cleared very rapidly from the circulation. A better understanding of the metabolism of precursor proteins in each of the amyloid deposition diseases will give insight into the mechanisms of fibril formation and pathogenesis of amyloidosis.

1996 The nature and origin of amyloid fibrils. Wiley, Chichester (Ciba Foundation Symposium 199) p 104–118

The amyloidoses are a group of diseases defined by the synthesis and deposition of protein fibrils having specific characteristics. For the systemic forms of amyloidosis (and presumably most forms of localized amyloidosis)

this process involves the transition of physiologically soluble precursor proteins into aggregated or polymerized macromolecular structures which we call the amyloid fibril. Obviously, there are many amyloid diseases, each defined by the subunit protein of the amyloid fibril in that particular condition. What these diseases share in common is the formation of fibril structures, i.e. the transition from soluble protein to insoluble fibrils. The cause or aetiology (for example, mutation in plasma proteins such as transthyretin, apolipoprotein AI, fibrinogen), is known for many forms of amyloidosis. What is largely unknown are the mechanisms, i.e. pathogenesis, of the amyloid fibril-forming process.

Obvious factors which may be involved in amyloid fibrillogenesis include: (1) structure of the precursor protein; (2) function of the precursor protein; and (3) metabolism of the precursor protein. There is strong but indirect evidence that structure of precursor proteins is important in the immunoglobulin, reactive and transthyretin amyloidoses. There is less compelling, but still suggestive, evidence that function of some of the precursor proteins may be pertinent to fibrillogenesis. Here we present the evidence that metabolism of amyloid precursor proteins is a significant factor in fibrillogenesis of many of the amyloid diseases.

Results and discussion

The strongest case for the involvement of protein metabolism in amyloid fibrillogenesis can be made for the hereditary amyloidoses. These diseases, which mostly involve single amino acid substitutions in soluble amyloid precursor proteins, show definite alterations in metabolic parameters. In hereditary amyloidosis associated with mutations in apolipoprotein AI (apoAI), amyloid deposits contain N-terminal fragments of apoAI, indicating that proteolysis is part of the fibrillogenic process (Nichols et al 1988, Soutar et al 1992). In addition, individuals with the Gly26Arg mutation of apoAI have significantly lowered plasma concentrations of high density lipoprotein (HDL) cholesterol, suggesting a more rapid turnover of apoAI, a major constituent of HDL particles (Rader et al 1992). *In vivo* metabolic studies using ^{131}I-labelled normal apoAI and ^{125}I-labelled Arg26 apoAI showed a decreased plasma residence time for the variant protein, confirming that the metabolic alteration was one of increased catabolism rather than production (Fig. 1). These data were generated from studies in individuals who had the variant apoAI, but had not yet shown any clinical manifestation of amyloidosis.

We have initiated similar studies to investigate the transthyretin (TTR) amyloidoses. Several investigators have demonstrated depressed plasma levels of TTR in both clinically affected subjects and asymptomatic carriers of amyloid-associated TTR gene mutations (Benson & Dwulet 1983, Skinner et al 1985, Westermark et al 1985). Preliminary studies using ^{131}I-labelled normal TTR and ^{125}I-labelled Met30 TTR demonstrated increased plasma clearance of

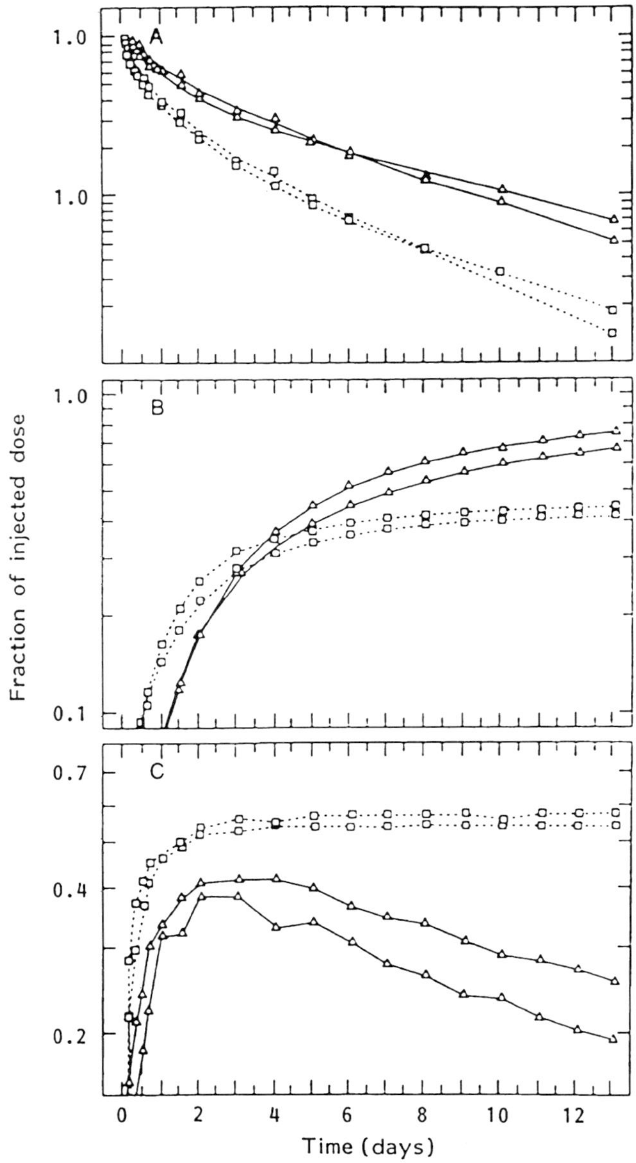

FIG. 1. Metabolism of $apoAI_{Iowa}$ (squares and dotted lines) and normal apoAI (triangles and solid lines) in two $apoAI_{Iowa}$ subjects. (A) Whole plasma decay curves; (B) cumulative urinary excretion; (C) extravascular accumulation in the body (Rader et al 1992).

the variant protein in both TTR Met30 affected subjects and normal volunteers (Fig. 2). The decreased plasma residence time of variant TTR in a normal subject (16 h) as well as an affected subject (12 h) demonstrated that this is a property of the variant protein and is not due to the presence of amyloidosis. These data also indicate that the plasma half-life ($t_{1/2}$) of TTR is somewhat less than the half-life determined approximately 25 years ago using similar radiolabelling techniques (Oppenheimer et al 1965, Vahlquist et al 1973). A plasma residence time of 26 h for wild-type TTR can be expressed as an approximate plasma $t_{1/2}$ of 18 h. This is significantly different from the 45 h reported by Oppenheimer et al (1965) and 48 h reported by Vahlquist et al (1973). A plasma residence time of 12–16 h for Met30 TTR corresponds to $t_{1/2}$ of 8.3–11 h and is significantly different from the residence time of wild-type TTR. These findings are consistent with an alteration in metabolism of the variant TTR, presumably secondary to the structural change caused by the amino acid substitution. On the basis of these data a kinetic model for metabolism of TTR has been proposed using SAAM (simulation, analysis and modelling) (Berman & Weiss 1978) (Fig. 3). Definition of the various compartments in this kinetic model may indicate the major pathways of TTR catabolism and identify pathogenic mechanisms of amyloid formation.

Other hereditary forms of amyloidosis in which there is some evidence for metabolic derangement include fibrinogen α-chain amyloidosis (Uemichi et al 1994) and hereditary cerebral haemorrhage with amyloid, Icelandic type (Abrahamson et al 1992). In subjects with one of the newly discovered mutations of fibrinogen α-chain gene, there is significant depression of plasma fibrinogen concentration and prolongation of the reptilase time, indicating that function of the protein may be affected as well as an increased catabolism which lowers the circulating plasma level. In hereditary cerebral haemorrhage with amyloidosis (HCAWA)-I, significantly depressed cerebral spinal fluid (CSF) levels of cystatin C in affected subjects suggest that processes similar to those for apoAI and TTR may be at play in the metabolism of this protein (Jensson et al 1986).

In reactive amyloidosis, which occurs in humans and most other mammalian species, metabolism is a prime factor in amyloid pathogenesis. From the synthetic aspect it has been shown that only those isoforms of serum amyloid A (SAA) which are subject to the acute-phase response with marked elevation of synthesis participate in the formation of fibril product. In addition, in almost all species, proteolysis of the SAA precursor protein occurs so that only the N-terminal portion of the protein is present in the fibrils. Classically, the first 76 residues of SAA were isolated from reactive amyloid fibrils (Levin et al 1972); however, we now know that proteolytic fragments as short as 45 amino acid residues, often 50–60 residues, and occasionally greater than 80 may be incorporated into the fibrils (Liepnieks et al 1995). This heterogeneity of the amyloid fibril subunit protein suggests less importance for the C-terminal

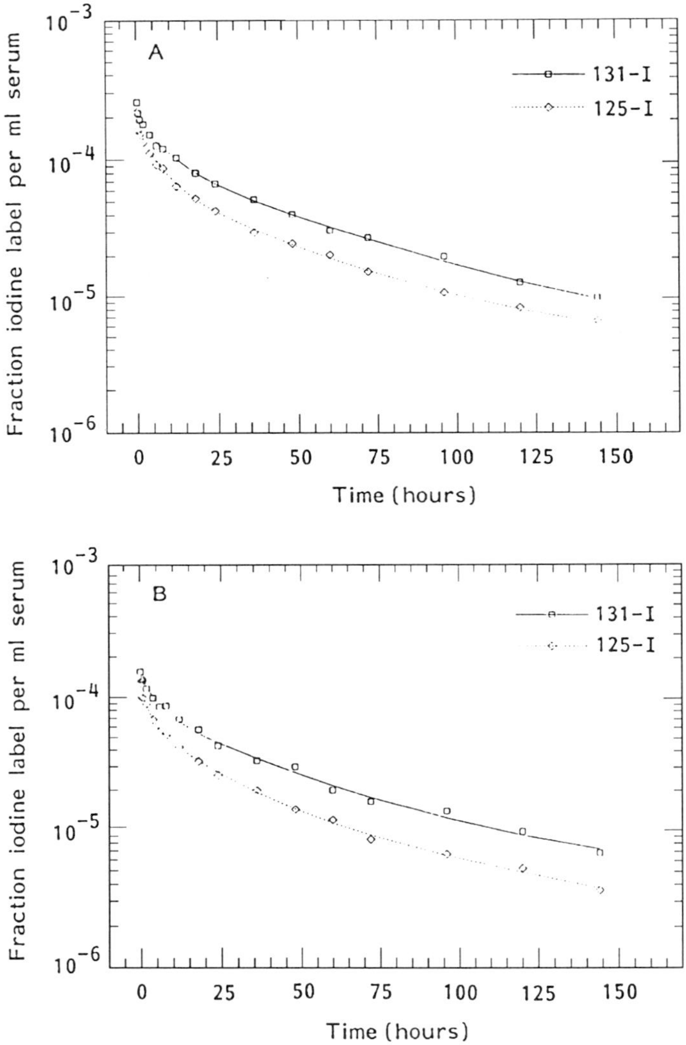

FIG. 2. Metabolism of normal transthyretin (TTR) (squares and solid lines) and Met30 TTR (diamonds and dotted lines). (A) Plasma clearance curve for [^{131}I]normal TTR and [^{125}I]Met30 TTR in a normal subject. (B) Plasma clearance curve for [^{131}I]normal TTR and [^{125}I]Met30 TTR in a patient with familial amyloidotic polyneuropathy.

portion of the molecule and enhanced importance of the N-terminal portion of the SAA molecule in amyloid fibrillogenesis. The studies of mouse SAA_1 and SAA_2 which have shown changes in conformation when the protein comes in contact with heparan sulfate also suggest that some destabilization or

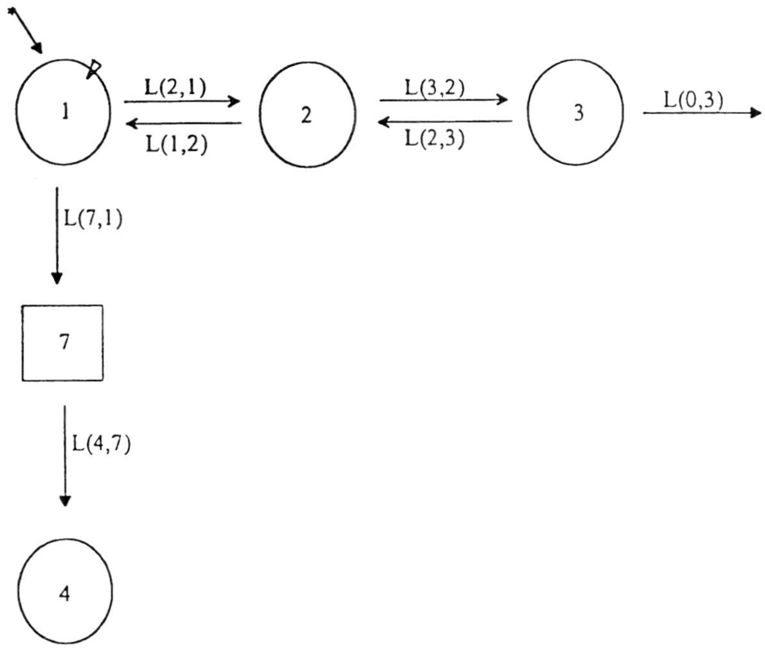

FIG. 3. Kinetic model for [^{131}I] and [^{125}I] plasma decay and urinary excretion derived from data as depicted in Fig. 2. Compartment 1 represents plasma, compartment 7 a delay compartment, compartment 4 urine, and compartments 2 and 3 undetermined.

alteration in the protein may alter metabolism and fibril formation (de Beer et al 1993).

Studies in the murine model of reactive amyloidosis have suggested differences in metabolism of murine SAA_1 and murine SAA_2 (Meek et al 1986). First, it has been shown (and used in the argument for the involvement of structure in amyloid formation) that murine SAA_2, but not murine SAA_1, is incorporated into amyloid fibrils (Hoffman et al 1984). Recent studies in our laboratory show that the plasma clearance of SAA_1 and SAA_2 differ. Using biosynthetically ^{35}S-labelled SAA proteins reconstituted with HDL, we have shown that SAA_2 is cleared from plasma significantly faster than SAA_1 (Fig. 4). In addition, it would appear that SAA clearance is modified by the overall composition of the HDL and the status of the animal re-inflammation. In mice undergoing an acute-phase response, SAA_2 clearance is slower than in normal mice but still faster than the clearance of SAA_1 under the same conditions. How these metabolic differences relate to AA fibrillogenesis is not yet clear but their recognition may well give new insight into pathogenesis of reactive amyloidosis.

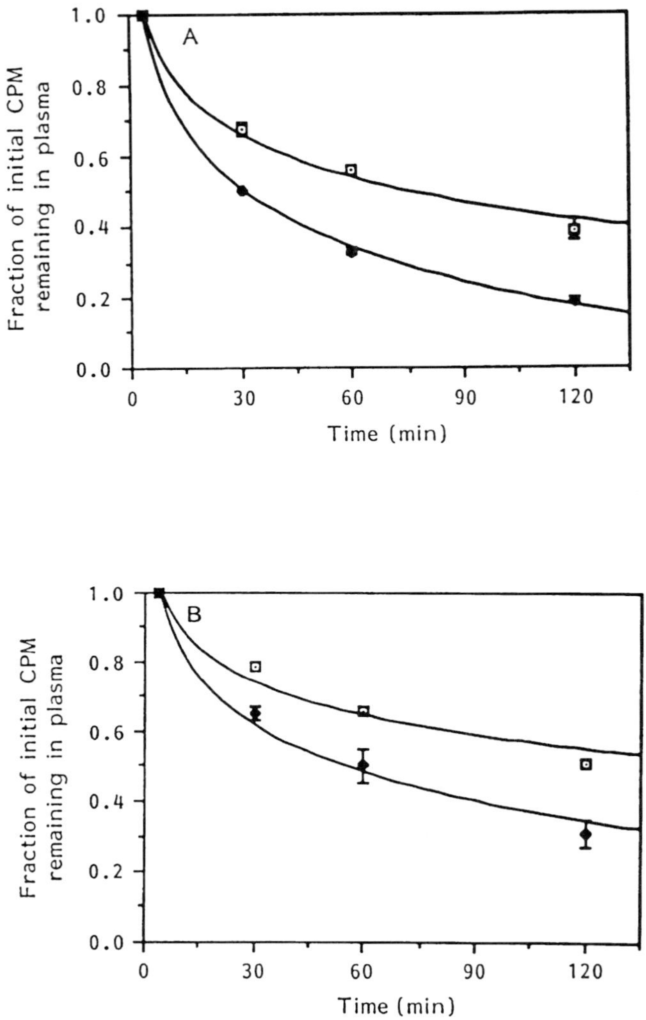

FIG. 4. Metabolism of murine SAA_1 (squares) and SAA_2 (diamonds). (A) Plasma clearance curve for [^{35}S]SAA-HDL in normal mice. (B) Plasma clearance curve for [^{35}S]SAA-HDL in mice undergoing acute-phase response. CPM, counts per minute.

Metabolism of immunoglobulin light-chain proteins in AL-type amyloidosis has not been studied. It is obvious that for immunoglobulin amyloidosis to occur, a monoclonal light chain protein must be synthesized; it is usually presumed that excess quantities of this light chain protein are produced. In addition, some degree of light chain protein processing appears to be important since most AL fibril subunit proteins are composed of V_L, but only part of the contiguous C_L (Glenner 1980a,b). Presumably, the amyloid fibril-forming subunit—the light chain dimer—is an unnatural species in the plasma in an uncoupled form, since the corresponding monoclonal heavy chain is often not present in the plasma of amyloid patients. Also, it has been calculated that normally only approximately 60% of synthesized light chains are coupled to heavy chains. Therefore, the light chain dimer would be the intermediate for amyloid fibril formation. Studies done 30 years ago suggested a very short plasma half-life for Bence–Jones proteins in patients with plasma cell dyscrasias (Solomon et al 1964, Waldmann et al 1972). Radiolabelled light chain proteins were cleared very rapidly by the kidney and metabolized within minutes to hours unless the nephrotic syndrome was present, in which case a significant proportion of light chain protein was cleared into the urine. Only in the presence of renal failure would prolonged plasma half-life of Bence–Jones proteins occur. I know of no such studies in recent times in patients with amyloidosis. This is a subject which should be addressed but, because of the unique aspects of amyloidosis in each patient with AL disease, these studies will not be easy.

Metabolic changes associated with localized forms of amyloidosis have been noted. In Alzheimer's disease associated with mutations of β-amyloid precursor protein (APP), there is evidence for increased generation of the fibril subunit amyloid β-peptide (Citron et al 1992, Mullan et al 1992, Suzuki et al 1994). Whether this is a significant factor in amyloid plaque formation is not known. In medullary carcinoma of the thyroid, a peptide precursor of calcitonin is incorporated into the fibrils, indicating aberrations in protein processing (Sletten et al 1976). Amyloid fibril formation in adult-onset diabetes mellitus has not been studied in detail.

Summary

There is good evidence that metabolic processing of amyloid precursor proteins may be important in fibrillogenesis in many of the amyloid diseases. Whether there is a common thread amongst these diseases can only be hypothesized in general terms, since they are all separate diseases and a variety of pathogenic processes are involved in the final outcome in each—formation of the amyloid fibril.

Acknowledgements

Supported by Veterans Affairs Medical Research (MRIS 583-0888), grants from RR-00750 (GCRC), the United States Public Health Service (DK49596, DK42111, AR20582, AG10608), the Marion E. Jacobson Fund and the Machado Family Research Fund.

References

Abrahamson M, Jonsdottir S, Olafsson I, Jensson O, Grubb A 1992 Hereditary cystatin C amyloid angiopathy: identification of the disease-causing mutation and specific diagnosis by polymerase chain reaction based analysis. Hum Genet 89:377–380

Benson MD, Dwulet FE 1983 Prealbumin and retinol binding protein serum concentrations in the Indiana type hereditary amyloidosis. Arthritis & Rheum 26:1493–1498

Berman M, Weiss M 1978 SAAM manual. US Department of Health, Education and Welfare. Washington, DC. (Publication no. (NJH) 78–180)

Citron M, Oltersdorf T, Haass C et al 1992 Mutation of the β-amyloid precursor protein in familial Alzheimer's disease increases β-protein production. Nature 360:672–674

de Beer MC, de Beer FC, McCubbin WD, Kay CM, Kindy MS 1993 Structural prerequisites for serum amyloid A fibril formation. J Biol Chem 268:20606–20612

Glenner GG 1980a Amyloid deposits and amyloidosis. The β-fibrilloses. 1. N Engl J Med 302:1283–1292

Glenner GG 1980b Amyloid deposits and amyloidosis. The β-fibrilloses. 2. N Engl J Med 302:1333–1343

Hoffman JS, Ericsson LH, Eriksen N, Walsh KA, Benditt EP 1984 Murine tissue amyloid protein AA: NH_2-terminal sequence identity with only one of 2 serum amyloid protein (ApoSAA) gene products. J Exp Med 159:641–646

Jensson O, Thorsteinsson L, Bots GTAM et al 1986 Immunohistochemical comparison between the Dutch and the Icelandic form of hereditary central nervous system amyloid angiopathy. Acta Neurol Scand 73:312–313

Levin M, Franklin EC, Frangione B, Pras M 1972 Amino acid sequence of a major nonimmunoglobulin component of some amyloid fibrils. J Clin Invest 51:2773–2776

Liepnieks JJ, Kluve-Beckerman B, Benson MD 1995 Characterization of amyloid A protein in human secondary amyloidosis: the predominant deposition of serum amyloid A1. Biochem Biophys Acta 1270:81–86

Meek RL, Hoffman JS, Benditt EP 1986 Amyloidogenesis: one serum amyloid A isotype is selectively removed from the circulation. J Exp Med 163:499–510

Mullan M, Crawford F, Axelman K et al 1992 A pathogenic mutation for probable Alzheimer's disease in the APP gene at the N-terminus of β-amyloid. Nat Genet 1:345–347

Nichols WC, Dwulet FE, Liepnieks JJ, Benson MD 1988 Variant apolipoprotein A-I as a major constituent of a human hereditary amyloid. Biochem Biophys Res Commun 156:762–768

Nichols WC, Gregg RE, Brewer HB Jr, Benson MD 1990 A mutation in apolipoprotein A-I in the Iowa type of familial amyloidotic polyneuropathy. Genomics 8:318–323

Oppenheimer JH, Surks MI, Bernstein G, Smith JC 1965 Metabolism of Iodine-131-labeled thyroxine-binding prealbumin in man. Science 149:748–750

Rader DJ, Gregg RE, Meng MS et al 1992 *In vivo* metabolism of a mutant apolipoprotein, ApoA-I_{IOWA}, associated with hypoalphalipoproteinemia and hereditary systemic amyloidosis. J Lipid Res 33:755–763

Skinner M, Connors LH, Rubinow A, Libbey C, Sipe JD, Cohell AS 1985 Lowered prealbumin levels in patients with familial amyloid polyneuropathy (FAP) and their non-affected but at risk relatives. Am J Med Sci 289:17–21

Sletten K, Westermark P, Natvig JB 1976 Characterization of amyloid fibril proteins from medullary carcinoma of the thyroid. J Exp Med 143:993–998

Solomon A, Waldmann TA, Fahey JL, McFarlane AS 1964 Metabolism of Bence Jones proteins. J Clin Invest 43:103–117

Soutar AK, Hawkins PN, Vigushin DM et al 1992 Apolipoprotein AI mutation Arg-60 causes autosomal dominant amyloidosis. Proc Natl Acad Sci USA 89:7389–7393
Suzuki N, Cheung TT, Cai X-D et al 1994 An increased percentage of long amyloid β protein secreted by familial amyloid β protein precursor (βAPP_{717}) mutants. Science 264:1336–1340
Uemichi T, Liepnieks JJ, Benson MD 1994 Hereditary renal amyloidosis with a novel variant fibrinogen. J Clin Invest 93:731–736
Vahlquist A, Peterson PA, Wibell L 1973 Metabolism of the vitamin A transporting protein complex. 1. Turnover studies in normal persons and in patients with chronic renal failure. Eur J Clin Invest 3:352–362
Waldmann TA, Strober W, Mogielnicki RP 1972 The renal handling of low molecular weight proteins. J Clin Invest 51:2162–2174
Westermark P, Pitkanen P, Benson L, Vahlquist A, Olofsson BO, Cornwell GG III 1985 Serum prealbumin and retinol-binding protein in the prealbumin-related senile and familial forms of systemic amyloidosis. Lab Invest 52:314–318

DISCUSSION

Merlini: I would like to present briefly our data and a hypothesis concerning the possible role of light chain dimers in the pathogenesis of immunoglobulin light chain-related (AL) amyloidosis. Since amyloidosis is a disease of protein conformation, we investigated the structural aspects of amyloid light chains and fibrils using murine monoclonal antibodies (MoAb). We selected a monoclonal anti-idiotope antibody raised against λ-chain dimers isolated from the urine of a patient (DEP) with AL amyloidosis that binds a conformational idiotype also present on the monoclonal DEP IgAλ immunoglobulin. When tested by ELISA, this antibody does not recognize the DEP λ monomer or the 15–17 kDa amyloid fibrillar light chain fragments, although they have the same N-terminal sequence as the urinary light chains, or different IgAλ or other immunoglobulins whose light chains belong to the same λ III subgroup as λ DEP. The non-reactivity of this MoAb with amyloid fibrils was confirmed by immunohistochemical examination of the patient's tissue. Cryostatic sections of the DEP amyloidoma, while positive with anti-λ and anti-P-component antisera, were not stained by the MoAb or by the anti-κ antibody used as a negative control. These data suggest that light chain dimers are not deposited in the amyloid. Structural studies showed that the light chains constituting the amyloid fibrils were fragments which lacked about 70 residues at the C-terminus (Bellotti et al 1992). The absence of these residues may prevent formation of the light chain dimer (and, consequently, creation of the conformational epitope recognized by the MoAb). The asymmetric dimer could have, as occurs with other proteins (Salemme 1983), a 'protective' role in the prevention of polymerization; the loss of a portion of the constant region may prevent its formation, thus priming the polymerization of fragments into amyloid fibrils (Fig. 1 [*Merlini*]).

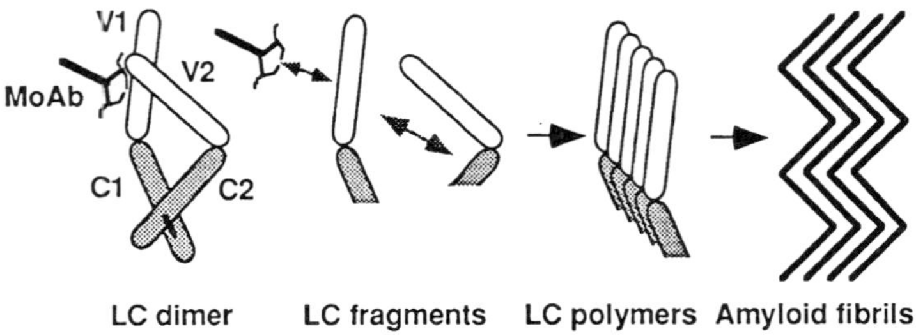

FIG. 1. *(Merlini).* Proposed model of monoclonal antibody (MoAb) epitope recognition and molecular events leading to amyloid formation. The asymmetric full-length light chain (LC) dimer is self-limiting: interaction between two variable regions (V) creates the epitope recognized by MoAb. The disulfide bond (indicated with a bold line) in the C-terminal region (C) is crucial for dimer stability. The partially proteolysed LC fragments cannot reconstitute the dimer, causing loss of the epitope recognized by the MoAb, and polymerize into amyloid fibrils. The polymerization of light chain fragments into amyloid fibrils does not reconstitute the epitope recognized by the MoAb on the light chain dimers. (From Merlini & Bellotti 1994.)

J. N. Buxbaum: Merril Benson, do you have any idea where the catabolism is taking place?

Benson: With regard to the immunoglobulin light chains, metabolic studies suggest that the body makes far more light chains than heavy chains. These light chains enter the plasma as dimers and go to the kidneys where they are absorbed by the kidney tubule cells. Their metabolism most likely occurs in the kidney, and it's only when you have a nephritic syndrome that there is so much protein going through the kidney that the tubules can't absorb and digest it.

A theme that I hoped would come from our discussion of metabolism is that in amyloid formation, of whatever type, probably what we are often looking at is normal metabolism. The amyloid is something that is freezing this metabolism at a particular stage. In other words, it's like a chemical reaction where you have $A + B \rightarrow C + D$. If C is insoluble, the equation goes to the right very rapidly, and C may be the fibril. This is a normal chemical reaction, and all we're seeing is the fibril, the end product, because it's freezing out metabolism over a sort of period of time.

J. N. Buxbaum: But is it fair to say that you don't have any data on where transthyretin (TTR) is catabolized?

Benson: Yes. It would appear not to be in the plasma phase. If we are to believe Jeff Kelly, it probably has to be in some place where pH is lowered to about 4.5. It obviously can't be outside the cell. I think labelling studies will be of value, but they are most likely going to have to be in species other than human.

Saraiva: Makover et al (1988) have studied the catabolism of TTR in rats, using the ligand trapped method. These studies have indicated that TTR is mainly catabolized in the liver, followed by the kidneys and, to a small extent, the skin.

Benson: Unfortunately the rat doesn't get TTR amyloid.

Saraiva: It would most probably get amyloid if the human mutant TTR were circulating. But the question here concerns where TTR is catabolized. I believe that as with the rat TTR, human TTR is catabolized in the liver; my assumption is based on the uptake of human TTR by human hepatomas (Divino & Schussler 1990), a cell line that also synthesizes and secretes TTR (Blaner et al 1991).

Sipe: I was interested in the data you showed on SAA clearance in the mouse: you showed faster clearance of the SAA_2 isoform. I have analysed a large number of acute-phase mouse sera. Protein levels as measured by isoelectric focusing or even mRNA levels in liver suggest roughly an equimolar ratio of SAA_1: SAA_2. Do you think there is faster translation of SAA_2 mRNA to keep up the concentration of SAA_2 protein in plasma?

Benson: I think that SAA_2 is cleared faster, not translated faster.

Sipe: Then why is there no evidence for it in plasma during acute inflammation? You see roughly equimolar SAA_1 and SAA_2 if you do the biochemical separation.

Benson: Not after 72 h.

Sipe: SAA_1 and SAA_2 do appear to be equal in concentration during the first 24 h following inflammatory stimulation.

Pepys: I found your clearance data very interesting, but I want to sound a note of caution. An *in vivo* clearance study is the most sensitive way to detect the most minor modifications in proteins. Any protein which is not in its native physiological form will be cleared more rapidly *in vivo* than its totally normal counterpart. We've done extensive clearance studies in humans of serum amyloid P component (SAP) (Hawkins et al 1990) and C-reactive protein (CRP) (Vigushin et al 1993) in which we have tried to make sure that our labelled tracer is absolutely physiological. The most rigorous test is to compare the clearance in animals of the labelled tracer molecules that we're going to use in humans with the clearance of the totally unlabelled unpurified SAP and CRP provided by whole human serum. The whole human serum is injected into mice and the clearance of the untouched proteins is then monitored by immunoassay. Before we do a clearance study with the radiolabelled purified proteins in humans we make sure they are cleared, in mice, in precisely the same way as those untouched control molecules.

Saraiva: Have you done metabolic studies comparing homozygous Met30 TTR from serum with heterozygous TTR?

Benson: So far we have only used homozygous normal or homozygous Met30 TTR.

Saraiva: When you draw your conclusions it is worth bearing in mind that the majority of TTR patients are heterozygous. Furthermore, if you have different ratios of mutant monomers in heterozygotic TTR circulating in familial amyloidotic polyneuropathy patients, the results on catabolism using homozygous TTR can be difficult to extrapolate.

Benson: I think you can appreciate the problem of having three normal and one variant monomer and three variants and one normal, and then, as one of my postdocs pointed out, what about the six species where the variants are in the *trans* rather than the *cis* position? I think that's an experiment that's going to take a bit of thought.

Saraiva: So it may be difficult to draw conclusions from catabolism.

Benson: That's true: I just presented data, and I'm letting you draw the conclusions.

J. N. Buxbaum: Per Westermark, have you looked at the local forms of amyloid, for instance the procalcitonin or the islet amyloid polypeptide, from the perspective of local turnover and synthesis versus catabolism versus secretion?

Westermark: No.

Benson: Perhaps we should have some comment from those who have studied amyloid precursor protein (APP), because a fair number of metabolic studies have been carried out on this protein.

Masters: I don't believe there's any general evidence of increased synthesis of APP in Alzheimer's disease. However, there is one paper from Selkoe's group showing that the chromosome 14 families have increased rates of transcription (Querfurth et al 1995).

Goldgaber: There are a number of papers showing an enormous increase in the level of APP mRNA in Down's syndrome and Alzheimer's disease (Palmert et al 1988, Neve et al 1988, Johnson et al 1990).

Westermark: In deposits of most systemic amyloidoses not only is the major protein fragment present, but so also is the uncleaved precursor protein. Is this also true for apolipoprotein AI (apoAI)? Is uncleaved apoAI found in the amyloid deposits?

Pepys: In all the patients we have studied, we find trace amounts of a species that is immunoreactive with anti-apoAI antibodies and which is the size of whole apoAI, but we haven't had enough of it to be able to purify and sequence it. The question is still open as to whether amyloidogenesis involves aggregation and precipitation of the whole apoAI, followed by cleavage of this N-terminal fragment which is the main species you find in the mature fibril, or whether amyloidogenesis involves cleavage between positions 88 and 93 and then aggregation of the cleaved fragment.

Benson: Are those data from kidney and spleen fibrils, or liver fibrils?

Pepys: They are from spleen, liver and heart.

Benson: We did spleen and kidney and found no full apoAI. I worry a little about findings from the liver, because that is where it is synthesized.

Pepys: It is also quite a sticky protein and is abundant in the plasma. Its presence on fibrils could reflect a *post facto* event rather than anything to do with pathogenesis. Hopefully experiments with recombinantly expressed amyloidogenic apoAI variants will resolve this question.

J. N. Buxbaum: Most of the patients we have seen with light chain amyloid have low serum levels of light chain. My interpretation of these data is that clearance is very rapid. In a substantial proportion of the patients we found light chain fragments intracellularly, yet deposition was at a distance from the site of synthesis. On the one occasion when we were able to look at both the bone marrow cells and the deposited fibrils, the fibril subunit was the same size and had the same amyloidogenicity as the smallest intracellular fragment. Although we were not able to get mRNA from that particular case, in other cases we have found a small message corresponding to a small protein. I would caution that observations in the immunoglobulin system are not likely to be uniform with respect to every monoclonal cell population or every precursor protein. Some fragments that you find in deposits have a circulating phase complexed with a normal size light chain. In the published reports, 90% of the deposits have fragments and only 5 or 10% have intact chains. There are usually a family of fragments with one size dominant. It is not clear precisely where cleavage is occurring—whether it occurs inside the synthesizing cell or in some other compartment.

Goldgaber: The Aβ story is very similar. Aβ fragments of different sizes have been described in deposits. It is not clear whether Aβ fragments of different length were first generated and then deposited, or whether longer Aβ fragments were first deposited and then shortened into fragments of varying lengths.

Maury: In gelsolin-derived amyloidosis (Finnish type of familial amyloidosis), abnormal proteolysis appears to be an important step in fibrillogenesis. We have identified a circulating gelsolin fragment (65 kDa) in the circulation of patients with Finnish-type amyloidosis that is cleaved post-translationally from full-length gelsolin (83 kDa) by abnormal proteolysis (Maury & Rossi 1993). During further degradation of this fragment the amyloid subunit protein is released and polymerizes to amyloid. Alan Weeds' group in Cambridge has provided an explanation for the generation of the abnormal proteolysis site: the substitution of the normal Asp with Asn at residue 187 would leave an arginine charge uncompensated and consequent local rearrangement to solvate this charge could easily generate the novel proteolysis site at residues 172–173 (McLaughlin et al 1993).

References

Bellotti V, Stoppini M, Perfetti V et al 1992 Use of an anti-idiotypic monoclonal antibody in studying amyloidogenic light chains in cells, urine and fibrils: pathophysiology and clinical implications. Scan J Immunol 36:607–615

Blaner W, Bonifácio MJ, Feldman HD, Piantedosi R, Saraiva MJ 1991 Studies on the synthesis and secretion of transthyretin by the human hepatoma cell line Hep G2. FEBS Lett 287:193–196

Divino CM, Schussler GC 1990 Receptor-mediated uptake and internalization of transthyretin. J Biol Chem 265:1425–1429

Hawkins PN, Wooton R, Pepys MB 1990 Metabolic studies of radioiodinated serum amyloid P component in normal subjects and patients with systemic amyloidosis. J Clin Invest 86:1862–1869

Johnson SA, McNeill T, Cordell B, Finch CE 1990 Relation of neuronal APP-751/APP-695 mRNA ratio and neuritic plaque density in Alzheimer's disease. Science 248:854–857

Makover A, Moriwaki H, Ramakrishman R, Saraiva MJ, Blaner W, Goodman D 1988 Plasma TTR: tissue sites of degradation and turnover in the rat. J Biol Chem 263:8598–8603

Maury CPJ, Rossi H 1993 Demonstration of a circulating 65 K gelsolin variant specific for familial amyloidosis, Finnish type. Biochem Biophys Res Commun 191:41–44

McLaughlin PJ, Gooch JT, Mannherz HG, Weeds AG 1993 Structure of gelsolin segment-1–actin complex and the mechanism of filament severing. Nature 364:685–692

Merlini G, Bellotti V 1994 Pathogenetic aspects of AL amyloidosis. In: Dammacco F, Barlogie B (eds) Multiple myeloma and related disorders. Ares-Serono Symp, Rome, 4:165–173

Neve RL, Finch EA, Dawes LR 1988 Expression of the Alzheimer amyloid precursor gene transcripts in the human brain. Neuron 1:669–677

Palmert MR, Golde TE, Cohen ML et al 1988 Amyloid protein precursor messenger RNAs: differential expression in Alzheimer's disease. Science 241:1080–1084

Querfurth HW, Wijsman EM, St George-Hyslop PH, Selkoe DJ 1995 βAPP mRNA transcription is increased in cultured fibroblasts from the familial Alzheimer's disease-1 family. Mol Brain Res 28:319–337

Salemme RF 1983 Anatomy of protein structure. In: Zubay G (ed) Biochemistry, 1st edn. Addison-Wesley, Reading, MA, p 69–129

Vigushin DM, Pepys MB, Hawkins PN 1993 Metabolic and scintigraphic studies of radioiodinated human C-reactive protein. J Clin Invest 91:1351–1357

Alzheimer's disease: genesis of amyloid

Konrad Beyreuther, Gerd Multhaup and Colin L. Masters*

*ZMBH, Center for Molecular Biology, University of Heidelberg, 282 Im Neuenheimer Feld, D-69120 Heidelberg, Germany and *Department of Pathology, The University of Melbourne, Parkville, Victoria 3052, Australia*

Abstract. Much of the present knowledge on the genes and genetic processes involved in the genesis of amyloid formation in Alzheimer's disease (AD) has come directly or indirectly from the retrospective molecular and genetic analysis of amyloid β-protein (Aβ or βA_4) deposits and from the identification of genes involved in inherited susceptibility to the disease. This analysis shows that the release and aggregation of the Aβ fragment from the amyloid precursor protein (APP) is involved in APP (AD1), chromosome 14 (AD3), 1 (AD4) and 19 (AD2) families as well as in the sporadic forms of AD, suggesting that AD is a single disease with a common APP/Aβ amyloid pathogenesis. Synthetic Aβ protein readily forms β sheets, filaments and amyloid at micromolar concentrations. The principle to inhibit this process has been worked out by our groups with Aβ variants. The N-terminal and C-terminal Aβ sequences, oxidative radicals, membrane integrity and metal ions also affect the aggregation of Aβ. Amino acid substitutions within the Aβ sequence, as occur in rodents, alter Aβ release and change the degree to which oxidation of the peptides occurs. Transgenic approaches resulting in overexpression of human APP have confirmed that Aβ sequence and concentration are critical prerequisites to amyloid deposition *in vivo*.

1996 The nature and origin of amyloid fibrils. Wiley, Chichester (Ciba Foundation Symposium 199) p 119–131

As we approach the end of this century, dementia is the most common neurological diagnosis in old age and the third leading cause of natural death. One condition dominates the dementia field: Alzheimer's disease (AD) accounts for over two thirds of all cases (Ott et al 1995). More than half of the patients living in nursing homes of the Western world suffer from dementia. In Germany, 200 000 demented patients live in these institutions (Bickel & Cooper 1994). These institutionalized patients account for only 60% of the demented patients needing care. Demented patients remain institutionalized in the nursing home until death, which usually occurs less than two years after admission. Together with those patients who stay at home, over 250 000 deaths annually must be attributed to dementia as a primary cause (Bickel & Cooper 1994). We estimate that for Germany the daily costs for institutionalized demented patients alone approximate US$22 million. In theory, postponement of institutionalization of these patients by an average of only ten days would save a sum corresponding to the entire budget of the US National Institute of Aging that is spent annually for dementia research on AD. How can such a delay in the onset of disease be achieved? It is generally accepted that the most direct therapeutic approach will be to target the cause or causes of dementia.

Preclinical Alzheimer's disease

Because rational therapeutic strategies for chronic diseases aim at the prevention or postponement of the onset of clinical symptoms, we determined the duration of preclinical amyloid deposition in AD. From necropsy examinations we estimate that in Trisomy 21 (Down's syndrome) and AD, before clinical recognition, a thirty-year period of amyloid β-protein (Aβ or βA_4) accumulation follows the initiation of this process (Rumble et al 1989). Similarly, a long clinically silent period of amyloid deposition probably precedes AD. Provided it can be diagnosed, this preclinical period would be the ideal time to institute therapeutic intervention.

Function of the amyloid precursor protein

The amyloid precursor protein (APP) is the source of the Aβ deposits found in Alzheimer brains. APP (Fig. 1) constitutes a family of eight transmembrane glycoproteins generated by alternative splicing of the three APP exons 7, 8 and 15 (Sandbrink et al 1994). Exon 15 is inserted within a signal sequence ENEGSG for xylose transferase. Alternative splicing of this exon 15 leads to L-APP molecules carrying chondroitin sulfate glycosaminoglycan side chains (Pangalos et al 1995) which have a function in growth regulation. Secretory forms of APP are produced by two pathways: a non-amyloidogenic pathway involving proteolytic cleavage within the Aβ region (Esch et al 1990), and an amyloidogenic pathway leading to the release of the Aβ subunit (Haass & Selkoe 1993). In neurons, these two pathways appear to not be mutually exclusive (Dyrks et al 1994). APP has non-overlapping binding sites for Zn^{2+} and Cu^{2+} which control the homophilic dimerization of APP and APP metabolism (Bush et al 1993, Hesse et al 1994). In addition, APP binds to cell surface receptors and to molecules of the extracellular matrix, such as heparan sulfate proteoglycans, collagen and laminin, which suggests a function in cell interaction (Bush et al 1993, Hesse et al 1994).

Neurons, the primarily affected cells in AD, are the only cells in the brain that constitutively express APP: microglia and astrocytes express high levels of APP, but only upon activation. The interaction of microglia with the extracellular environment, particularly components of the extracellular matrix, affects APP secretion as well as intracellular APP biogenesis and catabolism

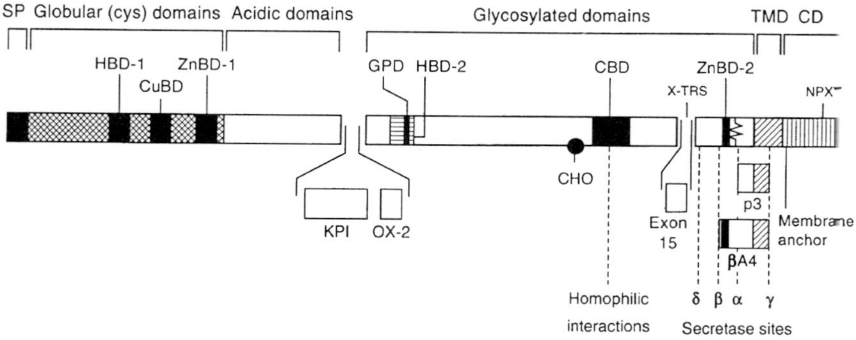

FIG. 1. Diagrammatic representation of APP domains and the secretase cleavage products. APP is composed of a signal peptide (SP), a large extracellular domain, a transmembrane domain (TMD) which spans the phospholipid bilayer once, and a short cytoplasmic domain (CD). The extracellular domain is complex and consists of: a globular region rich in cysteine residues which includes binding sites for heparin (HBD-1), copper (CuBD) and zinc (ZnBD-1); the acidic domain, a region rich in Glu, Asp and Thr residues; the glycosylated domains, which consist of a growth-promoting region (GPD) and another binding site for heparin (HBD-2), followed by an *N*-linked carbohydrate site (CHO) which may also subserve homophilic interactions or binding to collagen (collagen binding domain; CBD). The exon products which are alternatively spliced (exon 7, Kunitz protease inhibitor domain [KPI]; exon 8, OX-2 domain; and exon 15) are shown. At the splice junction of exon 15, a xylosyl transferase site (X-TRS) is created when exon 15 is not used—this enables the attachment of a chondroitin sulfate glycan side chain. The locations of the Aβ (βA4) domain and the p3 fragment as well as the secretase cleavage sites are indicated. There is a region in the βA4 segment that has been shown to interact with zinc (ZnBD-2). The TMD is anchored into the lipid bilayer by three charged residues. The short CD contains an NPXY recognition motif which could direct internalization.

(Mönning et al 1995). Fibronectin enhances APP secretion and decreases the level of transmembrane APP, whereas laminin and collagen causes a decrease in secretion and an accumulation of cellular full-length APP molecules and amyloidogenic APP fragments (Mönning et al 1995). Axotomy studies have shown that APP participates in immune responses of the CNS. The high expression of APP in activated microglia seen in concert with the release of free radicals and proteases by these cells make Aβ amyloid formation in Alzheimer's disease reminiscent of chronic inflammatory processes (Banati et al 1993).

In neurons, newly synthesized APP is first delivered from the cell body to the axon but later appears also in the dendrites (Simons et al 1995). This provides evidence for transcytosis of APP from the axonal to the dendritic plasma and synaptic membrane and suggests that the APP ligands Zn^{2+} and Cu^{2+} can be transported from the presynaptic to postsynaptic membrane of a neuron. The latter may be critical to the initiation and spread of the amyloid pathology in AD. Because APP occurs at the pre- and postsynaptic membrane (Schubert et al 1991, Simons et al 1995), we propose that APP participates in the regulation and repair/modulation of cell interactions such as at synapses and that APP is involved in brain plasticity and formation of long-term memory (Bush et al 1992, Schubert et al 1991). Formation of Aβ amyloid appears to occurs in the synaptic cleft, between synaptic terminals. This could interfere with the normal synaptic function of APP and lead to neuronal deafferentation by a mechanism resembling 'synaptic stripping' mediated by activated microglia (Blinzinger & Kreutzberg 1968). The consequence of such a process would be that neurons respond in transporting more APP to the lesioned site. Delivery of more APP also means more Aβ protein is released into the extracellular space, which could bind to the existing Aβ aggregates, thus contributing to the chronic growth of the amyloid deposits. If a critical size and compaction of these Aβ deposits are reached, these lesions could begin to interfere with synaptic plasticity and finally neuronal signalling.

Aβ amyloid in the causation of AD

The molecular and genetic analysis of AD has revealed that at the molecular level the deposition of Aβ amyloid protein is a necessary and, most likely, sufficient cause for the synaptic dysfunction and loss in AD (Bush et al 1992). All known risk factors for AD appear to influence either the concentration of the Aβ protein (Haass & Selkoe 1993, Levy-Lahad et al 1995, Rumble et al 1989, Sherrington et al 1995), the amount of the longer form of the Aβ protein (Aβ1–42) (Suzuki et al 1994) which is highly amyloidogenic (Hilbich et al 1992), or the initiation of Aβ aggregation to amyloid (Hyman et al 1995, Schmechel et al 1993). The evidence is as follows. First, both overexpression of APP, as in Trisomy 21 (Down's syndrome; Rumble et al 1989) as well as rare familial mutations in the AD1 gene of chromosome 21 (which turn out to be within or at the N- and C-terminal borders of the Aβ part of the APP gene; Hardy 1992), affect the release of Aβ or its length in favour of the longer, more amyloidogenic forms (Aβ1–42). The same appears to be the case for mutations in the AD3 gene (S182 gene) on chromosome 14 (Sherrington et al 1995). Mutations in the AD4 gene of chromosome 1 which affect a gene homologous to S182 are postulated also to increase the release of the longer Aβ forms (referenced in Levy-Lahad et al 1995). These genetic predispositions are the only causes of early onset for AD (between age 30 and 60). Second, the AD2 gene (the apolipoprotein E ε4 allele on chromosome 19) increases the risk of developing the disease after age 60 (Corder et al 1993). Patients carrying this genetic risk factor have more Aβ deposits (Hyman et al 1995, Schmechel et al 1993). Third, the amyloid deposition in the major form of AD, the late-onset and sporadic cases, cannot be distinguished from that of familial AD cases.

This suggests that the amyloidogenic processing of APP may be the final common pathway for the pathogenesis of AD.

Genesis of Aβ amyloid

If it turns out that the final common pathway underlying the neurodegeneration in AD is indeed the amyloidogenic processing of APP, inhibition of the genesis of Aβ amyloid would be the most direct therapeutic approach (Beyreuther & Masters 1995, Evin et al 1994, Whyte et al 1994). The development of such therapeutic approaches, however, requires the understanding of the mechanisms controlling the conversion of APP into its soluble breakdown product Aβ, the aggregation of Aβ and its conversion into insoluble deposits, and finally the compaction of these aggregates into amyloid plaques or congophilic angiopathy.

The Aβ domain (Fig. 2) encompasses parts of both the extracellular and transmembrane domains of APP. Consequently, the first step in the genesis of Aβ amyloid is the release of the Aβ fragment from the parent APP molecules. This implies the existence of two distinct proteolytic events to generate the N- and C-termini of Aβ. At least two secretory mechanisms exist which can release APP from the membrane and generate the soluble, C-truncated forms of APP (APP_{sec}). Any proteases that release APP and its fragments from the membrane are known as 'secretases' in the current literature. Most APP_{sec} is released by a putative α-secretase, which cleaves within the Aβ domain to release α-APP_{sec}, and precludes the release of intact Aβ (Esch et al 1990). A minor portion of APP_{sec} is released by a β-secretase, which cleaves near the N-terminus of Aβ and produces C-terminal fragments containing the whole Aβ domain (Seubert et al 1993). The finding of intact Aβ and other fragments of the Aβ domain (p3) in the extracellular compartment suggests that other proteolytic activities (γ-secretases) exist under normal conditions which can generate the C-terminus of Aβ after release of the transmembrane domain from the lipid bilayer (Haass & Selkoe 1993). Neither the identity nor the precise subcellular localization of the three secretases α, β and γ are known. Treatment with methylamine and ammonium chloride, inhibitors interfering with intracellular transport mechanisms, inhibits β-secretase activity without influencing the physiological cleavage by α-secretase activity (De Strooper et al 1993, Dyrks et al 1993a,b, Haass & Selkoe 1993). The calpain proteinase inhibitor (MDL 28170) has also been shown to block formation of the Aβ peptide and to prevent cleavage by γ-secretase, but this does not necessarily imply that this protease is a thiol protease or a Ca^{2+}-activated thiol protease (Higaki et al 1995). All these inhibitors prevent amyloidogenic but not non-amyloidogenic APP processing, suggesting the feasibility of targeting the inhibition of β- or γ-secretase.

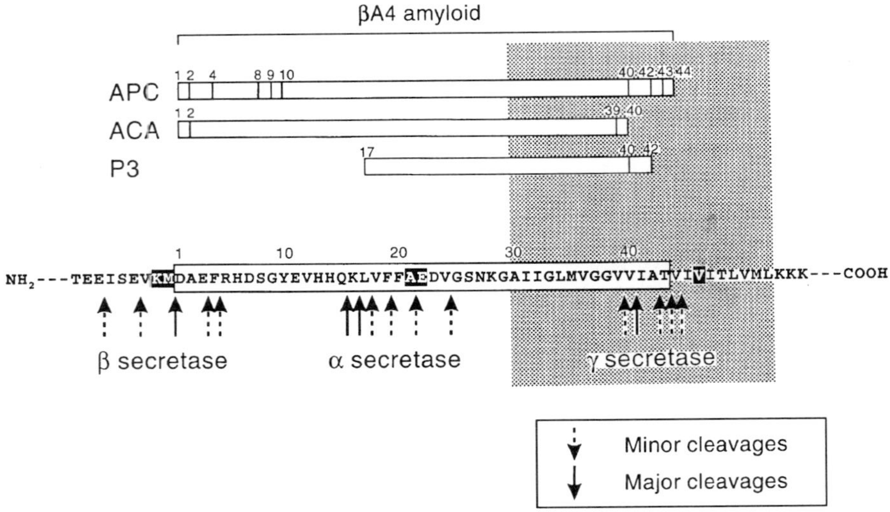

FIG. 2. Primary structure of Aβ (βA4) amyloid and the surrounding region of the secretase cleavage sites. The top part of the figure represents the components of native Aβ. The amyloid plaque cores (APC) show ragged N- and C-termini; the amyloid congophilic angiopathy (ACA) is less ragged, and ends at residue 40; the third bar represents the p3 sequence which may be a component of diffuse amyloid. In the partial sequence around the Aβ domain (lower part of figure), numbering is according to Aβ sequence. The Aβ domain is boxed; the mutated residues which cause Alzheimer's disease are highlighted (black boxes); arrows represent the various secretase cleavage sites identified in cultured cell lines (α- and β-secretases) or derived from sequencing of amyloid components (γ-secretase). The shaded area represents the transmembrane region.

The Aβ peptide is partially soluble (Hilbich et al 1991). Its clearance appears possible, and agents that interfere with or disrupt the process of Aβ amyloid aggregation are likely to alter the disease course. The transition of α-helical Aβ into the β conformation with the subsequent formation of β-sheets may be the rate-limiting step in amyloid formation (Hilbich et al 1991, 1992, Sticht et al 1995). Peptides inhibiting β-sheet formation of Aβ have been designed and are being evaluated (Hilbich et al 1992).

Oxidative radicals, membrane integrity and metal ions also affect the aggregation of Aβ, with clear implications for drug design (Bush et al 1994, Dyrks et al 1992). Substitutions of amino acids within the Aβ sequence, as occurs in rodents, can alter the tendency of Aβ peptides to aggregate by changing the degree to which oxidation of the peptides occurs (Dyrks et al 1993a).

To understand the influence of APP expression and turnover on Aβ genesis will require an in-depth appreciation of APP function, particularly in brain, where the restricted deposition of Aβ amyloid is characteristic. Risk factors for

AD that influence Aβ amyloid formation are likely to act on APP directly or on APP function. Because a gene dosage effect is likely to be the cause of premature AD in Down's syndrome, manipulation of APP expression and metabolism is a prime therapeutic target in sporadic AD. The expression and metabolism of APP has been shown to be affected by a number of potential pharmacologically active agents and manipulations, including interleukin 1, transforming growth factor β1, phorbol esters, tissue plasminogen activator, nerve growth factor, fibroblast growth factor, retinoic acid, components of the extracellular matrix, glucose, oestrogens, metal ions such as Zn^{2+} and Cu^{2+}, oxidative stress, long-term potentiation and the activation of neurotransmitter receptors (for review from our groups see Beyreuther & Masters 1995, Evin et al 1994, Whyte et al 1994).

Therapeutic strategies

Although a rational drug design program for AD would place the APP–Aβ conversion and Aβ amyloid pathway at the top of any list for therapeutic strategies, this is not to downgrade efforts currently under way in other areas. However, drugs that do not address the pathogenesis directly can be expected to give rise to only a transient effect.

Targeting events remote from the APP–Aβ pathway, which besides anti-inflammatory agents may include growth factors and intracellular Ca^{2+} levels, will prove to be extremely challenging. A transgenic mouse model that parallels the development of the Aβ amyloid lesions of AD but not of the intraneuronal deposits of neurofibrillary tangles (Games et al 1995) may well prove to have a direct application in the evaluation of anti-amyloid therapeutics.

It remains to be shown which of the varied strategies have the best future prospect of delivering some rational therapy for both the postponement of the progression of the structural lesions and the clinical course of AD, where today none has been proven to exist.

Acknowledgements

We gratefully acknowledge financial support by grants from the Deutsche Forschungsgemeinschaft through SFB 317 and 258, the BMBF of Germany, the Forschungsschwerpunkt Baden-Württemberg, the Metropolitan Life Foundation, the Fonds der Chemischen Industrie (to K. B.); and the National Health and Medical Research Council of Australia and the Victorian Health Promotion Foundation (to C. L. M.).

References

Banati RB, Gehrmann J, Czech C et al 1993 Early and rapid de novo-synthesis of Alzheimer βA4-amyloid precursor protein (APP) in activated microglia. Glia 9: 199–210

Beyreuther K, Masters CL 1995 Neurodegeneration and dementia: Alzheimer's disease as a model. Drug Res 45:347–350
Bickel H, Cooper B 1994 Incidence and relative risk of dementia in an urban elderly population: findings of a prospective field study. Psychol Med 24:179–192
Blinzinger K, Kreutzberg G 1968 Displacement of synaptic terminals from regenerating motoneurons by microglial cells. Z Zellforsch Mikrosk Anat 85:145–157
Bush AI, Beyreuther K, Masters CL 1992 βA4 amyloid protein and its precursor in Alzheimer's disease. Pharmacol Ther 56:97–117
Bush AI, Multhaup G, Moir RD et al 1993 A novel zinc (II) binding site modulates the function of the βA4 amyloid protein precursor of Alzheimer's disease. J Biol Chem 268:16109–16112
Bush AI, Pettingell WH Jr, Multhaup G et al 1994 Rapid induction of Alzheimer Aβ amyloid formation by zinc. Science 265:1464–1467
Corder EH, Saunders AM, Strittmatter WJ et al 1993 Gene dose of apolipoprotein E type 4 allele and the risk of Alzheimer's disease in late-onset families. Science 261:921–923
De Strooper B, Umans L, Van Leuven F, Van Den Berghe H 1993 Study of the synthesis and secretion of normal and artificial mutants of murine amyloid precursor protein (APP): cleavage of APP occurs in a late compartment of the default secretion pathway. J Cell Biol 121:295–304
Dyrks T, Dyrks E, Hartmann T, Masters CL, Beyreuther K 1992 Amyloidogenicity of βA4 and βA4-bearing APP fragments by metal catalysed oxidation. J Biol Chem 267:18210–18217
Dyrks T, Dyrks E, Masters CL, Beyreuther K 1993a Amyloidogenicity of rodent and human βA4 sequences. FEBS Lett 324:231–236
Dyrks T, Dyrks E, Mönning U, Urmoneit B, Turner J, Beyreuther K 1993b Generation of βA4 from the amyloid protein precursor and fragments thereof. FEBS Lett 335:89–93
Dyrks T, Mönning U, Beyreuther K, Turner J 1994 Amyloid precursor protein secretion and βA4 amyloid generation are not mutually exclusive. FEBS Lett 349:210–214
Esch FS, Keim PS, Battie EC et al 1990 Cleavage of amyloid β peptide during constitutive processing of its precursor. Science 248:1122–1124
Evin G, Beyreuther K, Masters CL 1994 Alzheimer's disease amyloid precursor protein (AβPP): proteolytic processing, secretases and βA4 amyloid production. Amyloid: Int J Exp Clin Invest 1:263–280
Games D, Adams D, Alessandrini R et al 1995 Alzheimer-type neuropathology in transgenic mice overexpressing V717F β-amyloid precursor protein. Nature 373:523–527
Haass C, Selkoe DJ 1993 Cellular processing of β-amyloid precursor protein and the genesis of amyloid β-peptide. Cell 75:1039–1042
Hardy J 1992 Framing β-amyloid. Nat Genet 1:233–234
Hesse L, Beher D, Masters CL, Multhaup G 1994 The βA4 amyloid precursor protein binding to copper. FEBS Lett 349:109–116
Higaki J, Quon D, Zhong ZY, Cordell B 1995 Inhibition of β-amyloid formation identifies proteolytic precursors and subcellular site of catabolism. Neuron 14:651–659
Hilbich C, Kisters-Woike B, Reed J, Masters CL, Beyreuther K 1991 Aggregation and secondary structure of synthetic amyloid βA4 peptides of Alzheimer's disease. J Mol Biol 218:149–163
Hilbich C, Kisters-Woike B, Reed J, Masters CL, Beyreuther K 1992 Substitutions of hydrophobic amino acids reduce the amyloidogenicity of Alzheimer's disease βA4 peptides. J Mol Biol 228:460–473

Hyman B, West HL, Rebeck GW et al 1995 Quantitative analysis of senile plaques in Alzheimer disease: observation of log-normal size distribution and molecular epidemiology of differences associated with apolipoprotein E genotype and trisomy 21 (Down syndrome). Proc Natl Acad Sci USA 92:3586–3590

Levy-Lahad E, Wasco W, Poorkaj P et al 1995 Candidate gene for the chromosome 1 familial Alzheimer's disease locus. Science 269:973–977

Masters CL, Simms G, Weinman NA, Multhaup G, McDonald BL, Beyreuther K 1985 Amyloid plaque core protein in Alzheimer's disease and Down syndrome. Proc Natl Acad Sci USA 82:4245–4249

Mönning U, Sandbrink R, Weidemann A, Banati R, Masters CL, Beyreuther K 1995 Extracellular matrix influences the biogenesis of amyloid precursor protein in microglial cells. J Biol Chem 270:7104–7110

Ott A, Breteler MMB, van Harskamp F et al 1995 Prevalence of Alzheimer's disease and vascular dementia: association with education. The Rotterdam study. Br Med J 310:970–973

Pangalos MN, Efthimiopoulos S, Shioi J, Robakis NK 1995 The chondroitin sulfate attachment site of Appican is formed by splicing out exon 15 of the amyloid precursor gene. J Biol Chem 270:10388–10391

Rumble B, Retallack R, Hilbich C et al 1989 Amyloid A4 protein and its precursor in Down's syndrome and Alzheimer's disease. N Engl J Med 320:1446–1452

Sandbrink R, Masters CL, Beyreuther K 1994 Amyloid protein precursor mRNA isoforms without exon 15 (L-APP mRNAs) are ubiquitously expressed in rat tissues including brain but not in neurons. J Biol Chem 269:1510–1517

Schmechel DE, Saunders AM, Strittmatter WJ et al 1993 Increased amyloid β-peptide deposition in cerebral cortex as a consequence of apolipoprotein E genotype in late-onset Alzheimer's disease. Proc Natl Acad Sci USA 90:9649–9653

Schubert W, Prior R, Weidemann A et al 1991 Localization of Alzheimer βA4 amyloid precursor protein at central and peripheral synaptic sites. Brain Res 563:184–194

Seubert P, Oltersdorf T, Lee MG et al 1993 Secretion of β-amyloid precursor protein cleaved at the amino terminus of the β-amyloid peptide. Nature 361:260–263

Sherrington R, Rogaev EI, Liang Y et al 1995 Cloning of a gene bearing missense mutation in early-onset familial Alzheimer's disease. Nature 375:754–760

Simons M, Ikonen E, Tienari PJ et al 1995 Intracellular routing of human amyloid protein precursor: axonal delivery followed by transport to the dendrites. J Neurosci Res 41:121–128

Sticht H, Bayer P, Willbold D et al 1995 Structure of amyloid A4-(1–40)-peptide of Alzheimer's disease. Eur J Biochem 233:293–298

Suzuki N, Cheung TT, Cai X-D et al 1994 An increased percentage of long amyloid β protein secreted by familial amyloid β-protein precursor (βAPP_{717}) mutants. Science 264:1336–1340

Whyte S, Beyreuther K, Masters CL 1994 Rational therapeutic strategies for Alzheimer's disease. In: DB Calne (ed) Neurodegenerative diseases. Saunders, Philadelphia, PA, p 647–664

DISCUSSION

Frangione: Is soluble Aβ increased in the circulation of individuals with Down's syndrome?

Masters: Those data are not available yet. The only people with sensitive assays are using the Japanese monoclonal antibodies (Suzuki et al 1994), and data relating to Down's syndrome are not available.

Pepys: Steve Younkin, at the recent FASEB meeting (Copper Mountain, August 1995), reported that both the chromosome 14 and the chromosome 1 familial Alzheimer's disease individuals had significantly higher levels of Aβ1–42 in the plasma than controls.

Masters: As I mentioned earlier (p 116), one group has shown increased transcription of APP in fibroblasts from what was thought to be a chromosome 14-linked family (Querfurth et al 1995), but this was before the presenilin (PS-2) mutations were described. I'm not sure whether these data have been re-analysed in the light of the more recent discoveries.

Kelly: Are the β-secretases a family of enzymes, or one enzyme that is not very specific?

Masters: That's the big question with all of the secretase activities. The evidence is leading towards the idea that it is not one specific enzyme that is performing these cuts. The problem is, how does one prove that any particular enzyme is *the* secretase? One can do a knockout *in vitro* or *in vivo*, but then if some other enzyme comes in to take over the missing function, it would be impossible to determine the levels of biological restriction.

Goldgaber: A number of enzymes have been purified and have been shown to possess secretase activities.

Masters: We're putting our money on calpain-like enzymes and cathepsin D-like activities (Li et al 1995, Evin et al 1995).

Hendriks: When do you think γ-secretase cuts? Before or after β-secretase?

Masters: Most of the evidence suggests that it is cutting after β-secretase. There is at least one report (Wallace et al 1995) suggesting that a γ-secretase cut can occur and release that form of a molecule, sAPPγ, with the Aβ still attached, but I think these data need to be confirmed. Most of the evidence is that an α or a β cut occurs, and then somehow the γ cut is made (for reviews see Evin et al 1994, Checler 1995). The other interesting observation is that we know that there are intracellular forms of Aβ (Fuller et al 1995), but the major problem is the extracellular release of this material—it is not clear how it gets from an intracellular to an extracellular compartment.

Kisilevsky: Are people interested in this area concerned at all about the lack of complete specificity of the secretases, given the variable cleavage points? I would have thought that enzymes that had a very specific physiological function would be pretty restrictive in how they attack these molecules.

Masters: We've been working now for three or four years trying to pin this down. It's very frustrating.

Caughey: But if they are lysosomal enzymes you might not expect that sort of specificity.

Pepys: What's your problem with this, Bob?

Kisilevsky: The problem I see is that if Aβ1–40 or 1–42 is going to be considered as a physiological product, and the Aβ amyloid is then derived from this physiological product, I would have expected that the enzymes involved in cleaving Aβ out of APP would be much more restrictive in where they would cut the APP. The raggedness of the N- and C-termini of Aβ needs to be better explained.

Pepys: I disagree; Aβ just happens to be a physiological breakdown product which, if you live long enough, causes the unfortunate side effect of forming amyloid in the brain. If you have a mutation that makes that physiological product more abundant, whether it's in the APP gene or elsewhere, you get the disease earlier. Aβ hasn't got a physiological function, unlike angiotensin which must be cleaved in a specific place for it to have its physiological function—it is just a degradation product.

Masters: Certainly, Aβ appears to be a minor metabolic pathway. The major product, p3, which is the cut made by α-secretase, may be the normal constitutive mechanism. However, we have a strong suspicion that the α and β cleavages are less important than the γ cleavage. The other aspect to keep in mind is that the half-life of APP varies between different compartments. The compartmentalization of this protein may determine which proteolytic enzymes have an opportunity to act on it.

Lundgren: You mentioned that you saw increased APP expression in activated lymphocytes. Could you give more details?

Masters: T cells and macrophages utilize a spliced APP product which lacks exon 15. If you activate these cells the amount of APP mRNA and protein increases. If the cells become adherent to a substratum, they also vary the amount of APP they produce.

Maury: Could you comment on the observation that there is some accumulation of Aβ in the skin in AD? This finding, if confirmed, could have potential diagnostic significance.

Masters: I don't know if Blas Frangione has more up to date information on this, but the initial promising reports have not been confirmed.

Frangione: There is no amyloid deposition in the skin. What has been reported is just non-fibrillar immunoreactive material detected with anti-Aβ antibodies. Furthermore, this deposition occurs in many tissues, not just in the skin.

Masters: It largely depends on how specific the antibody is; those used to date do not distinguish Alzheimer's patients from aged-matched controls.

Frangione: It was done two ways: by skin biopsy and rectal biopsy, and the results were negative in both instances.

Pepys: We've lately studied a group of Alzheimer's patients by radiolabelled serum amyloid P component (SAP) scintigraphy, which is a sensitive tool for detecting systemic amyloid (Hawkins et al 1988, 1990, Hawkins 1994). The results were completely negative. This doesn't exclude the possibility of there being microscopic deposits, because histology is more sensitive than scintigraphy, but it does exclude there being any major amyloid elsewhere in the body outside the brain. This contrasts, for example, with the cystatin C Icelandic type of hereditary cerebral amyloid angiopathy, which was previously thought to be a brain-localized disease: SAP scans on these patients reveal massive amyloid deposits in the spleen and lymphoid organs (Hawkins et al 1991).

Benson: Cystatin C was originally isolated in sequence from the urine: is Aβ ever found in the urine?

Frangione: Yes (unpublished results).

Masters: So is the precursor, APP. We still do not know whether it is derived from the plasma or from the renal system itself.

J. N. Buxbaum: Do you think that the entire zinc effect is transcriptional?

Masters: No, we think it is far more complex. For example, we see this change in the plasma where there's evidence that zinc affects the stability of platelets.

Westermark: We have done some studies concerning the effects of zinc on islet amyloid polypeptide, because there is a lot of zinc in the β cell granules. Certainly, zinc strongly promotes fibrillogenesis *in vitro* (Westermark et al 1996). Has anyone looked at the effects of zinc or other metals on accumulation of other amyloidogenic proteins?

J. N. Buxbaum: Joe Herbert showed that zinc is associated with transthyretin fibrils (Martone & Herbert 1994). He's currently doing some studies with chelating agents for zinc, but I don't think there are any results yet.

Masters: There are various histochemical methods for looking at the distribution of free zinc in the brain. In the rat brain at least, there is a very striking predominance of free zinc in the hippocampus and in very selected regions of the cerebral cortex in a distribution roughly parallel to where we see plaques and tangles. In contrast, some of the subcortical structures and the cerebellum have almost no free vesicular zinc. This is another reason why we're interested in the interactions of APP with zinc.

Pepys: What effect does zinc have on the cognitive performance of people with other sorts of dementia apart from Alzheimer's disease, or even normal people?

Masters: We are now studying some of these questions. In particular, a large cohort of normal ageing persons is being assessed.

References

Checler F 1995 Processing of the β-amyloid precursor protein and its regulation in Alzheimer's disease. J Neurochem 65:1431–1444

Evin G, Beyreuther K, Masters CL 1994 Alzheimer's disease amyloid precursor protein (AβPP): proteolytic processing, secretases and βA4 amyloid production. Amyloid: Int J Exp Clin Invest 1:263–280

Evin G, Cappai R, Li Q-X et al 1995 Candidate γ-secretases in the generation of the carboxyl terminus of the Alzheimer's disease βA4 amyloid: possible involvement of cathepsin D. Biochemistry 34:14185–14192

Fuller SJ, Storey E, Li Q-X, Smith AI, Beyreuther K, Masters CL 1995 Intracellular production of βA4 amyloid of Alzheimer's disease: modulation by phosphoramidon and lack of coupling to the secretion of the amyloid precursor. Biochemistry 34:8091–8098

Hawkins PN 1994 Studies with radiolabelled serum amyloid P component provide evidence for turnover and regression of amyloid deposits *in vivo*. Clin Sci 87:289–295

Hawkins PN, Myers MJ, Epentos AA, Caspi D, Pepys MB 1988 Specific localization and imaging of amyloid deposits *in vivo* using labelled I_{123} serum amyloid P component. J Exp Med 167:903–913

Hawkins PN, Lavender JP, Pepys MB 1990 Evaluation of systemic amyloidosis by scintigraphy with ^{123}I-labeled serum amyloid P component. N Engl J Med 323: 508–513

Hawkins PN, Tyrrell P, Jones T et al 1991 Metabolic and scintigraphic studies with radiolabeled serum amyloid P component in amyloidosis: applications to cerebral deposits and Alzheimer disease with positron emission tomography. Bull Clin Neurosci 56:178–190

Li Q-X, Evin G, Small DH, Multhaup G, Beyreuther K, Masters CL 1995 Proteolytic processing of Alzheimer's disease βA4 amyloid precursor protein in human platelets. J Biol Chem 270:14140–14147

Martone RL, Herbert J 1994 Metallo–protein interactions in TTR amyloidogenesis: therapeutic interactions. In: Kisilevesky R, Benson MD, Frangione B, Gaudie J, Muckle TJ, Young ID (eds) Amyloid and amyloidogenesis 1993. Parthenon Park Ridge, NJ, p 517–519

Querfurth HW, Wijsman EM, St George-Hyslop PH, Selkoe DJ 1995 βAPP mRNA transcription is increased in cultured fibroblasts from the familial Alzheimer's disease-1 family. Mol Brain Res 28:319–337

Suzuki N, Cheung TT, Cai X-D et al 1994 An increased percentage of long amyloid β protein secreted by familial amyloid β-protein precursor (βAPP_{717}) mutants. Science 264:1336–1340

Wallace WC, Lieberburg I, Schenk D, Vigo-Pelfrey C, Davies KL, Haroutunian V 1995 Chronic elevation of secreted amyloid precursor protein in subcortically lesioned rats, and its exacerbation in aged rats. J Neurosci 15:4896–4905

Westermark P, Li Z-C, Westermark GT, Leckström A, Steiner DF 1996 Effects of β cell granule components on human islet amyloid polypeptide fibril formation. FEBS Lett 379:203–206

Apolipoprotein E and amyloidogenesis

Blas Frangione, Eduardo M. Castaño, Thomas Wisniewski* Jorge Ghiso, Frances Prelli and Ruben Vidal

*Department of Pathology and *Neurology, New York University Medical Center, 550 1st Avenue TH 427, New York, NY 10016, USA*

Abstract. Alzheimer's amyloid β-protein (Aβ) is a modified, pathogenic form of a constitutive host protein, soluble amyloid β-protein (sAβ). Both are conformational isomers encoded by the gene for the β-amyloid precursor protein (APP), located on chromosome 21. sAβ and Aβ have identical sequence but are thought to differ in their secondary structure and physicochemical properties, hence they are conformational isomers. sAβ is easily degraded, while Aβ is partially resistant. Aβ has a high β-pleated sheet content, while sAβ is thought to be more random-coil and/or α-helical. Aβ, unlike sAβ, adopts an amyloidogenic conformation, forms aggregates and gives rise to fibrils. Most early-onset forms of Alzheimer's disease (AD) have been linked to mutations of the presenilin 1, presenilin 2 or APP genes, located on chromosomes 14, 1 and 21, respectively. Their relationship to amyloidogenesis is being investigated. On the other hand, the major risk factor for the most common form, sporadic and familial late-onset AD, is the presence of the apoE ε4 allele. Recent studies have shown that a 10 kDa C-terminal fragment of apoE is complexed to Aβ in neuritic plaques and that apoE isoforms can modulate amyloid formation *in vitro*. Moreover, thrombin cleavage of apoE generates a similar C-terminal fragment that can form amyloid-like fibrils. Thus neuritic plaques may contain both Aβ and apoE amyloid fibrils. AD can be neuropathologically defined by the presence of several interacting proteins that can adopt an amyloidogenic conformation. This has led us to hypothesize that in AD, amyloidosis may be reactive rather than causative.

1996 The nature and origin of amyloid fibrils. Wiley, Chichester (Ciba Foundation Symposium 199) p 132–145

Amyloidoses and prionosis are disorders of protein conformation. In amyloidosis, the deposition of soluble peptides as insoluble fibrils leads to cell death and organ dysfunction. These fibrils are large polymers that result from the assembly of precursor peptides, which adopt a β-pleated sheet secondary structure. Regardless of the primary structure, all amyloids have a similar morphological appearance under the electron microscope and an affinity for dyes such as Congo red or thioflavines (Castaño & Frangione 1995). Much of what we know about the mechanisms involved in amyloid fibril formation is based on *in vitro* studies with synthetic peptides homologous to amyloid precursors. Among these peptides, synthetic analogues of the amyloid β-protein (Aβ), the main constituent of senile plaques and vascular amyloid of Alzheimer's disease (AD) (Glenner & Wong 1984, Masters et al 1985), have provided most of the information regarding the physicochemical factors that affect amyloidogenesis *in vitro* (Castaño et al 1986). The role of a critical concentration above which amyloid assembly proceeds rapidly, the importance of pH and amino acid substitutions in the precursors, and the effect of metal ions such as Zn or Al in the modulation of this process have been established (Burdick et al 1992, Bush et al 1994, Exley et al 1993). Also likely to be important are the origin, transport and clearance of soluble Aβ, all of which are currently under study. Immunohistochemical and biochemical methods have long shown that amyloid deposits *in vivo* are complex structures composed not only of amyloid proteins but also of a set of amyloid-associated proteins that are consistently present regardless of the identity of the amyloid subunit. Sulfated proteoglycans (Snow et al 1987), amyloid P component (Coria et al 1988), apolipoprotein J (Choi-Miura et al 1992) and apolipoprotein E (apoE) (Wisniewski & Frangione 1992) are the most well known. Recent efforts to elucidate the mechanisms of amyloid formation have focused on the interaction between amyloid precursors and their associated proteins. Among these, apoE has come under special scrutiny owing to its presence in senile plaques, vascular amyloid and neurofibrillary tangles of AD and the recently described genetic relationship of the apoE $\varepsilon4$ allele with this major human disease. ApoE is a 34 kDa product of a four-exon gene located on the long arm of chromosome 19, which is central to cholesterol metabolism (Mahley 1988). In addition to its function in cholesterol transport, apoE is important in local circuits of lipid turnover that are involved in membrane repair. This is especially relevant to the nervous system, in which apoE has been shown to participate in cholesterol redistribution during membrane remodelling after injury both in peripheral nerves and brain (Mahley 1988, Poirier 1994). In humans, the apoE gene is polymorphic, leading to three major apoE isoforms, namely E2, E3 and E4. ApoE3, the most common isoform, has a cysteine at position 112 and an arginine at position 158; apoE2 is the least frequent isoform, with cysteine at both positions whereas apoE4 presents arginine at both sites (Mahley 1988).

Recently, a strong association between the inheritance of the apoE $\varepsilon4$ allele and AD has been described (Corder et al 1993, Strittmatter et al 1993). These studies have shown that: (1) carriers of the $\varepsilon4$ allele have an increased risk of developing AD in an allele-dose dependent manner; (2) the apoE $\varepsilon4$ genotype modulates the age of onset of the disease; and (3) the inheritance of the $\varepsilon4$ allele correlates with increased deposition of Aβ in blood vessels and plaques and a greater density of senile plaques in the cerebral cortex (Rebeck et al 1993, Schmechel et al 1993). The apoE locus is not considered to be a causative gene but rather a susceptibility or modifying factor, because the presence of the $\varepsilon4$

allele is neither sufficient nor necessary for AD to develop. In an attempt to provide an explanation for the association of apoE with the neuropathology and genetics of AD, ourselves and others have studied the interaction of apoE and synthetic Aβ analogues *in vitro*. These proteins can form a complex that is partially resistant to SDS treatment; under certain conditions, apoE can enhance amyloid fibril formation by Aβ *in vitro* (Sanan et al 1994, Wisniewski et al 1994, Ma et al 1994).

Together, these data have strengthened the hypothesis that apoE, particularly apoE4, acts as a pathological chaperone (Wisniewski & Frangione 1992) and participates in the pathogenesis of AD by modulating Aβ conformation and its accumulation in the brain. However, there is evidence suggesting that apoE may have a general role in the process of amyloid formation regardless of the biochemical nature of the amyloid peptide or its localization. Immunohistochemistry has shown that apoE is associated with other types of cerebral amyloidosis, including: (1) Down's syndrome related to Aβ; (2) hereditary cerebral haemorrhage with amyloidosis, Dutch type, associated with the glutamine 22 variant of Aβ (Levy et al 1990); (3) hereditary cerebral haemorrhage with amyloidosis, Icelandic type, related to a cystatin C variant (Ghiso et al 1986); (4) spongiform encephalopathies such as Creutzfeldt–Jakob and kuru; (5) Gerstmann–Sträussler–Scheinker syndrome, associated with the prion amyloid (Namba et al 1991, Bugiani et al 1994); and (6) a newly described condition known as Hungarian amyloidosis. This disease is characterized by meningocerebrovascular amyloid deposition, which results in a massive vascular dementia. These deposits are associated with apoE. A novel transthyretin (TTR) missense mutation at codon 18 (D18G) is found in all affected individuals (Vidal et al 1996). This mutation has not previously been reported and is illustrated in Fig. 1. Interestingly, another kindred has recently been described in which there is TTR deposition in the brain, producing a dementia that is associated with a TTR V30G mutation (Peterson et al 1995). These two kindreds clearly establish that TTR is another protein that can be deposited as amyloid within the CNS and produce dementia.

Immunostaining has also identified apoE localized within amyloid deposits in systemic forms of the disease, such as immunoglobulin light chain-related (AL) primary amyloidosis, secondary amyloidosis and familial Mediterranean fever related to amyloid A (AA) and familial amyloidotic polyneuropathy caused by the accumulation of TTR variants (Saraiva 1995). Yet, little is known about the biochemical interactions underlying these apoE amyloid associations. ApoE is conformationally and functionally a two-domain protein which is represented by the two major fragments obtained after thrombin digestion. The 22 kDa N-terminal fragment is a stable four-helix bundle structure, as demonstrated by X-ray crystallography (Wilson et al 1991). This portion of the molecule contains the sequence that mediates low density

gttaacttctcacgtgtcttctctacacccag GGC ACC GGT GAA TCC AAG TGT CCT
Gly Thr Gly Glu Ser Lys Cys Pro

18
G
CTG ATG GTC AAA GTT CTA | GAT | GCT GTC CGA GGC AGT CCT
Leu Met Val Lys Val Leu | Asp | Ala Val Arg Gly Ser Pro
Gly

GCC ATC AAT GTG GCC GTG CAT GTG TTC AGA AAG GCT GCT
Ala Ile Asn Val Ala Val His Val Phe Arg Lys Ala Ala

GAT GAC ACC TGG GAG CCA TTT GCC TCT GG gtaagttgccaaagaaccctc
Asp Asp Thr Trp Glu Pro Phe Ala Ser Gl

ccacaggactt

FIG. 1. DNA sequence of exon 2 of the TTR gene. Capital letters give exon sequences and lower case letters designate flanking intron sequences. The underlined sequences are oligonucleotides used for PCR amplification. The broken line gives an *XbA*I restriction site. Box indicates the location of the G for A substitution at the second base of codon 18, resulting in the conversion of Asp to Gly found in Hungarian amyloidosis patients. (Vidal et al 1996.)

lipoprotein–receptor binding. By contrast, the 10 kDa C-terminal fragment is less stable and mediates binding to lipoprotein particles.

Recent work from our laboratory has shed some light on the biochemistry of the apoE–amyloid interaction. We had previously reported the finding of a tryptic peptide of apoE corresponding to residues 270–278 in association with two AA proteins. These observations were confirmed and extended by the characterization of apoE fragments that co-purified with amyloid subunits isolated from the spleen of systemic AA and AL amyloidosis (Prelli et al 1991, Castaño et al 1995). In both cases, microsequencing analysis identified C-terminal peptides similar to the 10 kDa fragment generated *in vitro* by thrombin digestion. In AL, two major apoE fragments starting at positions 225 and 227 and a minor one starting at position 216 were found, whereas in AA, a major fragment starting at position 199 was associated with the amyloid subunit. These findings suggest that the apoE fragments that co-purify with AA and AL are bound to these amyloid proteins *in vivo* and that the remainder of the apoE molecule is cleaved by thrombin or other serine proteases *in situ* either before or after the formation of the apoE–amyloid complex. A similar 10 kDa apoE fragment was purified from AD senile plaque in association with

Aβ (Wisniewski et al 1995a). This apoE fragment *in vitro* forms amyloid-like fibrils, suggesting that senile plaques may contain more than one biochemical type of amyloid (Wisniewski et al 1995a; Fig. 2). This result has been corroborated by another group (Näslund et al 1995). Interestingly, the purported binding region to synthetic Aβ analogues has been located between residues 244 and 272 of apoE (Strittmatter et al 1993), a portion of the molecule that is contained in the apoE fragments isolated with systemic amyloids. We have also shown that under *in vitro* conditions, apoE and AA form an SDS-resistant complex. Furthermore, the presence of apoE increased the polymerization and aggregation of the AA peptide, similar to its action on synthetic Aβ peptides (Castaño et al 1995). These results indicate that the binding of apoE and amyloids is not sequence-specific but rather reflects a hydrophobic interaction between apoE and a common conformation shared by amyloid proteins of diverse primary structure. Secondary structure analysis predicts that an amphipathic helix with high lipid affinity is located within the region of apoE that co-purifies with amyloids. It seems possible that other exchangeable apolipoproteins that share similar amphipathic helices (Segrest et al 1992) can also interact with amyloids. In this respect, apoAI has been found associated with senile plaques of AD (Wisniewski et al 1995b). Many examples underscore the intimate relationship between apolipoproteins and amyloids: (1) the soluble form of Aβ appears to be bound to apoJ and apoE in biological fluids (Ghiso et al 1993, Golabek et al 1995); (2) apoAI genetic variants can form amyloid in certain hereditary amyloidoses (Nichols et al 1988); (3) serum amyloid A (SAA), the precursor of AA, is itself an acute-phase reactant apolipoprotein associated with high density lipoproteins, and is capable of forming complexes with phospholipid vesicles and of binding cholesterol *in vitro* (Bausserman et al 1983, Liang et al 1995); and (4) apoAII is the amyloid precursor in the senescent mouse-related amyloidosis (Naiki et al 1993). Furthermore, we have recently demonstrated that the 10 kDa C-terminal fragment of apoE generated by thrombin digestion can assemble into amyloid-like fibrils, as assessed by electron microscopy and Congo red staining (Wisniewski et al 1995b). These findings indicate that just as there is a large number of amyloid precursors capable of forming amyloid fibrils, there is also a group of amyloidogenic apolipoproteins that participate in this process either as modulators of fibrillogenesis or as constituents of the amyloid deposits. Other proteins may also participate in this process, such as the non-Aβ component (NAC) of AD amyloid (Uéda et al 1993). In this scenario, it is possible that certain amyloid proteins can misfold due to changes in the local environment, adopting a β-pleated sheet conformation. This abnormal conformation can then be induced in other proteins with an unrelated primary structure. This 'conformational mimicry' may underlie the initiation or propagation of the amyloid cascade (Wisniewski et al 1995b). The absence of apoE and amyloid P component in the non-fibrillar deposits of light chain

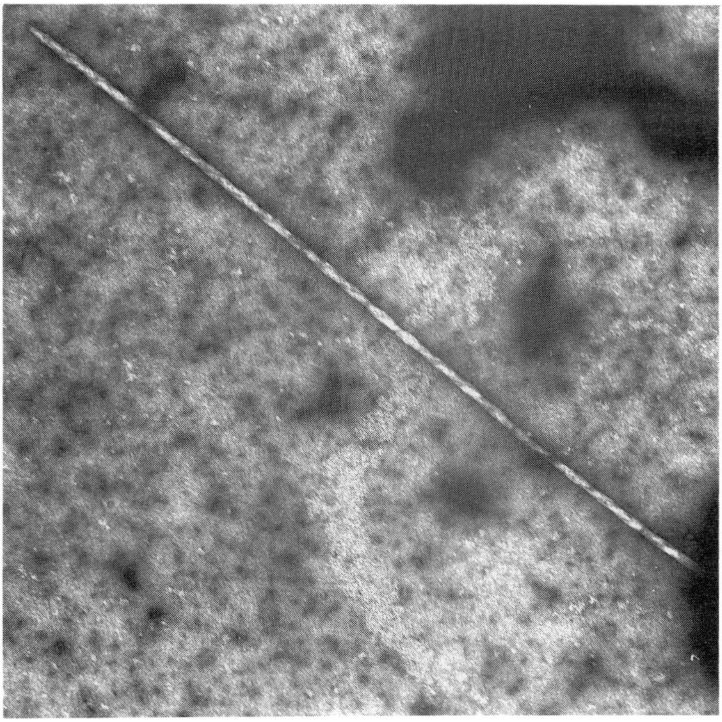

FIG. 2. Electron micrograph of negatively stained 'amyloid-like' fibrils produced by a thrombolytic C-terminal fragment of recombinant apoE (Wisniewski et al 1995a).

deposition disease and light and heavy chain deposition disease, which are considered pre-amyloid forms of AL disease, suggests that these two amyloid-associated proteins are essential components of the amyloidogenic response (Gallo et al 1994). Yet, other local reactants such as proteoglycans, to which apoE and amyloid proteins are known to bind, may influence apoE–amyloid interactions.

Despite this descriptive body of information regarding the close relationship between apoE and amyloids, the biological significance of apoE in the process of amyloidogenesis is unclear and controversial. The above data were generated through *in vitro* experiments and protein purification of post-mortem tissue. Although these are suitable means to raise hypotheses, they have a limited power to provide definitive answers to such dynamic and complex processes *in vivo*. The genetic association between AD and apoE alleles has strengthened the putative role of apoE in Aβ amyloidogenesis. However, it is possible that the apoE4 isoform may influence the pathogenesis of AD through a pathway that is unrelated to Aβ deposition. This possibility remains strong in light of the multiple and crucial functions of apoE related to lipid transport and membrane biology in the nervous system, especially those concerning neurite growth and repair (Nathan et al 1994). Should this be the case, then Aβ–apoE amyloid formation may reflect a response to unknown factors that lead to cell injury and membrane repair in the AD brain. The recent discoveries of presenilin 1 and 2 genes on chromosomes 14 and 1, respectively, that are linked to familial AD (Levy-Lahad et al 1995, Rogaev et al 1995, Sherrington et al 1995) raise the question of whether Aβ, APP, apoE or other factors interact with the products of these genes. Significantly, we have shown that at least a fragment of the presenilin 1 gene is found immunohistochemically in neuritic plaques of both chromosome 14-linked patients and sporadic AD cases, suggesting that this gene has a more general role in the pathogenesis of AD (Wisniewski et al 1995c).The development of transgenic mice carrying the cDNA of human mutated APP, which express a phenotype similar to AD in terms of plaque amyloid formation (Games et al 1995), will allow testing of many aspects of the amyloid hypothesis, including the role of apoE and presenilin 1 and 2, as well as that of the blood–brain barrier in Aβ amyloidogenesis (Zlokovic et al 1994). The availability of these suitable animal models together with knockout gene strategies will help to clarify whether apoE is an essential component for the amyloid cascade to develop both inside and outside the brain.

References

Abraham CR, Selkoe DJ, Potter H 1988 Immunohistochemical identification of the serine protease inhibitor alpha 1-antichymotrypsin in the brain amyloid deposits of Alzheimer's disease. Cell 52:487–501

Bausserman LL, Herbert PN, Forte T et al 1983 Interaction of the serum amyloid A proteins with phospholipid. J Biol Chem 258:10681–10688

Bugiani O, Giaccone G, Frigero L, Farlow MR, Ghetti B, Tagliavini F 1994 Apolipoproteins E and J immunoreactivity in Gerstmann–Sträussler–Scheinker disease. Neurobiol Aging (suppl 1) 15:156S

Burdick D, Soreghan B, Kwon M et al 1992 Assembly and aggregation properties of synthetic Alzheimer's A4/β amyloid peptides analogs. J Biol Chem 267:546–554.

Bush AI, Pettingell WH, Multhaup G et al 1994 Rapid induction of Alzheimer Aβ amyloid formation by zinc. Science 265:1464–1467

Castaño EM, Frangione B 1995 Non-Alzheimer's disease amyloidoses of the nervous system. Curr Opin Neurol 8:279–285

Castaño EM, Ghiso J, Prelli F, Gorevic PD, Migheli A, Frangione B 1986 *In vitro* formation of amyloid fibrils form two synthetic peptides of different lengths homologous to Alzheimer's disease β-protein. Biochem Biophys Res Commun 141:782–789

Castaño EM, Prelli F, Pras M, Frangione B 1995 Apolipoprotein carboxyl terminal fragments are complexed to amyloids A and L. Implications for amyloidogenesis and Alzheimer's disease. J Biol Chem 270:17610–17615

Choi-Miura NH, Ihara Y, Fukuchi K et al 1992 SP-40,40 is a constituent of Alzheimer's amyloid. Acta Neuropathol 83:260–264

Corder EH, Saunders AM, Strittmatter WJ et al 1993 Gene dose of apolipoprotein E type 4 allele and the risk of Alzheimer's disease in late-onset families. Science 261:921–923

Coria F, Castaño EM, Prelli F et al 1988 Isolation and characterization of amyloid P component from Alzheimer's disease and other types of cerebral amyloidosis. Lab Invest 58:454–457

Exley C, Price NC, Kelly SM, Birchall D 1993 An interaction of β-amyloid with aluminium *in vitro*. FEBS Lett 324:293–295

Gallo G, Wisniewski T, Choi-Miura NH, Ghiso J, Frangione B 1994 Potential role of apolipoprotein E in fibrillogenesis. Am J Pathol 145:526–530

Games D, Adams D, Alessandrini R et al 1995 Alzheimer-type neuropathology in transgenic mice overexpressing V717F β-amyloid precursor protein. Nature 373: 523–527

Ghiso J, Jensson O, Frangione B 1986 Amyloid fibrils in hereditary cerebral hemorrhage with amyloidosis of Icelandic type is a variant of gamma-trace basic protein (Cystatin C). Proc Natl Acad Sci USA 83:2974–2978

Ghiso J, Matsubara E, Koudinov A et al 1993 The cerebrospinal-fluid soluble form of Alzheimer's amyloid beta is complexed to SP-40,40 (apolipoprotein J), an inhibitor of the complement membrane-attack complex. Biochem J 293:27–30

Glenner GG, Wong CW 1984 Alzheimer's disease: initial report of the purification and characterization of a novel cerebrovascular amyloid protein. Biochem Biophys Res Commun 120:885–890

Golabek AA, Marques M, Lalowski M, Wisniewski T 1995 Amyloid β binding protein, *in vitro* and in normal human cerebrospinal fluid. Neurosci Lett 191:79–82

Levy E, Carman MD, Fernandez-Madrid IJ et al 1990 Mutation of the Alzheimer's disease amyloid gene in hereditary cerebral hemorrhage, Dutch type. Science 248:1124–1126

Levy-Lahad E, Wasco W, Poorkaj P et al 1995 Candidate gene for the chromosome 1 familial Alzheimer's disease locus. Science 269:973–977

Liang JS, Sipe JD 1995 Recombinant human serum amyloid A (apoSAAp) binds cholesterol and modulates cholesterol flux. J Lipid Res 36:37–46

Ma J, Yee A, Brewer HB Jr, Das S, Potter H 1994 Amyloid-associated proteins α_1-antichymotrypsin and apolipoprotein E promote assembly of Alzheimer β-protein into filaments. Nature 372:92–94

Mahley RW 1988 Apolipoprotein E: cholesterol transport protein with expanding role in cell biology. Science 240:622–629

Masters CL, Simms G, Weinman NA, Multhaup G, McDonald BL, Beyreuther K 1985 Amyloid plaque core protein in Alzheimer disease and Down syndrome. Proc Natl Acad Sci USA 82:4245–4249

Naiki H, Higuchi K, Shimada A, Takeda T, Nakakuki K 1993 Genetic analysis of murine senile amyloidosis. Lab Invest 68:332–337

Namba Y, Tomonaga M, Kawasaki H, Otomo E, Ikeda K 1991 Apolipoprotein E immunoreactivity in cerebral amyloid deposits and neurofibrillary tangles in Alzheimer's disease and kuru plaque amyloid in Creutzfeldt–Jakob disease. Brain Res 541:163–166

Näslund J, Thyberg J, Tjernberg LO et al 1995 Characterization of stable complexes involving apolipoprotein E and the amyloid β peptide in Alzheimer's disease brain. Neuron 15:219–228

Nathan BP, Bellosta S, Sanan DA, Weisgraber KH, Mahley RW, Pitas RE 1994 Differential effects of apolipoproteins E3 and E4 on neuronal growth *in vitro*. Science 264:850–852

Nichols WC, Dwulet FE, Liepnieks JJ, Benson MD 1988 Variant apolipoprotein A-I as a major constituent of a human hereditary amyloid. Biochem Biophys Res Commun 156:762–768

Peterson RB, Tressor NJ, Richardson SL, Gali M, Goren H, Gambetti P 1995 A family with oculomeningeal amyloidosis and dementia has a mutation in the transthyretin gene. J Neuropathol Exp Neurol 54:413(abstr)

Poirier J 1994 Apolipoprotein E in animal models of CNS injury and in Alzheimer's disease. Trends Neurosci 17:525–530

Prelli F, Pras M, Shtrasburg S, Frangione B 1991 Characterization of high molecular weight amyloid A proteins. Scand J Immunol 33:783–786

Rebeck GW, Reiter JS, Strickland DK, Human BT 1993 Apolipoprotein E in sporadic Alzheimer's disease: allelic variations and receptor interactions. Neuron 11:575–580

Rogaev E, Sherrington R, Rogaeva EA et al 1995 Familial Alzheimer's disease in kindreds with missense mutations in a gene on chromosome 1 related to the Alzheimer's disease type 3 gene. Nature 376:775–778

Sanan DA, Weisgraber KH, Russell SJ et al 1994 Apolipoprotein E associates with β amyloid peptide of Alzheimer's disease to form novel monofibrils. Isoform apoE4 associates more efficiently than apoE3. J Clin Invest 94:860–869

Saraiva MJM 1995 Transthyretin mutations in health and disease. Hum Mutat 5:191–196

Schmechel DE, Saunders AM, Strittmatter WJ et al 1993 Increased amyloid β-peptide deposition in cerebral cortex as a consequence of apolipoprotein E genotype in late-onset Alzheimer's disease. Proc Natl Acad Sci USA 90:9649–9653

Segrest JP, Jones MK, DeLoof H, Brouillette CG, Venkatachalapathi YV, Anantharamaiah GM 1992 The amphipathic helix in the exchangeable apolipoproteins: a review of secondary structure and function. J Lipid Res 33:141–166

Sherrington R, Rogaev EI, Liang Y et al 1995 Cloning of a gene bearing missense mutations in early onset familial Alzheimer's disease. Nature 375:754–760

Snow AD, Willmer J, Kisilevsky R 1987 Sulfated glycosaminoglycans: a common constituent of all amyloids? Lab Invest 56:120–123

Strittmatter WJ, Saunders AM, Schmechel D et al 1993 Apolipoprotein E: high-avidity binding to β-amyloid and increased frequency of type 4 allele in late-onset familial Alzheimer disease. Proc Natl Acad Sci USA 90:1977–1981

Uéda K, Fukushima H, Masliah E et al 1993 Molecular cloning of cDNA encoding an unrecognized component of amyloid in Alzheimer disease. Proc Natl Acad Sci USA 90:1282–1286

Vidal R, Garzuly F, Budka H et al 1996 Meningocerebrovascular amyloidosis associated with a novel transthyretin missense mutation at codon 18 (TTRD18G). Am J Pathol 148:361–366

Wilson C, Wardell MR, Weisgraber KH, Mahley RW, Agard DA 1991 Three-dimensional structure of the LDL receptor-binding domain of human apolipoprotein E. Science 252:1817–1822

Wisniewski T, Frangione B 1992 Apolipoprotein E: a pathological chaperone protein in patients with cerebral and systemic amyloid. Neurosci Lett 135:235–238

Wisniewski T, Castaño EM, Golabek A, Vogel T, Frangione B 1994 Acceleration of Alzheimer's fibril formation by apolipoprotein E *in vitro*. Am J Pathol 145:1030–1035

Wisniewski T, Lalowski M, Golabek A, Vogel T, Frangione B 1995a Is Alzheimer's disease an apolipoprotein E amyloidosis? Lancet 345:956–958

Wisniewski T, Golabek AA, Kida E, Wisniewski KE, Frangione B 1995b Conformational mimicry in Alzheimer's disease: role of apolipoproteins in amyloidogenesis. Am J Pathol 147:238–244

Wisniewski T, Pahla JA, Ghiso J, Frangione B 1995c S182 protein in Alzheimer's disease neuritic plaques. Lancet 346:1366
Zlokovic BV, Martel CL, Mackic JB et al 1994 Brain uptake of circulating apolipoproteins J and E complexed to Alzheimer's amyloid β. Biochem Biophys Res Commun 205:1431–1437

DISCUSSION

Pepys: It may not be possible to generalize the concept of conformational mimicry that you introduced whereby an amyloidogenic protein alters the conformation of another protein. In some of the hereditary systemic amyloidoses it is quite clear from detailed protein sequence and mass spectrometry studies that the only protein in the amyloid fibrils is the variant protein, even in cases where people have 50% wild-type protein.

Frangione: I would advise you to look again. We had a similar experience with our studies of apoE: we couldn't see it because we weren't looking for it. When you can't detect a protein it means one of three things: either it is not there, it degraded or your method is not sensitive enough. In general, the wild-type proteins are present in the amyloid alongside the variants. This is known in the Dutch variant of Alzheimer's disease (Prelli et al 1990) and in familial amyloidotic polyneuropathy (FAP), Finnish type related to gelsolin (Frangione et al 1991).

Pepys: Of course, one's failure to find the wild-type protein may be because of insufficient sensitivity of the methods. However, with the methods we've used, protein sequencing and electrospray mass spectrometry, we can't detect it in the fibrils from systemic amyloidoses.

Prusiner: What do you think triggers the conformational change that you're hypothesizing? Do you think that conformational change is occurring in the peptide or is it occurring in the whole protein which then gives rise to the peptide?

Frangione: In the case of Aβ, it is most likely that the conformational change is occurring in the peptide.

Prusiner: You can really separate this?

Frangione: We can separate at least two conformers by centrifugation (Soto et al 1995). One is called a non-amyloidogenic conformer (nac) and the other one is called an amyloidogenic conformer (ac). We can convert one into the other by changing the conditions, such as pH and temperature.

Prusiner: It could be that circular dichroism is not sensitive enough and you need to do nuclear magnetic resonance studies in order to understand fully the conformations.

Frangione: Yes.

Kirschner: Is there any correlation between apoJ and E isoform levels and animal strains or species that are resistant to amyloid formation?

Frangione: I don't have any data on this. Both are acute reactant proteins in the human brain, especially apoE. ApoJ and Aβ when complexed pass through the blood–brain barrier whereas apoE complexed to Aβ passes much less readily. These findings suggest that apoE is synthesized in the brain.

Masters: However, it could also go the other way—when Aβ is complexed to apoJ or E it may be going out of the brain. I would suggest that the pathological lesions are more consistent with it being caught going out rather than coming in.

Frangione: We did the following experiment: we infused the complex into the carotid artery in guinea-pig, and we infused Aβ intraventricularly in rats. This showed that Aβ is able to cross the blood–brain barrier from both directions (Zlokovic et al 1994, Strazielle et al 1995).

Goldgaber: You mentioned some interesting Hungarian cases of FAP with dementia and TTR amyloid depositions in brain parenchyma. Could you elaborate on this?

Frangione: This Hungarian family contains 56 members, spanning four generations. Affected members develop a vascular dementia, hearing loss, cerebellar dysfunction and bilateral pyramidal dysfunction with an onset from age 36 to 53. Death occurs between ages 51 and 60. There is extensive amyloid deposition in the subpial and subependymal regions as well as in the leptomeningeal vessels. This autosomal dominant condition is associated with a novel TTR D18G missense mutation (Vidal et al 1996). Another family has also been presented (Peterson et al 1995) with a different TTR mutation which is also associated with leptomeningeal amyloid and a dementia. This family also has extensive periventricular TTR-related amyloid deposition.

Goldgaber: Does it look like plaques?

Frangione: It is not like a typical AD neuritic plaque or prion plaque. There is diffuse infiltration in the periventricular parenchyma.

Benson: In our first publication on a Swedish Met30 TTR family, there are pictures of the amyloid in the parenchymal blood vessels of the brain. It wasn't possible to say whether they were in connection with blood vessels or not. These patients had no evidence of any dementia, but they did have fairly extensive TTR amyloid in the meninges and in the parenchymal blood vessels.

Goldgaber: There was also a paper from Japan several years ago which described deposition of TTR amyloid along the blood vessels in the brain, but I don't think there was pronounced dementia in those patients (Ushiyama et al 1991).

Frangione: Some accumulation in vessel walls has been reported before, although not associated with dementia. However, these two families reported in the last year are related to TTR with dementia and cerebrovascular amyloid.

J. D. Buxbaum: Do the different isoforms of apoJ differ in their amyloidogenicity?

Frangione: I don't know. ApoJ2 and apoJ3 are very rare isoforms and little is known about them.

J. D. Buxbaum: You showed that a 10 kDa C-terminal fragment of apoE generated by thrombin digestion can form fibrils. It has been suggested by several people that it is only the *de-lipidated* form of apoE that can make fibrils. Was the apoE you used in the thrombin experiment lipidated or non-lipidated?

Frangione: For our studies on the effect of apoE on Aβ fibrillogenesis, we used both lipidated and de-lipidated apoE. However, the fibril formation with the C-terminus of apoE was done with de-lipidated material (Wisniewski et al 1995a). Our unpublished work suggests a 1 : 1 stoichemistry between Aβ and apoE. We have also studied the stoichemistry of apoJ and Aβ. The latter is 1 : 1 (Matsubara et al 1995).

Prusiner: Has anyone produced transgenic mice that overexpress APP, making something that looks like a plaque in an apoE knockout mouse?

Frangione: A transgenic mouse model was published by the Athena Neuroscience group. It overexpresses APP V717F. These mice do develop amyloid plaques and I understand that these plaques are positive for apoE (Games et al 1995). They are now performing the same studies in apoE knockout mice.

Prusiner: When we inoculated apoE knockout mice with prions, we found that the incubation time was the same as in the untargeted controls (Tatzelt et al 1996). Our conclusion was that apoE doesn't play any role in prion formation. It is relatively simple to cross these mice, and the parallel experiment with APP would be very interesting.

Goldgaber: People are now doing that. Crossing of the transgenic mice expressing Aβ with apoE knockout mice is underway.

Frangione: ApoE doesn't only have a role in Aβ amyloid: we have seen the same fragment (a 10 kDa apoE C-terminus) in other types of amyloid such as light chain amyloid and amyloid A (Castaño et al 1995).

Kisilevsky: A comment on the apoE story. Mark Kindy and Fred de Beer have looked at AA amyloid formation in apoE knockout mice and they still get amyloid, but the rate at which it is deposited is significantly slower than in the presence of apoE. So it looks here as if, again, apoE is not necessary to initiate the process, but rather has something to do with its rate of progression.

Prusiner: How is the amyloid generated in that mouse?

Kisilevsky: Usually with an inflammatory stimulus and what we call 'amyloid enhancing factor'.

Merlini: You propose the hypothesis that the mutant APPs may serve as templates for the wild-type to trigger amyloid deposition. In what proportions are the mutant and wild-type precursors deposited *in vivo*?

Frangione: 60:40. In the patient you frequently have more of the mutated one, but I think this has something to do with the method we use to detect it. If you change the method, the numbers may change.

Merlini: Would you also expect this hypothesis to hold true in prion diseases?

Frangione: It is possible.

Masters: A note of warning on the significance of apoE as a risk factor: most of the studies reported to date are terribly biased in the populations they have sampled. New data are now coming out on population-based surveys of risk of dementia in the general community. My understanding is that if you look in an open population the risk factor is only about twofold.

Frangione: That is a very controversial point. However, the linkage studies from different populations indicate that it is true even if the risk has been exaggerated. Current evidence suggests that late-onset Alzheimer's is linked to apoE ε4.

Masters: Yes, apoE ε4 is involved, but it is probably not a major determinant.

Pepys: We've recently reported that there's no correlation between apoE isotypes and either the incidence or the age at the time of onset of AA amyloid or FAP. It doesn't seem that the apoE genotypes are a significant risk factor for those two types of amyloid (Lovat et al 1995).

Frangione: ApoE is linked to Alzheimer's disease, but not to Down's syndrome or FAP.

Pepys: I would like to suggest, perhaps as a sort of marker for the future, that the role of apoE in Alzheimer's disease is more likely to turn out to be related to the role of apoE in trophic functions, nerve cell regeneration, nerve cell survival under stress and so on, rather than being a key factor in amyloidogenesis. My suspicion is that it probably isn't a major factor in amyloidogenesis: because apoE is so abundant in the brain it is more likely to be related to how well cerebral neurons survive and re-grow under conditions of stress.

Frangione: You have to remember that in every amyloid deposit, there is more than one apolipoprotein. We are talking about apoE because it is fashionable. But the relationship between apolipoproteins and amyloidogenesis is very old. We know already of four apolipoproteins (serum amyloid A, apoAI, apoAII and apoE) that can form amyloid (Wisniewski et al 1995b). The main question concerns how they interact with each other and how they interact with other amyloidogenic proteins that are not lipoproteins.

References

Castaño EM, Prelli F, Pras M, Frangione B 1995 Apolipoprotein carboxyl terminal fragments are complexed to amyloids A and L. Implications for amyloidogenesis and Alzheimer's disease. J Biol Chem 270:17610–17615

Frangione B, Haltia M, Levy E, Ghiso J, Kiuru S, Prelli F 1991 Co-occurrence of two amyloid proteins in a patient with familial amyloidosis, Finnish type. In: Iqbal K, McLachlan DRC, Winblad B, Wisniewski HM (eds) Alzheimer's disease: basic mechanisms, diagnosis and therapeutic strategies. Wiley, Chichester p 255–264

Games D, Adams D, Alessandrini R et al 1995 Alzheimer-type neuropathology in transgenic mice overexpressing V717F β-amyloid precursor protein. Nature 373:523–527

Lovat LB, Booth SE, Booth DR et al 1995 Apolipoprotein E4 genotype is not a risk factor for systemic AA amyloidosis or familial amyloid polyneuropathy. Amyloid: Int J Exp Clin Invest 2:163–166

Matsubara E, Frangione B, Ghiso J 1995 Characterization of apolipoprotein J–Aβ interaction. J Biol Chem 270:7563–7567

Peterson RB, Tressor NJ, Richardson SL, Gali M, Goren H, Gambetti P 1995 A family with oculomeningeal amyloidosis and dementia has a mutation in the transthyretin gene. J Neuropathol Exp Neurol 54:413(abstr)

Prelli F, Levy E, Vanduinen SG, Bots GTAM, Luyendijk W, Frangione B 1990 Expression of normal and variant Alzheimer's β-protein gene in amyloid of hereditary cerebral hemorrhage, Dutch type: DNA and protein diagnostic assays. Biochem Biophys Res Commun 170:301–307

Soto C, Frangione B 1995 2 conformational states of amyloid β-peptide: implications for the pathogenesis of Alzheimer's disease. Neurosci Lett 186:115–118

Strazielle N, Ghersi-Egea J-F, Ghiso J et al 1995 Clearance of amyloid beta peptide from cerebrospinal fluid and brain. Soc Neurosci Abstr 2:1678

Tatzelt J, Maeda N, Pekny M et al 1996 Scrapie in mice deficient for apolipoprotein E or glial fibrillary acidic protein. Neurology, in press

Ushiyama M, Ikeda S, Yanagisawa N 1991 Transthyretin-type cerebral amyloid angiopathy in type I familial amyloid polyneuropathy. Acta Neuropathol 81:524–528

Vidal R, Garzuly F, Budka H et al 1996 Meningocerebrovascular amyloidosis associated with a novel transthyretin missense mutation at codon 18 (TTRD18G). Am J Pathol 148:361–366

Wisniewski T, Lalowski M, Golabeck A, Vogel T, Frangione B 1995a Is Alzheimer's disease an apolipoprotein E amyloidosis? Lancet 345:956–958

Wisniewski T, Golabeck AA, Kida E, Wisniewski KE, Frangione B 1995b Conformational mimicry in Alzheimer's disease: role of apolipoproteins in amyloidogensis. Am J Pathol 147:238–244

Zlokovic BV, Martel CL, Mackic JB et al 1994 Brain uptake of circulating apolipoproteins J and E complexed to Alzheimer's amyloid β. Biochem Biophys Res Commun 205:1431–1437

Interaction of transthyretin with amyloid β-protein: binding and inhibition of amyloid formation

Alexander L. Schwarzman and Dmitry Goldgaber

Department of Psychiatry, School of Medicine, State University of New York at Stony Brook, Stony Brook, NY 11794–8101, USA

Abstract. Aggregated amyloid β-protein (Aβ) is a key component of the amyloid depositions found in the brains of patients with Alzheimer's disease. In contrast, in cerebrospinal fluid (CSF), Aβ is found in a soluble form. The analysis of complexes of Aβ with CSF proteins in a KBr gradient revealed an association of Aβ only with free proteins and not with lipoprotein particles. Transthyretin (TTR), a second major CSF protein, formed SDS-stable complexes with Aβ and significantly decreased the rate of Aβ fibril formation. In physiological buffers and CSF, TTR exclusively decreased the level of Aβ pentamers. Endogenous TTR–Aβ complexes were detected in human CSF by immunoprecipitation. Using site-directed mutagenesis and computer-assisted modelling, we identified amino acid residues on the surface of the TTR monomer that interact with Aβ. Specific TTR immunoreactivity was detected in multiple cortical neurons and astrocytes in the human brain. We propose that Aβ binding proteins play a key role in the modulation of Aβ aggregation and normally prevent amyloid formation in biological fluids and in the brain.

1996 The nature and origin of amyloid fibrils. Wiley, Chichester (Ciba Foundation Symposium 199) p 146–164

In recent years, several hypotheses based on overproduction and self-aggregation of amyloid β-protein (Aβ) in the brains of Alzheimer's disease (AD) patients have been presented (Goldgaber et al 1987, Selkoe 1994). However, the finding that Aβ is continuously produced and secreted by cells under normal metabolic conditions and is present in a soluble form in biological fluids (Seubert et al 1992, Shoji et al 1992) suggested that new approaches for understanding of Aβ amyloidosis are required.

Our sequestration hypothesis suggests that normally produced Aβ is sequestered by certain extracellular proteins, thereby preventing amyloid formation and Aβ cytotoxicity. We propose that amyloid formation occurs when sequestration fails. Several conditions could potentially lead to such failure. These include Aβ overproduction, a decreased level of sequestering proteins, impairment or inability of sequestering proteins to interact with Aβ, defective clearance mechanisms, or a combination of the above (Goldgaber et al 1993).

Published experimental data support the sequestration hypothesis. Wisniewski et al (1993a) reported that cerebrospinal fluid (CSF) prevents amyloid formation *in vitro*. Several CSF proteins were found to bind Aβ and inhibit or facilitate Aβ aggregation. These include apolipoprotein E (apoE) (Strittmatter et al 1993, Wisniewski et al 1993b, 1994, Evans et al 1995), transthyretin (TTR) (Schwarzman et al 1994) and apoJ (Ghiso et al 1993). ApoE efficiently blocked Aβ cytotoxicity in cell culture experiments (Whitson et al 1994), while TTR prevented Aβ accumulation in cell cultures (Mazur-Kolecka et al 1995) and in transgenic *Caenorhabditis elegans* (Link 1995)

This chapter focuses on the possible role of TTR in Aβ amyloidosis. TTR is a 54980 Da protein composed of four identical subunits that is found in CSF and plasma (Benson & Wallace 1989, Jacobson & Buxbaum 1991). Plasma TTR is synthesized in liver hepatocytes and secreted into the plasma, where it plays a key role in the transport of retinol and thyroxine. TTR in CSF is synthesized in the choroid plexus and is the main transporter of retinol and thyroxine into the brain (Herbert et al 1986, Benson & Wallace 1989).

Almost 50 TTR variants have been documented (Jacobson & Buxbaum 1991, Saraiva 1995). Most of them were found in patients with familial amyloidotic polyneuropathy (FAP), an autosomal dominant inherited disease resulting from peripheral and cerebral TTR amyloid depositions. Several amyloidotic TTR variants were also found in patients with senile cardiac amyloidosis, familial carpal tunnel syndrome and amyloidotic vitreous opacities. Six TTR variants were not associated with amyloidoses, namely, Ser6, Asn90, Arg102, Thr109, Tyr116 and Met119 (Saraiva 1995). Some TTR variants reveal an increased affinity to thyroxine which could potentially lead to abnormalities in thyroid metabolism (Fitch et al 1991, Scrimshaw et al 1992, Murrel et al 1992).

It has been reported that the level of TTR in CSF is decreased in both AD and Down's syndrome (DS) (Elovaara et al 1986, Riisoen 1988). Consequently, we have examined experimentally the molecular nature of the interaction of TTR with Aβ. The results suggest a mechanism of inhibition of Aβ amyloid formation by TTR.

Methods

Density gradient centrifugation

We incubated 2 ml of human CSF from non-AD patients with radioiodinated Aβ1–28 (10^7 cpm) in 1 × PBS for 24 h at 37 °C. KBr was added to a density of

1.25 g/ml in a final volume of 4 ml. The samples were centrifuged at 110 000 **g** for 36 h at 12 °C in a SW-60 Ti rotor (Beckman, L5–65). We collected 0.25 ml fractions of the KBr gradient, measured their refractive indices, and dialysed them overnight against 150 mM NaCl/10 mM Na phosphate buffer, pH 7.4. The distribution of radioactivity was assayed by PAGE under non-denaturing conditions. The 4–20% gradient gels were dried and exposed to an X-ray film or were Western blotted to a 0.2 μm PVDF membrane (Bio-Rad) and probed with anti-apoE antibodies (Calbiochem).

Aβ radioassay

Aβ1–28 or 1–40 was labelled with [^{125}I]Bolton-Hunter reagent (Amersham) according to manufacturer's instructions. For the binding assay, we incubated 10 μl of human CSF with 10^5 dpm [^{125}I]Aβ1–28 or [^{125}I] Aβ1–40 (specific activity $3–6 \times 10^6$ dpm/mg) in a final volume of 20 μl PBS at 37 °C. Samples were analysed by SDS-PAGE. 12% Tris-Glycine gels were used for analysis of complexes of Aβ and CSF proteins, and 15% Tris-Tricine gels were used for analysis of Aβ oligomers. In order to detect TTR dimers, we did not boil the samples before electrophoresis. After electrophoresis, the gels were dried and exposed to X-Omat R film (Kodak).

Immunoprecipitation of the TTR–Aβ complexes

The 3.5 ml samples of human CSF were mixed with equal volumes of 2 × PBS, pH 7.4, containing 1% Triton X-100, 2 mM EDTA, 1 μg/ml leupeptin, 1 mM phenylmethanesulfonyl fluoride, 0.1 μg/ml pepstatin, 1 μg/ml tosyl-lysylchloromethan, 80 μl of rabbit anti-Aβ antibodies (SY2134; generously provided by Dr. S. Younkin), and 3.5 ml of 25% PEG 6000. After incubation at 20 °C for 16 h, samples were centrifuged at 2000 **g** for 20 min. Precipitated proteins were washed three times with PBS containing 0.5% Triton X-100 and 8% PEG 6000. SDS was added to 2% final concentration and the samples were boiled for 20 min before electrophoresis. Electrophoretic analysis was performed in 15% Tris/Tricine/SDS polyacrilamide gels. To identify TTR immunoreactivity, we used sheep anti-TTR antibodies (ICN) and the ECL Western blotting kit (Amersham).

Construction of recombinant TTR

Full-length human TTR cDNA cloned in pUC18 was obtained from ATCC. In order to remove the leader sequence by PCR, we designed two primers. The 'forward' primer contained 5′-clamp (cg), *BamH*1 cloning site and 5′-sequence corresponding to mature TTR (5′-cgggatccGGCCCTACGGGCACCGGT-GAATCCA). The 'reverse' primer incorporated 5′-clamp (gg), *Xho*1 cloning site and 3′-sequence of TTR cDNA starting from the stop codon (5′-ggcctcgagTCATTCCTTGGGATTGGTGACGACAG). The amplified PCR fragment was isolated from a low-melting 1% agarose gel (NuSieve GTG agarose, FMC) according to manufacturer's instructions. In order to direct the recombinant protein into periplasm and to secrete the protein into the media, we cloned the modified leaderless TTR cDNA into pET-22b(+) plasmid vector (Novogen) containing the N-terminal bacterial *pelB* leader. The PCR product with flanking restriction sites and the vector DNA were digested with *BamH*1 and *Xho*1 restriction endonucleases. The digested vector and the PCR product were ligated and the ligation product was transformed into competent cells (*Escherichia coli* XL1-Blue). Ampicillin-resistant colonies were screened for the presence of the vector with the TTR insert by 1% agarose gel electrophoresis. To avoid PCR-derived errors, we sequenced the cloned TTR cDNA. A DNA fragment of 33 bp between the end of the *pelB* leader and the first codon of mature TTR was then deleted using site-directed mutagenesis (Kunkel 1985). The same method of site-directed mutagenesis was used to generate TTR mutants with deletions and substitutions. Plasmids, carrying cDNA of 35 TTR mutants were expressed in the *E. coli* strain BL21 (DE3). After 3 h induction by 1 mM IPTG, the recombinant TTR was detected in the media by electrophoresis and Western blotting.

Purification of recombinant TTR

Cells were grown at 37 °C in 50 ml of LB broth until they reached an optical density of 0.7–0.8 OD_{600}. Induction of TTR synthesis was performed by 1 mM IPTG with gentle shaking. After 3 h induction, the cultures were centrifuged at 5000 ***g*** and pelleted cells were discarded. After a second centrifugation, the supernatants containing secreted TTR were subjected to ion-exchange chromatography on 2 ml column with DEAE-Sephacel (Pharmacia) which was equilibrated with 20 mM Tris-HCl (pH 7.2) and 10 mM NaCl. The peak of recombinant TTR was eluted at 0.3 M NaCl and concentrated in PBS using Centricon 30 concentrators (Amicon). Purified proteins were analysed by PAGE and Western blot analysis with anti-TTR antibody and ECL kit (Amersham), and by staining with Coomassie Briliant Blue R-250 (Sigma). Sequencing of recombinant TTR which was immobilized on PVDF membranes (Bio-Rad) was performed by automated Edman degradation with an Applied Biosystem 477A sequencer.

Electron microscopy

Samples of 100 μM Aβ1–40 were incubated with 15 μM TTR for 24 h at 37 °C, applied to carbon-coated copper grids, negatively stained with 2% uranyl acetate, and visualized in the JEOL 200cx transmission electron microscope operating at 80 kV. Samples were examined and photographed at a magnification of ×60 000.

Congo red-based spectrophotometric assay of Aβ aggregation

We incubated 20 μl samples of synthetic 100 μM Aβ plus 200 μg/ml recombinant TTR at 37 °C in microplate wells (Corning-Costar). After incubation, 150 μl of PBS and 2 μl of 5 μM Congo red were added to each sample and incubation continued in the dark at room temperature for 10 min. The microplates were then spun at 3000 rpm for 40 min. The supernatants were discarded, and the absorbance of red pellets was measured in a microplate reader at 490 nm. We determined percentage absorbance by comparing the average of duplicate samples to Congo red blanks.

Immunocytochemical detection of TTR in the human brain

We immunostained 40 μm Vibratom brain sections using rabbit anti-TTR antibody (Boehringer Mannheim) at 1:1600 dilution and horseradish-conjugated anti-human secondary antibody. Diaminobenzidine was used as a chromogenic substrate. A postmortem brain was obtained from a non-demented 100 year-old woman. Immunostaining was performed by Dr. D. Schmechel from Duke University.

Results

Aβ has been shown to form specific complexes with free apoE and apoJ *in vitro* (Strittmatter et al 1993, Wisniewski et al 1993b, Ghiso et al 1993). However, more than 90% of apolipoprotein is associated with lipoprotein particles (Roheim et al 1979). We therefore initially tested whether Aβ would associate with lipoprotein particles in CSF. We subjected CSF samples that were incubated with radioiodinated Aβ to ultracentrifugation in a KBr density gradient that is widely used to float and separate lipoprotein particles. Fractions of the gradient were analysed by PAGE, autoradiography and Western blot analysis with the anti-apoE antibody (Fig. 1a). Fractions from the lower half of the gradient consisting primarily of lipid-free proteins contained complexes of CSF proteins with [^{125}I]Aβ1–28. A peak of [^{125}I]Aβ1–28 complexes was found at a density of 1.27 g/ml. Unbound [^{125}I]Aβ1–28 was detected throughout the gradient with a major peak at the density 1.30 g/ml (Fig. 1a). No Aβ complexes were found at the top of the gradient where lipoprotein particles floated. Western blot analysis revealed that, as expected, most of the apoE immunoreactivity was colocalized with lipoprotein particles at the top of gradient, d = 1.09–1.10 g/ml (Fig. 1b). A small amount of apoE immunoreactivity was found in a lipoprotein-free area of the gradient and appeared as bands at 34 and 68 kDa, which correspond to apoE monomers and dimers. However, apoE-containing fractions lacked detectable complexes of apoE with [^{125}I]Aβ1–28. Similar results were obtained for [^{125}I]Aβ1–40 (data not shown). Although we did not detect complexes of [^{125}I]Aβ with apoE in CSF, apoE3 or E4 purified from human plasma did bind [^{125}I]Aβ1–28 and [^{125}I]Aβ1–40 in PBS. Complexes with an apparent molecular weight of 37 kDa were detected after incubation of [^{125}I]Aβ1–28 with purified apoE3 and E4 (Fig. 1c, lanes 3 and 4). The migration of these complexes is clearly distinct from 30 kDa and 50 kDa Aβ complexes that were formed by the TTR dimer and albumin under non-denaturing conditions (see Schwarzman et al 1994 and Fig. 1c, lanes 1 and 2). A minor band of 80 kDa probably represents complexes of Aβ with apoJ (Fig. 1c, lane 1).

To determine whether TTR forms complexes with Aβ in CSF *in vivo*, we immunoprecipitated samples of CSF obtained from non-AD patients with the rabbit anti-Aβ antibody SY2134. The immunoprecipitates were subjected to PAGE and Western blot analysis with sheep anti-TTR antibodies. As shown in Fig. 1d, TTR co-precipitated with Aβ. The electrophoretic mobility of the retrieved TTR corresponds to that of the TTR–Aβ complex.

To understand the interaction of Aβ and TTR, we built a computer-assisted model of TTR–Aβ complexes (Schwarzman et al 1994). The model predicts a putative Aβ binding domain on the surface of each TTR monomer and identifies four key amino acid residues—Asp38, Glu42, Glu62 and Glu66. To test this model, we utilized a highly efficient expression system for the production of recombinant mature TTR secreted into the media. The secretion of TTR is mediated by a bacterial *pelB* leader sequence in the pET-22b(+) plasmid. The main advantage of this system is a very high concentration of secreted recombinant TTR in cell culture media. While the total yield of the unpurified protein in the conditioned media reached 10–50 mg/l, the level of secreted TTR reached 70–80% of the total protein (Fig. 2). Purified TTR was analysed by N-terminal sequencing. The first 10 amino acids of the recombinant TTR showed a complete match with the amino acid sequence of mature TTR.

Using this expression system, we produced 25 recombinant TTR mutants and tested their ability to bind Aβ. We either deleted or substituted several negatively charged amino acid residues of TTR for uncharged or positively charged ones. TTR mutants with different combinations of these substitutions and deletions were also produced. (Table 1). Analysis of these recombinant TTRs shows that mutants with alterations in amino acids 38 and 42 either partially or completely failed to bind Aβ and inhibit Aβ aggregation. Alterations of amino acid residues E62 and E66 had no effect on binding, and therefore these amino acids cannot be considered as contact sites. Multiple deletions in the region containing residues 46–51 resulted in rapid degradation of TTR. Thus, the protrusion on the surface of the TTR monomer which is formed by amino acid residues 38–42 is the key structure of the Aβ binding domain.

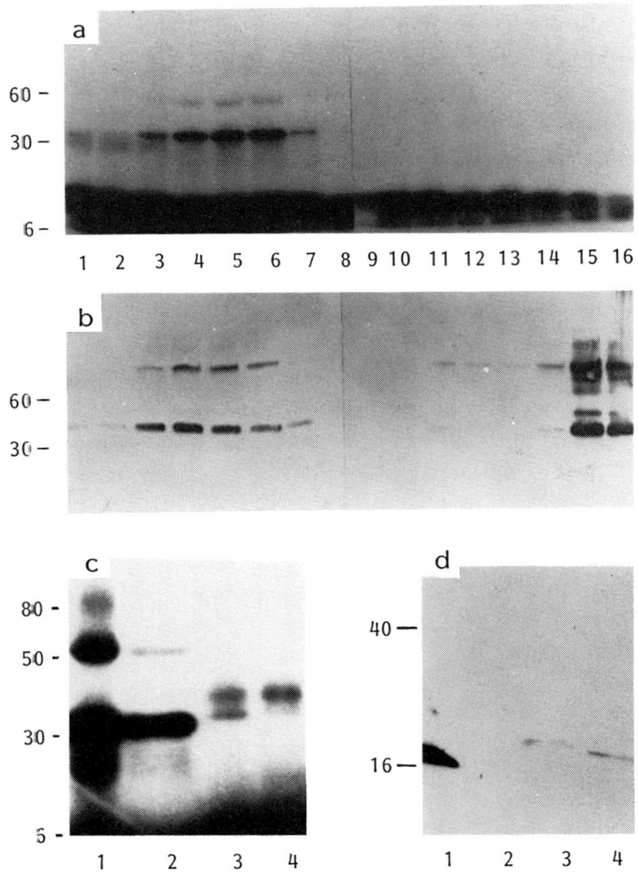

FIG. 1. Analysis of complexes of Aβ with CSF proteins. (a) Distribution of [^{125}I]Aβ1–28 after incubation for 24 h in CSF in KBr gradient. Gradient fractions were analysed by non-denaturing gradient PAGE (4–20%). (b) Distribution of apoE immunoreactivity in the same KBr gradient. (c) Analysis of [^{125}I]Aβ1–28 complexes with CSF proteins in 12% SDS-PAGE (Tris-Glycine). [^{125}I]Aβ1–28 (0.25 nM) was incubated for 24 h with: lane 1, CSF; lane 2, lipoprotein free fraction of CSF; lane 3, apoE3; lane 4, apoE4. (d) Immunoprecipitation of TTR–Aβ complexes from human CSF. Electrophoretic analysis was done in 12% Tris-Glycine SDS-PAGE. Immunostaining was done using ECL kit for Western blotting and rabbit anti-TTR polyclonal antibody. Lane 1, recombinant TTR (50 ng); lane 2, immunoprecipitation of the purified recombinant TTR (700 ng) with anti-Aβ antibody SY2134; lanes 3 and 4, immunoprecipitation of TTR–Aβ complexes from two different CSF samples obtained from patients without AD.

The mechanism of inhibition of Aβ aggregation by TTR is unknown. To determine whether TTR inhibits fibril formation or disrupts already-formed fibrils, we analysed aggregation of Aβ1–40 by electron microscopy in the presence or absence of TTR. After 24 h of incubation of Aβ1–40 at 100 μM, we observed the fibrillar structures shown in Fig. 3A. The fibrils were long and twisted around each other. They were concentrated in clusters that probably represent fibrillar structures of a higher order. Short or single fibrils were not observed. The addition of TTR to Aβ after Aβ was incubated for 24 h did not change these fibrillar structures. However, the presence of 15 μM TTR during incubation resulted in drastic changes of fibril formation. Only very short single fibrils and centres of fibril growth were found.

Analysis of the electron microscopic pictures of the fibrils suggested that TTR significantly decreased the rate of fibril formation but did not disrupt preformed fibrillar structures.

According to the nucleation theory of amyloid formation, the rate limiting step in the formation of Aβ fibrils is the formation of nuclei which consist of an ordered array of Aβ molecules. These nuclei must consist of oligomeric species of Aβ and, according to the theory, represent thermodynamically stable complexes of Aβ multimers. While postnucleation aggregation of nuclei into fibrils is very fast, the nuclei reach the critical size during the slow 'lag-period' (Eaton & Hofrichter 1990, Jarrett & Lansbury 1993, Vitek et al 1994).

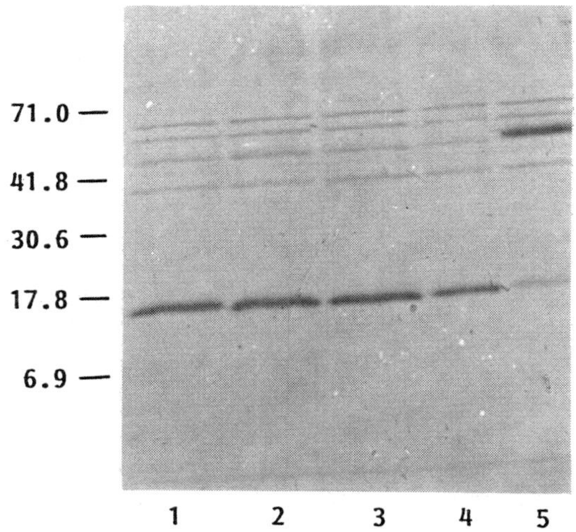

FIG. 2. Secreted recombinant TTR in conditioned media. Electrophoretic analysis of purified recombinant TTR using 12% non-denaturing PAGE. Lanes 1, 2, 3 and 4 represent wild type recombinant TTR from four different clones. Samples were boiled for 5 min in 2% SDS before electrophoresis. Lane 5, recombinant TTR. This sample was boiled in a sample buffer without SDS.

TABLE 1 Interaction of TTR mutants with Aβ

TTR	*Aggregation (binding)*	*TTR*	*Aggregation (binding)*
No TTR	100%	ΔE62ΔE66	ND (+)
TTR (wt)	17.7% (+)	H38Q62	24.8% (+)
ΔE38	48.2% (±)	R3839	71.9% (−)
ΔE42	87.5% (−)	H38Q42	82.2% (−)
ΔE62	24.8% (+)	N38Q42	75.8% (±)
ΔE66	29.6% (+)	N38N39	66.6% (±)
H38	41.4% (±)	Q62Q66	19.2% (+)
Q42	89.9% (−)	Q61Q62Q63Q66	41.5% (+)
Q62	21.1% (+)	N38Q42Q62Q66	ND (+)
Q66	27.2% (+)	N38Q42Q62Q66	ND (+)
ΔE38ΔE42	ND (−)	ΔS46ΔG47ΔK48	ND (−)
ΔE42ΔE62	ND (−)	ΔT49ΔS50ΔE51	ND (−)

Aβ1–40 aggregation was measured by Congo red binding assay (see 'Methods'). Concentration of TTR was 200 μg/ml. Data represent the mean of two independent duplicate experiments. Standard deviation did not exceed ±7%. Aβ1–40 binding to TTR was detected by non-denaturing 4–20% gradient PAGE (Bio-Rad). +, strong binding; ±, weak binding; −, no binding; ND, not determined.

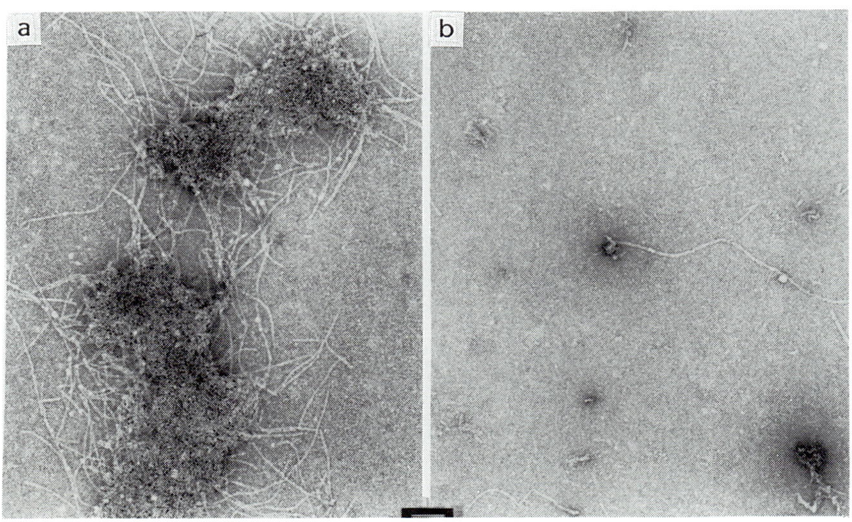

FIG. 3. Electron micrographs of Aβ1–40 fibrils formed in the presence of TTR. Aβ1–40 (100 μM) was incubated for 24 h at 37 °C in PBS (a) without or (b) with 15 μM TTR and analysed as described in 'Methods'.

In order to investigate the effect of TTR on Aβ nucleation, we analysed the kinetics of the formation of Aβ multimers in the presence of TTR. In these experiments, we used 5 nM of [^{125}I]Aβ1–42, which is the physiological concentration of Aβ in CSF. After 2 h incubation in PBS with or without TTR, the samples were analysed by PAGE followed by autoradiography. Aβ was detected as a mixture of monomers and oligomers (Fig. 4a, lanes 1 and 2). Aβ multimers of a maximum size appeared as a band with an apparent molecular mass of 18–22 kDa, which corresponds to the calculated size of the Aβ pentamer. Incubation of Aβ with TTR resulted in the selective inhibition of Aβ pentamer formation (Fig. 4a, lanes 3–7). In order to better resolve Aβ multimers, we used experimental conditions under which complexes of Aβ with TTR and apoE were detected at the top of gel. When radiolabelled Aβ was incubated in CSF instead of PBS, it did not form high molecular weight multimers. Prolonged incubation had no effect on the pattern of Aβ multimers and complexes of Aβ with CSF proteins (Fig. 4b, lanes 2–4). A major band with an apparent molecular weight of 18–21 kDa corresponding to Aβ pentamers was the maximum size of Aβ multimers. This pattern of Aβ distribution in CSF was drastically different from the pattern of Aβ incubated in PBS where Aβ formed a series of aggregates, the highest of which was found at the top of the gel (Fig. 4b, lane 1). When we increased the concentration of TTR in CSF samples by adding purified TTR, we observed an increased amount of TTR–Aβ complexes in parallel with the decreased amount of Aβ pentamers (Fig. 4b, lanes 5–9).

The identification of TTR as a protein that sequesters Aβ in human CSF suggested that TTR could play a similar role in the brain. Published reports describe TTR immunoreactivity primarily in the choroid plexus with some other cells scattered in different parts of the brain. We used polyclonal anti-TTR antibodies which were absorbed and not absorbed with TTR and verified the completeness of absorption by Western blot analysis. We found that TTR immunoreactivity was distributed along blood vessels and in multiple cortical neurons in the visual cortex (Fig. 5). Some neurons revealed a prominent intranuclear staining. It should be noted that many adjacent neurons were unstained. In the hippocampus, prominent staining of astrocytes (arrow) was detected near and around plaques. The heterogeneous pattern of TTR immunoreactivity suggests a complex regulation of TTR uptake into brain cells.

Discussion

The deposition of fibrillar Aβ amyloid in the brains of AD patients and aged individuals is surprising considering what we currently know about the aggregation of Aβ into amyloid (Selkoe 1994). Although the exact mechanism of amyloid formation is unknown, a number of studies have demonstrated that

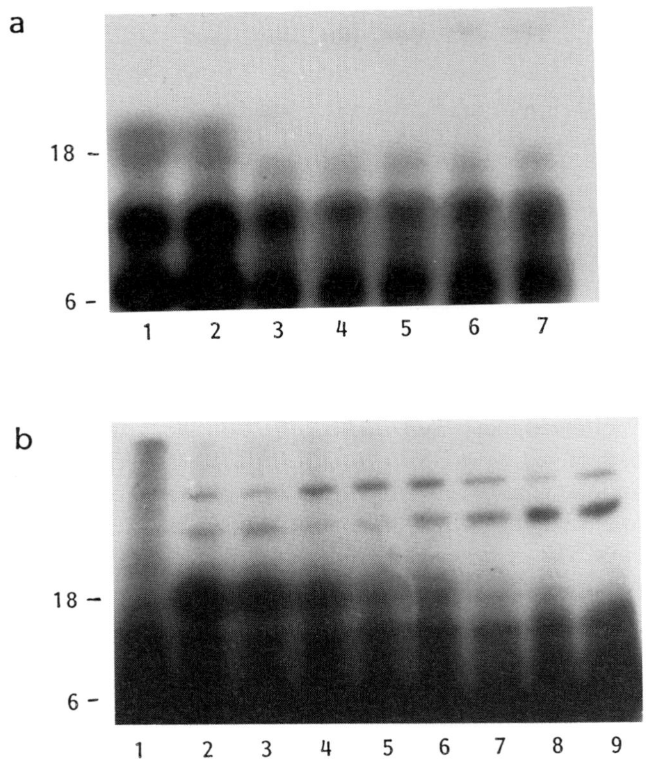

FIG. 4. Inhibition of Aβ1–42 multimer formation by TTR. Aβ multimers were analysed using 15% SDS-Tris-Tricine PAGE as described in 'Methods'. (a) Lane 1, [^{125}I]Aβ1–42 (5 nM) after 2 h incubation in PBS; lanes 2–7, [^{125}I]Aβ1–42 incubated with 15 μM TTR in CSF; lanes 2–7 correspond to 2, 6, 12, 24 and 36 h incubation. (b) [^{125}I]Aβ1–42 was added to CSF and incubated with various concentrations of TTR for 24 h at 37 °C. [^{125}I]Aβ multimers were analysed using 15% SDS-Tris Tricine PAGE and autoradiography as described in 'Methods'. In order to identify the position of TTR dimers, samples were not boiled in SDS before electrophoresis. Lane 1, [^{125}I]Aβ1–42 (5 nM) after incubation for 24 h in PBS; lanes 2–4, 5 nM of [^{125}I]Aβ1–42 after incubation for 24 h with three different CSF samples; lanes 5–9, 5 nM [^{125}I]Aβ1–41 after 24 h incubation with increasing quantities of added TTR (lane 5, 0.25 μg; 6, 0.5 μg; 7, 1 μg; 8, 2.0 μg; 9, 5.0 μg).

synthetic Aβ spontaneously aggregates in physiological buffers, forming β-amyloid fibrils similar to those found in the brains of AD patients (Selkoe 1994).

Several lines of evidence obtained *in vitro* and *in vivo* suggest that Aβ binding proteins inhibit the formation of Aβ amyloid. We previously demonstrated that TTR binds Aβ and inhibits Aβ fibril formation *in vitro* (Schwarzman et al 1994). Prevention of intracellular accumulation of Aβ by TTR was also observed in two model systems: cultured vascular smooth muscle cells (Mazur-Kolecka et al 1995) and transgenic *C. elegans* (Link 1995). Contradictory results regarding stimulation or inhibition of Aβ amyloid formation *in vitro* were reported for apoE (Schwarzman et al 1994, Evans et al 1995, Wisniewski et al 1994) and α_1-antichymotrypsin (Ma et al 1994, Frazer et al 1993). The

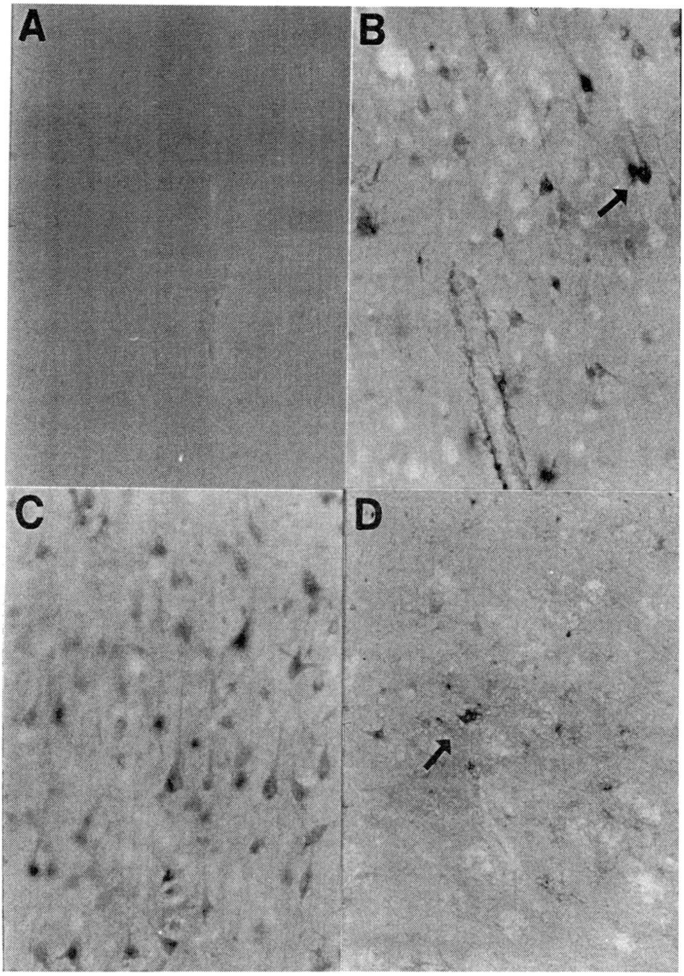

FIG. 5. TTR immunoreactivity in the visual cortex of a human brain. (A) Control section of visual cortex stained with TTR antibody absorbed with human TTR. (B) TTR immunoreactivity in visual cortex along blood vessels and in multiple cortical neurons (example is shown by arrow). (C) TTR immunoreactivity in a region a few millimetres from (B) showing a sector where nearly all neurons are stained with some prominent intranuclear staining. (D) TTR immunoreactivity in hippocampus showing prominent astrocytic staining (arrow) near and around plaques.

most compelling evidence that Aβ binding proteins are involved in AD amyloidosis is the strong association of the apoE ε4 allele with increased vascular and plaque Aβ deposits in the brains of late-onset AD patients (Schmechel et al 1993).

In this study we have found that TTR inhibits the formation of Aβ pentamers in physiological buffers and CSF. From the point of view of the nucleation theory of amyloid formation (Eaton & Hofrichter 1990, Jarrett & Lansbury 1993, Vitek et al 1994), this subclass of Aβ multimers most likely represents 'nucleus' or 'pre-nucleus' structures in the cascade of Aβ amyloid formation. The largest Aβ multimers detected at physiological conditions in cell culture media were pentamers (Podlisny et al 1995).

There are two ways to inhibit or delay formation of amyloid. The first is to decrease the critical concentration of Aβ monomers. The interaction of Aβ binding proteins with Aβ monomers at, or close to, a molar ratio of 1:1 of Aβ binding protein to Aβ would result in a sufficient decrease of Aβ monomer concentration. ApoJ, which binds Aβ with a K_d of 5 nM, represents a good example of such an interaction. ApoJ was found to inhibit amyloid formation at a ratio of 1:1 (J. Ghiso, personal communication). The second way is to inhibit amyloid fibril formation by direct interaction with Aβ nuclei, pre-nuclei or higher order Aβ structures. In this second case, the molar ratio of Aβ binding protein to Aβ will be significantly lower than 1:1. We previously described an example of such an interaction showing that a significant suppression of Aβ amyloid formation was detected at a molar ratio of 1:300 of TTR to Aβ and 1:3000 of apoE to Aβ (Schwarzman et al 1994).

Since TTR has been shown to inhibit Aβ aggregation *in vitro*, the biological implications for its interaction with Aβ should be investigated under physiological conditions. Our results indicate that TTR forms complexes with Aβ in human CSF. TTR immunoreactivity was found in the cytoplasm of the epithelial cells of the choroid plexus (Herbert et al 1986), in the leptomeningeal amyloid depositions and subependymal parenchyma of patients with cerebral amyloid angiopathy (Ushiyama et al 1991) and in human cortical neurons (Kunicki et al 1995). Our results, together with those already published, suggest that either TTR is transported from CSF into neurons and astrocytes or is produced in these cells at significantly lower levels than in the choroid plexus. Detection of TTR immunoreactivity in neurons and astrocytes suggests that this protein may inhibit amyloid formation in the human brain.

Acknowledgements

This research was supported in part by NIH, Alzheimer's Association and American Health Assistance Foundation. We are grateful to Audrey Wang, Maria Tsiper, Henning Wente and Gregory Rudamen for their excellent technical support and Dr Michael P. Vitek for critical comments.

References

Benson MD, Wallace MR 1989 Amyloidosis, the metabolic basis of disease. In: Scriver CP, Beaudet AL, Sly WS, Valles D (eds) The metabolic and molecular basis of inherited disease. McGraw-Hill, New York, p 2439–2460

Eaton WA, Hofrichter J 1990 Sickle cell hemoglobin polymerization. Adv Protein Chem 40:63–279

Elovaara IJ, Maury CP, Palo J 1986 Serum amyloid A, albumin and prealbumin in Alzheimer's disease and in demented patients with Down's syndrome. Acta Neurol Scand 74:245–250

Evans KC, Berger EP, Cho C-G, Weisgraber KH, Lansbury PT Jr 1995 Apolipoprotein E is a kinetic but not a thermodynamic inhibitor of amyloid formation. Proc Natl Acad Sci USA 92:763–776

Fitch NJS, Akbari MT, Ramsden DB 1991 An inherited non-amyloidogenic transthyretin variant, [Ser6]-TTR, with increased thyroxine-binding affinity, characterized by DNA sequencing. J Endocrinol 129:309–313

Fraser PE, Nguyen JT, McLachlan DR, Abraham CR, Kirschner D 1993 α1-Antichymotrypsin binding to Alzheimer Aβ peptides is sequence specific and induces fibril disaggregation *in vitro*. J Neurochem 61:298–306

Ghiso J, Matsubara E, Koudinov A et al 1993 The cerebrospinal-fluid soluble form of Alzheimer's amyloid beta is complexed to SP-40,40 (apolipoprotein J), an inhibitor of the complement membrane-attack complex. Biochem J 293:27–30

Goldgaber D, Lerman MI, McBride OW, Saffiotti U, Gajdusek DC 1987 Characterization and chromosomal localization of a cDNA encoding brain amyloid of Alzheimer's disease. Science 235:877–880

Goldgaber D, Schwarzman AL, Bhasin R et al 1993 Sequestration of amyloid beta-peptide. Ann N Y Acad Sci 695:139–143

Herbert J, Wilcox JN, Pham KTC et al 1986 Transthyretin: a choroid plexus-specific transport protein in human brain. Neurology 36:900–911

Jacobson DR, Buxbaum JN 1991 Genetic aspects of amyloidosis. Adv Hum Genet 20:69–123

Jarrett JT, Lansbury PT Jr 1993 Seeding 'one-dimensional crystallization' of amyloid: a pathogenic mechanism in Alzheimer's disease and scrapie? Cell 73:1055–1058

Kunicki S, Zorychta E, Richardson J 1995 Biondi ring protein is found in the human cortex and cerebrospinal fluid. Mol Biol Cell 6:94A(abstr 548)

Kunkel TA 1985 Rapid and efficient site-specific mutagenesis without phenotypic selection. Proc Natl Acad Sci USA 82:488–492

Link CD 1995 Expression of human β-amyloid peptide in transgenic *Caenorhabditis elegans*. Proc Natl Acad Sci USA 92:9368–9372

Ma J, Yee A, Brewer HB Jr, Das S, Potter H 1994 Amyloid-associated proteins α_1-antichymotrypsin and apolipoprotein E promote assembly of Alzheimer β-protein into filaments. Nature 372:92–95

Mazur-Kolecka B, Frackowiak J, Wisniewski HM 1995 Apolipoproteins E3 and E4 induce and transthyretin prevents accumulation of the Alzheimer's β-amyloid peptide in cultured vascular smooth muscle cells. Brain Res 698:217–222

Murrell JR, Schoner RG, Liepnieks JJ, Rosen HN, Moses AC, Benson MD 1992 Production and functional analysis of normal and variant recombinant human transthyretin proteins. J Biol Chem 267:16595–16600

Podlisny MB, Ostaszewski BL, Squazzo SL et al 1995 Aggregation of secreted amyloid beta-protein into sodium dodecyl sulfate-stable oligomers in cell culture. J Biol Chem 270:9564–9570

Riisoen H 1988 Reduced prealbumin (transthyretin) in CSF of severely demented patients with Alzheimer's disease. Acta Neurol Scand 78:455–459

Roheim PS, Carey M, Forte T, Vega GL 1979 Apolipoproteins in human cerebrospinal fluid. Proc Natl Acad Sci USA 76:4646–4649

Saraiva MJM 1995 Transthyretin mutations in health and disease. Hum Mutat 5: 191–192

Schmechel DE, Saunders AM, Strittmatter WJ et al 1993 Increased amyloid β-peptide deposition in cerebral cortex as a consequence of apolipoprotein E genotype in late-onset Alzheimer's disease. Proc Natl Acad Sci USA 90:9649–9653

Schwarzman AL, Gregori L, Vitek MP et al 1994 Transthyretin sequesters amyloid β protein and prevents amyloid formation. Proc Natl Acad Sci USA 91:8368–8372

Scrimshaw BJ, Fellowes AP, Palmer BN, Croxson MS, Stockigt JR, George PM 1992 A novel variant of transthyretin (prealbumin), Thr119 to Met, associated with increased thyroxine binding. Thyroid 2:21–26

Selkoe DJ 1994 Normal and abnormal biology of the beta-amyloid precursor protein. Annu Rev Neurosci 17:489–517

Seubert P, Vigo-Pelfrey C, Esch F et al 1992 Isolation and quantification of soluble Alzheimer's β-peptide from biological fluids. Nature 359:325–327

Shoji M, Golde TE, Ghiso J et al 1992 Production of the Alzheimer amyloid β protein by normal proteolytic processing. Science 258:126–129

Strittmatter WJ, Saunders AM, Schmechel D et al 1993 Apolipoprotein E: high-avidity binding to β-amyloid and increased frequency of type 4 allele in late-onset familial Alzheimer disease. Proc Natl Acad Sci USA 90:1977–1981

Ushiyama M, Ikeda S, Yanagisawa N 1991 Transthyretin-type cerebral amyloid angiopathy in type I familial amyloid polyneuropathy. Acta Neuropath 81:524–528

Vitek MP, Bhattacharya K, Glendening JM et al 1994 Advanced glycation end products contribute to amyloidosis in Alzheimer disease. Proc Natl Acad Sci USA 91:4766–4770

Whitson JS, Mims MP, Strittmatter WJ, Yamaki T, Morrisett JD, Appel SH 1994 Attenuation of the neurotoxic effect of Aβ amyloid peptide by apolipoprotein E. Biochem Biophys Res Commun 199:163–170

Wisniewski T, Castaño E, Ghiso J, Frangione B 1993a Cerebrospinal fluid inhibits Alzheimer beta-amyloid fibril formation *in vitro*. Ann Neurol 34:631–633

Wisniewski T, Golabek A, Matsubara E, Ghiso J, Frangione B 1993b Apolipoprotein E: binding to soluble Alzheimer's β-amyloid. Biochem Biophys Res Commun 192:359–365

Wisniewski T, Castaño EM, Golabek A, Vogel T, Frangione B 1994 Acceleration of Alzheimer's fibril formation by apolipoprotein E *in vitro*. Am J Pathol 145:1030–1035

DISCUSSION

Palha: We have obtained exactly the opposite results. We found that recombinant TTR promoted rather than inhibited Aβ amyloid formation, as measured in a thioflavine assay. Might a contaminant in your commercial TTR preparation be responsible for the inhibition observed?

Goldgaber: I don't know how pure the TTR preparation is. However, when we tried to use recombinant TTR we had difficulties which we think were related to contamination by material in the growth medium.

Palha: Do you have any idea of the K_d of the Aβ peptides with TTR?

Goldgaber: I don't know: this is difficult to determine for Aβ because of its tendency to aggregate.

Palha: When you did the CSF experiment and you immunoprecipitated with an anti-Aβ antibody, did you only check these fractions for TTR or did you also look for other amyloid-related proteins, such as apoE?

Goldgaber: We tested for TTR alone.

Palha: If TTR does sequester Aβ in the CSF, mutations in the TTR molecule could alter TTR conformation and therefore release the bound Aβ, as you have suggested. Because of the possible association between TTR and Aβ in AD we screened for TTR mutations in 60 AD patients. Ser6 occurs in 12% of the normal population (Jacobson et al 1995) and we found the Ser6 polymorphic mutation at exactly the same frequency (Palha et al 1996). Therefore, a link between TTR and AD seems unlikely.

Goldgaber: After we found that TTR binds Aβ, we analysed the TTR gene in patients with AD. We found the Ser6 variant in 12% (6 out of 50) families from Allen Roses' collection of families with late-onset AD patients. Linkage analysis of this variant revealed a weak positive LOD score which did not exclude the possibility that the TTR gene is associated with AD, but was not strong enough for us to conclude anything else. We also found that 12% of spouses of AD patients who were used as controls also had the Ser6 variant. This figure is very close to that reported by Joel Buxbaum from a general population sample (Jacobson et al 1995). At present, we do not have data allowing us to say whether TTR is linked to AD in some families. Moreover, because AD is a heterogeneous disease, it will not be an easy question to answer. We have begun a collaboration with Richard Mayeux from Colombia University to analyse the TTR gene in a large sample of AD patients in his community study.

J. D. Buxbaum: You suggest that the TTR 42 and 58 mutations don't bind Aβ. Wouldn't you expect these patients to have amyloidosis very early on, irrespective of AD?

Goldgaber: I don't think that TTR alone can explain amyloid depositions in Alzheimer's brain. Although I'm fairly convinced that TTR plays an important role in prevention of amyloid formation in CSF and serum, the situation in the brain might be quite different. Tabaton et al (1994) have assayed soluble Aβ in different regions of AD patients' brains which were either populated by plaques or devoid of insoluble Aβ. They compared these data to those they generated using the same analysis for normal age-matched controls. Surprisingly, they were only able to detect soluble Aβ in areas of Alzheimer's brains which were heavily populated by insoluble amyloid. This suggests that the amount of Aβ detectable in the brain is beyond the level of sensitivity of their method, and is raised dramatically only in focal points where amyloid is already formed or is being formed. This means that the normal mechanism preventing amyloid formation, whether it is TTR, apoE or numerous other molecules which can inhibit amyloid formation, fails to prevent amyloid formation in those regions where you find amyloid.

Saraiva: Did you try the binding assay with different TTR mutations using unlabelled Aβ to rule out a possible effect of labelling on the binding properties?

Goldgaber: No we did not.

Frangione: Dr A. Roher has done an ELISA study showing that soluble Aβ is present both in normal and AD brains (Kuo et al 1996).

Goldgaber: Tabaton and colleagues used a very sensitive ELISA which was developed by Steve Younkin's group. However, I think that what is important is the difference in the amounts of soluble Aβ in regions of the brain with plaques versus regions without. I am not saying that soluble Aβ is not present in all areas of the brain that are devoid of plaques. When Aβ was not detected it was obviously because it was below the sensitivity of the assay. However, the level of soluble Aβ was dramatically increased in brain regions containing insoluble amyloid.

Frangione: So far the sequence of brain 'soluble' Aβ has not been reported. The published studies have only shown ELISA, Western blot and SDS-PAGE data.

Goldgaber: They described the solubilization procedure in the paper.

Frangione: It is very important to know the sequence of the protein.

Kelly: While I agree that the Zagorski structure is correct, it is not relevant, because it was recorded in trifluoroethanol. There's a more recent paper by Maggio, which is a very careful study of Aβ10–35 (Lee et al 1995). He shows through a number of experiments that this peptide is as representative as one can get in an NMR of Aβ1–40. There's absolutely no evidence for a helical structure, which sort of makes sense on the basis of the data that other people have reported. So I think your modelling is interesting, but I'm not sure that it is relevant, because it's my conviction that this peptide is not α-helical in its circulating state. It is only partially a β-hairpin and the rest is basically unstructured.

We've confirmed your data in the sense that TTR does bind to Aβ, but the dissociation constant is so high that I don't think it's physiologically relevant. However, we were working with recombinant protein, and basically anything else we used that binds to Aβ, bound much better to TTR. I would not trust the Calbiochem TTR.

Blake: I would like to add a structural gloss to what you say, which doesn't mean I endorse this idea, but was merely something that occurred to me while we were talking. I'm usually rather concerned about models in the absence of data, but we do have some, namely the positions of residues 42 and 58 of TTR. It occurred to me that 58 is located on the D strand, and residue 42 is on the C strand, so each is on the edge of the two β-sheets in TTR. The natural way in which a molecule might interact in this region, would be if it were to form a

β-sheet structure complementary to the existing one so, as it were, it extended the β-sheets, maybe by one or two strands. In that sense TTR might be a sort of template for converting the Aβ into a β-sheet kind of structure and binding to it. Even more interestingly, this is the region of the hot spot in TTR for the natural amyloidogenic mutants. Here we have the involvement of strands C and D again. In my model, these two edge strands of the β-sheets are the area where TTR molecules might come together to form the fibrils. So if these regions in TTR were inhibited by Aβ binding, it might inhibit formation of amyloid of the TTR type. Or, indeed, it could work the other way round and the TTR could inhibit the Aβ from forming amyloid. This is just, as I said, a structural gloss: there may be nothing in it, but it might explain some of your observations.

Kirschner: If I could address Colin Blake's hypothesis about the interaction between TTR and Aβ in amyloid formation. Francisco Domingues in my laboratory did some experiments in which he attempted to co-crystallize Aβ with TTR under conditions where both molecules exist as monomers. In many cases he obtained crystals of TTR simultaneously with fibres of Aβ. Although he started out with monomers and not a TTR–Aβ complex, the results suggest that under these crystallization conditions neither molecule prevents the other type from aggregating in its usual way.

Blake: But that could be a matter of the actual conditions that you were using.

Kirschner: These were not very extreme conditions.

Goldgaber: The purpose of our model was simply to find a binding site on the TTR for Aβ. We modified it when Mike Zagorski came up with new coordinates, and we now have a new model of Aβ, and we will see how that model fits the complex formation.

Kelly: My major point is that is really not appropriate to put a peptide in trifuoroethanol and draw conclusions about its structure in aqueous solution.

Goldgaber: I'm not arguing about that. This model is useful only for experimental purposes.

Kelly: If you map in the binding site which is now known for the retinol binding protein, what happens when you add retinol binding protein or thyroxine to these interactions?

Goldgaber: We haven't done those competition experiments yet, but we will.

Arvinte: I would like to ask about the fibrillation mechanism you proposed. Can you comment about the critical nucleus for Aβ amyloid formation? Is it a pentamer?

Goldgaber: At the moment it is only speculation. During the incubation of Aβ with TTR we were able to see first the disappearance and then the reappearance of the Aβ tetramer. This process took place without fibril formation. Therefore one can speculate that these data suggest that the pentamer is the critical size of the nucleus.

Arvinte: In your experiments you showed that bovine serum albumin had no effect on the fibrils, and that ApoE and TTR influence the fibrillation process. Have you also tried other proteins that are water insoluble?

Goldgaber: No, we have not.

Arvinte: Do apoE, low-density lipoprotein or high-density lipoprotein bind or interact in a similar way to Aβ?

Goldgaber: We will look at that. In fact, we have already used ultracentrifugation in a potassium iodide gradient to analyse the distribution of radioiodinated Aβ1–28 in CSF. This procedure is a standard way to separate lipoprotein particles, which float to the top of the gradient.

References

Jacobson DR, Alves IL, Saraiva MJ, Thibodeau SN, Buxbaum JN 1995 Transthyretin Ser6 gene frequency in individuals without amyloidosis. Hum Genet 95:308–312

Kuo YM, Emmerling MR, Vigo-Pelfry C et al 1996 Water-soluble Aβ (N-40, N-42) oligomers in normal and Alzheimer disease brains. J Biol Chem 271:4077–4081

Lee JP, Stimson ER, Ghilardi JR et al 1995 H-1 NMR of Aβ amyloid peptide congeners in water solution: conformational changes correlate with plaque competence. Biochemistry 34:5191–5200

Palha JA, Moreira P, Wisinewski T, Frangione B, Saraiva MJ 1996 Transthyretin gene in Alzheimer's disease patients. Neurosci Lett 204:212–214

Tabaton M, Nunzi MG, Xue R, Usiak M, Autillo-Gambetti L, Gambetti P 1994 Soluble amyloid β protein is a marker of Alzheimer amyloid in brain but not in cerebrospinal fluid. Biochem Biophys Res Commun 200:1598–1603

General discussion III

Apolipoprotein E, TTR and Alzheimer's disease

Pepys: The majority of experiments that have been done with apolipoprotein E (apoE) with regard to interactions with amyloid β-protein (Aβ) fibrillogenesis have been done with isolated, purified, delipidated, denatured apoE. Those that have been done with apoE expressed in transfected cells or reconstituted into phospholipid particles tend to give rather different results. Do these denatured delipidated apoEs reflect the physiological form in which this molecule exists *in vivo*?

Frangione: We use purified apoE from human plasma because recombinant apoE doesn't have the same effect. We have also used high-density lipoproteins, and they act similarly.

Pepys: Mary Jo LaDu, from Chicago, has used apoE reconstituted into phospholipid particles or expressed in the supernatant of transfected cells, and she gets rather different results (LaDu et al 1994, 1995).

Frangione: ApoE3 binds better than E4.

Pepys: Which one is physiologically meaningful?

Frangione: ApoE3 is the most abundant.

Pepys: The question is not which of the isoforms is most abundant, but rather which of the forms of apoE used in these experiments has physiologically relevant effects on fibrillogenesis.

Frangione: We have used a number of different apoE preparations, including heterologous human apoE purified from human plasma, apoE from homozygous apoE3 or E4 patients, and recombinant apoE2, E3 and E4 from both *Escherichia coli* and baculovirus. The best results were obtained with the purified human apoE.

An important difference between our studies and those of others is the concentration of apoE. Most other studies have used a concentration of apoE equivalent to that found in the circulation where there is a 100-fold excess of apoE to Aβ. We did not use this ratio since it is obvious that amyloid fibrils do not form in the circulation. We used an apoE to Aβ ratio of 1 : 100, which is close to that found within tissue in Alzheimer's disease patients (Wisniewski et al 1995).

Pepys: But there's still quite a lot of apoE in the brain.

Frangione: Yes, because apoE is an acute reactive protein. There is very little in the extracted material, but in the supernatant there is plenty of apoE.

Goldgaber: It has been shown that in plasma, apoE is always associated with lipoprotein particles. So-called 'free' apoE appeared as a result of the experimental manipulation of samples. The exact status of apoE in cerebrospinal fluid (CSF) is not known in part because only a few groups have studied apoE in CSF. Estimates tend to suggest that in CSF, as in plasma, most apoE is associated with lipoprotein particles. However, nobody knows what is happening to apoE in the brain. So far the studies of apoE in the brain have involved immunocytochemical localization or biochemical extraction, which disrupt the tissue. Therefore, at this stage, it is not possible to determine whether there is free apoE in the brain.

Pepys: But a lot is known about this and other similar apolipoproteins. They don't exist in physiological saline, for example, as soluble proteins. They aggregate and precipitate.

Goldgaber: The are no results on the state of apoE in the brain.

J. D. Buxbaum: ApoE which has been produced in the baculovirus expression system, in which there is very high expression and no appropriate lipidation, is in an aggregated form from the outset. In contrast, it is very unlikely that whatever you might find in the brain is similarly de-lipidated and aggregated.

Goldgaber: That is speculation; we really don't know. From our experience of studies of apoE in plasma or in CSF, we would suggest that apoE is also in association with lipids in the brain. We don't know what happens to it when it gets inside cells, nor how it gets into amyloid depositions.

Frangione: If apoE does prevent fibrillogenesis, as you have postulated, none of us will develop Alzheimer's, because there is plenty of apoE in the brain.

Kelly: In a test tube it might be an inhibitor if the protein is prepared in a certain way, but *in vivo* it could be totally different. So both sides could be right.

Arvinte: Terzi et al (1995) recently showed that Aβ interacts with the negatively charged liposome membrane and changes its conformation, i.e. Aβ adopts a β-sheet structure at the lipid membrane surface. This suggests that the lipid membrane might act as a nucleation site for the formation of fibrils. It will be interesting to see whether the lipids in apoE also influence the fibrillation process.

Goldgaber: A couple of recent papers have suggested that the interaction of transthyretin (TTR) with Aβ could have biological significance in inhibiting amyloid formation. Mazur-Kolecka et al (1995) showed that apoE3 can prevent accumulation of Aβ amyloid in smooth muscle cells. They used cultured vascular smooth muscle cells from dog brains. After several days in culture they saw Aβ amyloid deposition, which they could inhibit by TTR.

In addition, Link (1995) has created the first transgenic *Caenorhabditis elegans* model of Aβ amyloid formation. Link crossed these animals with other worms producing human TTR, and the hybrids thus generated showed drastically reduced Aβ amyloid deposition, whereas the levels of both TTR and Aβ stayed the same.

Don Schmechel from Duke University has raised antibodies directly against TTR. Immunoreactivity for TTR was detected in numerous cells in the brain, but amyloid plaques were not stained. In some cells, the immunoreactivity for TTR was in the nuclei. This reminded us of the suggestion of Colin Blake, who came up with the first model of TTR structure. He suggested that TTR could be a DNA binding protein. I'm not aware of anyone who has reported that TTR can bind DNA. However, it is not clear how TTR gets into cells and then when it has got into the cell, whether it goes to the nucleus or not. This is surprising, because TTR mRNA has only been detected in the brain in the choroid plexus and the meninges. However, TTR immunoreactivity has also been detected in a number of cells in the rat brain.

Pepys: Of course, immunohistochemistry is an exquisitely sensitive technique identifying antibodies and antigens that sometimes you can't detect by almost any other method. What was the source of the TTR you used to absorb your anti-TTR and what were the criteria for the purity of the antibody? For example, if you are using commercial TTR to absorb the antiserum and you get a negative result, how sure are you that there's nothing in that preparation except TTR? Such prevalent nuclear staining for a cytoplasmic protein is quite a remarkable finding.

Goldgaber: We used commercial preparations of both TTR and antibodies. We did adsorptions which we checked on Western blots using the same TTR.

Pepys: I'm not denying that you have anti-TTR there. The question is: are you sure that you haven't got any other antibody or that there isn't another antigen in the TTR preparation used for adsorption?

Goldgaber: We did Coomassie blue staining of the preparations and we did Western blot analysis of this preparation only. We did not do any sequencing. I would be interested to know whether anyone has stained adult human brain for TTR, because when I looked in the literature there were many papers on the detection of mRNA and a few papers looking at protein in the rat and fetal human brain, but I couldn't find any on protein in the adult human brain.

Masters: I can quote one reference where Shirahama et al (1982) took an antibody to prealbumin (TTR) and found immunoreactivity in the plaques.

Goldgaber: But another paper showed that there is no TTR in the plaques (Eikelenboom & Stam 1984). In fact, if you believe that this stain recognizes TTR, TTR is not in the plaques.

Pepys: There are plenty of monoclonal antibodies around to TTR. It would be quite easy to screen with a panel of these.

Benson: I have tried for a long time to make a monoclonal antibody that will stain TTR amyloid.

Saraiva: We have experience with monoclonal anti-TTR antibodies staining amyloid deposits. For instance, the antibodies referred to in my paper (Saraiva et al 1996, this volume) stain TTR amyloid perfectly.

Sipe: Is Aβ ever found in association with systemic TTR deposits?

Frangione: No one has looked.

Benson: We've looked very closely at the sequence: we have never sequenced the Aβ sequence out of TTR amyloid although we have sequenced other components like histones.

Kelly: A general question about the metabolism of TTR: is there any evidence for TTR crossing the blood–brain barrier?

Saraiva: The experience we have is with rat TTR. When you inject it intravenously it doesn't cross the barrier, but if you inject it intraventricularly, it does—that is, it appears in the circulation. It is one-way transport (Saraiva et al 1988).

Benson: I don't know how much 'one-way' it is. It is a matter of concentration. In the patients with liver transplant the variant is there in normal amounts in the CSF, but it is not detectable in the peripheral circulation, which is a much bigger pool. It could be coming out of the CSF but in insufficient quantities to make it detectable.

Saraiva: That agrees with my observation that brain-derived TTR crosses the blood–brain barrier into the vascular circulation.

Costa: A general question: how far away do you think an anti-amyloid therapy for Alzheimer's is?

Pepys: It must be a long way away. Even if you had a drug that could cure amyloid now, the pharmaceutical companies tell us it would take several years before such a drug would actually be on the market. The best you could hope for, even if the amyloid causes the dementia, is that you would arrest cognitive decline, and you would need difficult and very expensive clinical trials to prove this.

Kelly: Many of the proposals for potential anti-amyloid therapies are based around the concept of inhibition of protein–protein interactions. Short of neurotrophic factor action, these drugs have to bind to the protein and do something. A number of companies having been trying to do this in other contexts for at least 10 years and there are precious few success stories of small molecules inhibiting protein–protein interactions. It is a lot easier to stabilize a protein. That is one strategy that we can use in amyloid diseases, because it may not take too much to tweak the balance.

Pepys: The successful strategy may well involve a multipronged approach: a little bit of this and a little bit of that.

Kelly: Per Westermark raised the interesting point that actually stabilizing the fibril might not be such a bad move. It may not be the fibril itself that is toxic, but instead the small fragments that diffuse out of it. It would be interesting to see if stabilized fibrils would still kill nerve cells.

Pepys: It really depends whether you think that toxicity is important or not. If you have a patient with 100 g of amyloid stiffening their left ventricular wall, it might be best to get it out of there rather than stabilize it.

Kelly: I agree completely, but it is a proof of concept: is it the presence of the fibril that's killing the nerve cell? It is pretty hard to conceive how this could happen.

Benson: With Alzheimer's disease that is certainly a good question. However, I had a patient who died last month whose heart weighed 990 g: it is not too hard to know what the toxic factor was.

Masters: It is the exact reverse in Alzheimer's disease, because the total amyloid load in the Alzheimer's disease brain is probably in the order of only 10–100 mg.

Pepys: Neurons have been successfully cultured on top of amyloid plaques or slices of Alzheimer's brain, and they grow very happily. It certainly doesn't look as though the plaque itself has biochemical toxicity.

References

Eikelenboom P, Stam FC 1984 An immunohistochemical study on cerebral vascular and senile plaque amyloid in Alzheimer's dementia. Virchows Arch B Cell Pathol Incl Mol Pathol 47:17–25

LaDu MJ, Falduto MT, Manelli AM, Reardon CA, Getz GS, Frail DE 1994 Isoform-specific binding of apolipoprotein E to β-amyloid. J Biol Chem 269:23403–23406

LaDu MJ, Pederson TM, Frail DE, Reardon CA, Getz GS, Falduto MT 1995 Purification of apolipoprotein E attenuates isoform-specific binding to β-amyloid. J Biol Chem 270:9039–9042

Link CD 1995 Expression of human β amyloid peptide in transgenic *Caenorhabditis elegans*. Proc Natl Acad Sci USA 92:9368–9372

Mazur-Kolecka B, Frackowiak J, Wisniewski HM 1995 Apolipoproteins E3 and E4 induce and transthyretin prevents accumulation of the Alzheimer's β-amyloid peptide in cultured vascular smooth muscle cells. Brain Res 698:217–222

Saraiva MJM, Makover A, Moriwaki H, Blaner W, Costa PP, Goodman DS 1988 Studies on transthyretin metabolism in the nervous system. In: Isobe T (ed) Amyloid and amyloidosis. Plenum, NY, p 343–348

Saraiva MJM, Almeida MR, Alves IL et al 1996 Modulating conformational factors in transthyretin amyloid. In: The nature and origin of amyloid fibrils (Ciba Found Symp 199). Wiley, Chichester, p 47–57

Shirahama T, Skinner M, Westermark P, Rubinow A, Cohen AS 1982 Senile cerebral amyloid prealbumin as a common constituent in the neuritic plaque, in the neurofibrillary tangle, and in the neuropathological lesion. Am J Pathol 107:41–50

Terzi E, Hölzemann G, Seelig J 1995 Self-association of β-amyloid peptide (1–40) in solution and binding to lipid membranes. J Mol Biol 252:633–642

Wisniewski T, Lalowski M, Golabeck A, Vogel T, Frangione B 1995 Is Alzheimer's disease an apolipoprotein E amyloidosis? Lancet 345:956–958

β-amyloid precursor protein and early-onset Alzheimer's disease

Lydia Hendriks, Chris De Jonghe, Patrick Cras, Jean-Jacques Martin and Christine Van Broeckhoven

Neurogenetics Laboratory, Born-Bunge Foundation, University of Antwerp, Department of Biochemistry, Universiteitsplein 1, B-2610 Antwerp, Belgium

Abstract. One of the major pathological hallmarks of Alzheimer's disease is the deposition in the brain parenchyma and cerebral blood vessel walls of amyloid β-protein, a 4 kDa proteolytic product of the longer β-amyloid precursor protein (APP). Six different single base mutations in the APP gene have been reported causing early-onset Alzheimer's disease (age at onset $\leqslant$65 years) or related amyloidosis in a small number of families. Cell transfection experiments using wild-type and mutant APP cDNA indicated that APP mutations result in the production of more or longer, aggregation prone, Aβ peptides.

1996 The nature and origin of amyloid fibrils. Wiley, Chichester (Ciba Foundation Symposium 199) p 170–180

Alzheimer's disease, Down's syndrome and congophilic amyloid angiopathy

Alzheimer's disease (AD) is the major form of progressive senile dementia in the elderly. The first symptoms of the disease are short-term memory disturbances and disorientation. As the disease progresses, complete impairment of memory, judgement and reasoning follows. A definite diagnosis of the disease can only be obtained by post-mortem examination of the brain. AD pathology is characterized by extensive neuronal cell loss and by particular brain lesions in the neocortex, hippocampus and amygdala, i.e. the neurofibrillary tangles and senile plaques. The neurofibrillary tangles are intraneuronal inclusions of paired helical filaments composed of hyperphosphorylated tau, a microtubule-associated protein. The senile plaques are mainly composed of amyloid β-protein (Aβ) deposited in the brain parenchyma. Aβ is a 4 kDa proteolysis product of the β-amyloid precursor protein (APP). In brains from AD patients, congophilic amyloid angiopathy (CAA) is also present as a consequence of the accumulation of Aβ in the leptomeningeal and cortical blood vessel walls.

Older (aged 30–40) patients with Down's syndrome (trisomy 21) tend to develop neuropathological features similar to those seen in AD patients (Wisniewski et al 1985).

In CAA, Aβ is deposited in blood vessel walls where it provokes intracerebral haemorrhages. Most CAA cases occur sporadically, but a particular form of CAA, hereditary cerebral haemorrhage with amyloidosis of the Dutch type (HCHWA-D), is inherited as an autosomal dominant trait in a small number of Dutch families. HCHWA-D is typified by recurrent haemorrhagic strokes between ages 45–65 due to extensive Aβ deposition in the cerebral and leptomeningeal blood vessel walls. In contrast to AD, no dystrophic neurites or neurofibrillary tangles are present. HCHWA-D has been referred to as the vascular form of AD, because of its predominant vascular involvement (van Duinen et al 1987).

APP and Aβ

Structure of APP

Aβ is derived by the proteolytic processing of APP. The APP gene is localized on chromosome 21 at 21q21.2 (e.g. Kang et al 1987) and is encoded by 18 exons of which exon 16 and 17 encode in part the Aβ peptide (e.g. Yoshikai et al 1990). Three major splicing variants have been identified containing the Aβ sequence, i.e. APP695, APP751 and APP770 isoforms, of which APP695 is the major isoform found in brain. The two larger isoforms include exon 7 which encodes a domain homologous to a Kunitz protease inhibitor. The amino acid sequence of APP predicts that it is an integral membrane protein with a single transmembrane domain near the C-terminus (Fig. 1).

Processing of APP

APP is processed through different proteolytic pathways (reviewed by Haass & Selkoe 1993) (Fig. 2). The major pathway is the constitutive secretory pathway which cleaves APP within the extracellular portion of the Aβ sequence at APP codon 687 (codon numbering is referring to the APP770 isoform through the whole text) producing soluble APP (APP_s) and a membrane bound 10 kDa (p10) fragment containing only part of Aβ. Since this pathway does not produce intact Aβ, it is non-amyloidogenic and does not lead to AD pathology.

Several potential amyloidogenic pathways have been described. In an endosomal/lysosomal pathway APP is degraded producing Aβ-containing, 11 kDa (p11) C-terminal fragments of APP. In this pathway the membrane-bound APP may be reinternalized from the cell surface and is then degraded into potentially amyloidogenic fragments accumulating in the lysosomes. These

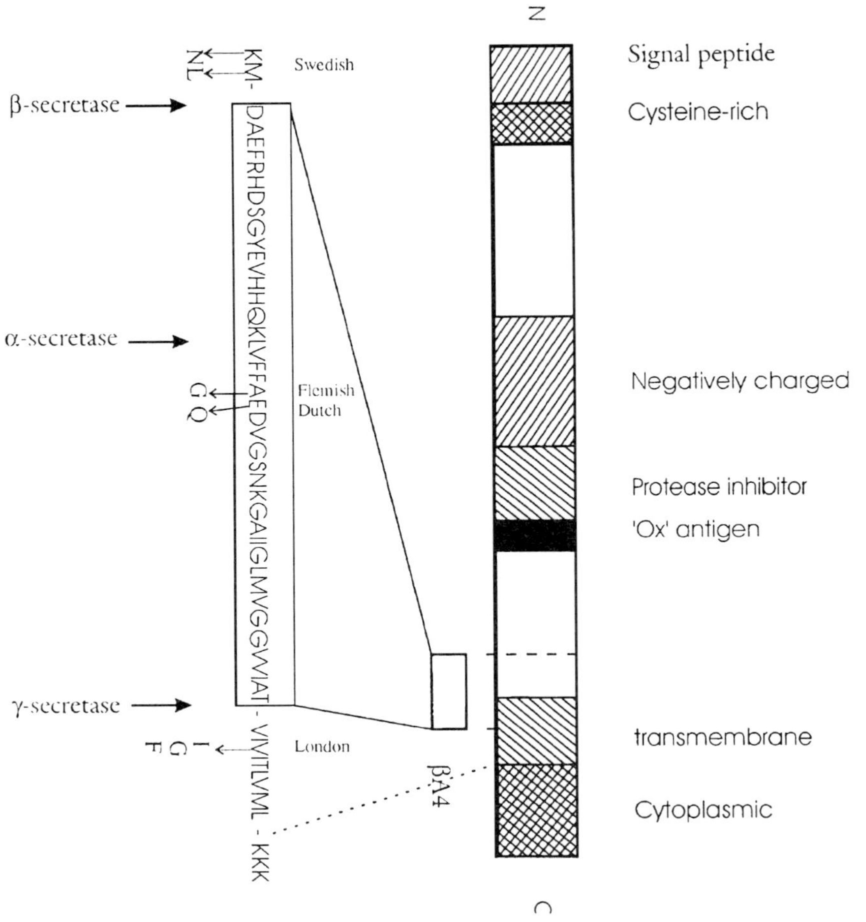

FIG. 1. Structure of APP. Proposed domain structure of APP as a cell-surface glycoprotein (Kang et al 1987): different shaded boxes present the distinct domains of the protein. The amyloid β-protein (βA4) sequence and the secretase cleavages sites of the amyloidogenic (β- and γ-secretases) and non-amyloidogenic (α-secretase) pathway are shown. The amino acid substitutions involving the different APP mutations are indicated.

amyloidogenic fragments are probably further processed by γ-secretase cutting at the C-terminal (APP codon position 711 to 714) side of Aβ, producing Aβ. APP has an NPXY consensus sequence in its cytoplasmic domain which can mediate the internalization of the protein. Further, it was shown that intact Aβ is secreted in the medium of different cell cultures and in cerebrospinal fluid of non-demented controls (Haass et al 1992, Seubert et al 1992, 1993). In this secretory pathway APP is cleaved between Met671 and Asp672 of APP, near the N-terminus of Aβ (Seubert et al 1993).

The proteolytic enzymes involved in the different APP metabolic pathways have not yet been identified. The enzymes have been termed α-secretase (cutting APP within Aβ), and β-secretase and γ-secretase (cutting APP at the N- and C-terminal sides of Aβ, respectively) (Fig. 2). The β-secretase is highly sequence specific while the α-secretase is not (Citron et al 1995). Recent data show that several proteases can cleave Aβ at or near to the N-terminus, resulting in Aβ peptides that are heterogeneous at their N-terminal side (Haass et al 1995).

APP mutations

So far six different mutations have been found in exons 16 and 17 of the APP gene. The mutations in the APP gene change amino acids at codon 717 of APP, i.e. Val to Ile (Goate et al 1991), Val to Phe (Murrell et al 1991) and Val to Gly (Chartier-Harlin et al 1991), and at codons 670/671 Lys to Asn and Met to Leu (Swedish mutation) (Mullan et al 1992). Only the APP717 (Val to Ile) London mutation has been observed in distinct early-onset AD families of different ethnic background and therefore is the most common APP mutation in AD. The prevalence of this mutation is 5.5% among familial early-onset AD patients (Van Broeckhoven 1995). In early-onset AD families in which mutations in the APP gene segregate, the mean age at disease onset is between 50 and 60 years.

A mutation in Aβ was also identified in patients with cerebral haemorrhages due to CAA and patients with AD belonging to the same Dutch family. Here an Ala to Gly mutation was detected at codon 692 of APP (Flemish mutation). The mean age at onset for all patients was 45.7 ± 7.3 years ($n = 11$). Histopathological examination of brain biopsy material of a patient suffering from a cerebral haemorrhage showed extensive deposition of Aβ in cerebral blood vessels and in the brain parenchyma. Dystrophic neurites were also present but no neurofibrillary tangles were seen (Hendriks et al 1992). Histopathological studies on brain autopsy material of a demented patient confirmed a diagnosis of AD. Numerous neurofibrillary tangles and extensive CAA were observed. Compared with the classical disease, this form of AD has a severe vascular component with more Aβ deposited in the senile plaques and blood vessels (Cras et al 1995). In HCHWA-D patients, a Glu to Gln mutation at APP codon 693 (Dutch mutation) was described (Levy et al 1990).

Effect of APP mutations on processing

The early-onset AD mutations APP717 and APP670/671 are located outside the Aβ sequence, with APP717 close to the C-terminal γ-secretase cleavage site

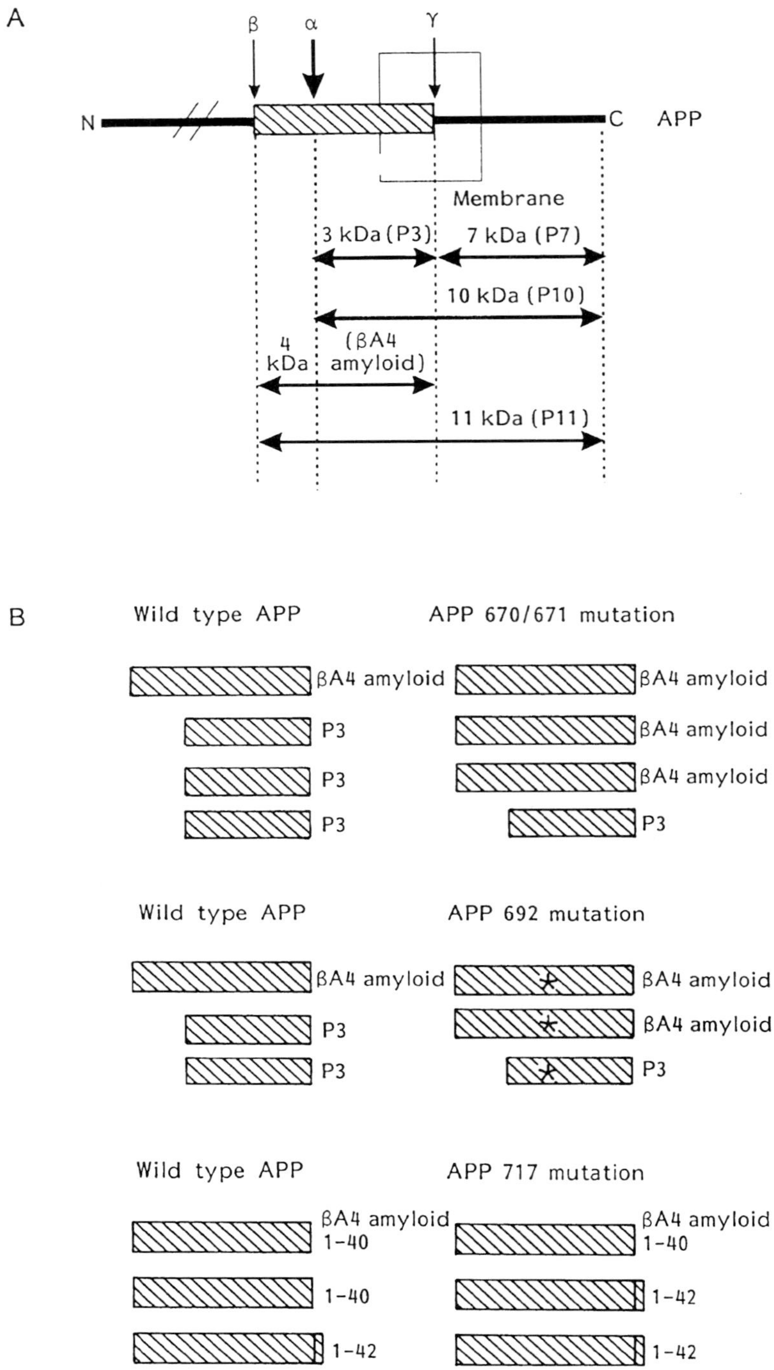
A
β
α
γ
N
C
APP
Membrane
3 kDa (P3)
7 kDa (P7)
10 kDa (P10)
4 kDa
(βA4 amyloid)
11 kDa (P11)
B
Wild type APP
APP 670/671 mutation
βA4 amyloid
P3
Wild type APP
APP 692 mutation
βA4 amyloid
P3
Wild type APP
APP 717 mutation
βA4 amyloid 1-40
1-40
1-42

within the transmembrane domain, and APP670/671 near the N-terminal β-secretase cleavage site within the extracellular part of APP. In contrast, the APP692 and APP693 mutations are located inside the Aβ sequence, next to the α-secretase cleavage site (Fig. 1). These localizations led to the hypothesis that these mutations might influence the activity of the respective secretases, resulting in an aberrant processing of APP. *In vitro* studies have already provided some evidence for this hypothesis.

APP670/671 (Swedish) mutation. The effect of the pathogenic APP mutations on the production of Aβ is depicted schematically in Fig. 2B. A three- to eightfold overproduction of Aβ has been observed in the medium of neuronal and non-neuronal cells transfected with the Swedish mutant APP670/671 cDNA (Citron et al 1992, Cai et al 1993, Felsenstein et al 1994, Hendriks et al 1995). Citron et al (1992) found that the APP671 (Met to Leu) substitution is responsible for this increase in Aβ secretion. These authors also showed that the 3 kDa (p3) fragment, the C-terminal subpeptide of Aβ resulting from both α- and γ-secretase activity (Fig. 1A), was decreased in the medium of cells transfected with the Swedish mutant APP cDNA. This increase results from a shift in the APP secretase activities favouring β-secretase cleavage in the mutant (Felsenstein et al 1994). It is likely that p11 is further processed into Aβ by γ-secretase. Citron et al (1994) and Johnston et al (1994) reported that fibroblasts of patients with the Swedish mutation also produce threefold more Aβ than fibroblasts from controls. The fact that the increase in Aβ production is detected in AD patients as well as in presymptomatic individuals carrying the Swedish mutation, suggests that Aβ overproduction is causal rather than secondary (Citron et al 1994).

The antibiotic bafilomycin A1, an agent which inhibits lysosomal protein degradation, has a differential effect on the processing of wild-type and Swedish mutant APP in transfected cells: Aβ secretion from wild-type APP increases whereas Aβ production from the Swedish mutant is decreased. After

FIG. 2. (*opposite*) β-amyloid precursor protein (APP) processing in wild-type and mutated APP. (A) Schematic representation of APP with the extracellular N-terminus and intracellular C-terminus. The amyloid β-protein (βA4) part is shown by the horizontal shaded box. The transmembrane domain is indicated by the vertical open box. The proteolytic cleavage sites of α-secretase in the non-amyloidogenic pathway and of β- and γ-secretases in the amyloidogenic pathway are indicated by arrows. The proteolytic products are shown together with their molecular mass and name as solid horizontal lines. (B) Influence of APP mutations on amyloid β-protein production. The main differences between the processing of wild-type APP (left) and mutated APP (right) are shown. The intra-amyloid β-protein mutation APP692 is denoted by an asterisk.

sequencing it became clear that in cells transfected with wild-type APP, an alternative secretase is used which cleaves Aβ at alternative positions. In cells expressing the Swedish mutant, no such alternative Aβ amyloid peptides could be formed. This differential effect of bafilomycin A1 is also seen in fibroblasts from patients bearing the Swedish mutation compared with fibroblasts from normal controls (Haass et al 1995).

APP692 (Flemish) and APP693 (Dutch) mutations. In vitro aggregation studies with synthetic Aβ amyloid comprising the APP693 mutation showed accelerated amyloid fibril formation (Wisniewski et al 1991, Clements et al 1993). For the APP692 mutation, however, no significant change in the rate of *in vitro* amyloid aggregation was detected. In fact, the aggregation of Aβ fibrils bearing the APP692 mutation was slightly slower than that of wild-type Aβ amyloid (Clements et al 1993). Recently, transfection experiments with a Flemish mutant APP cDNA demonstrated a relative increase in the secretion of Aβ amyloid and a decrease in p3 production (Haass et al 1994). These data suggested a lowered activity for the α-secretase due to the presence of the APP692 mutation. No increase in Aβ production was noticed in COS cells transfected with APP692 or APP693 cDNA (Hendriks et al 1995).

APP717 (London) mutations. In cells transfected with mutant APP717 cDNA (Val to Ile or Phe), the ratio of Aβ1–42/43 : Aβ1–40 is increased compared with cells transfected with wild-type APP (Suzuki et al 1994). The amount of secreted Aβ, however, remains the same (Cai et al 1993, Felsenstein et al 1994). *In vitro*, longer Aβ peptides tend to aggregate faster because the nucleation step is significantly accelerated (Jarrett et al 1993).

Aβ was also purified from brain of two unrelated patients with the APP717 (Val to Ile) mutation, and it was shown that the ratio of Aβ1–42,43 : Aβ1–40 was markedly increased compared with sporadic AD patients (Tamaoka et al 1994).

Discussion

It is widely accepted that AD is a complex disorder in which many genetic and environmental factors influence the pathogenesis. There is substantial evidence from the literature that Aβ deposition plays a central role in AD pathogenesis. The cascade hypothesis states that APP or, more likely, amyloidogenic derivatives of it, are neurotoxic and trigger the neuronal response, i.e. formation of neurofibrillary tangles and neuronal cell loss. The mechanisms by which this happens are mostly unknown (Hardy & Higgins 1992).

In AD patients APP is misprocessed and/or the deposition of Aβ is accelerated. Point mutations in the APP gene can mediate the preferential use of an amyloidogenic pathway compared with the non-amyloidogenic one. This leads to the production of longer and/or more Aβ peptides which aggregate faster. Other factors can act in the pathway leading to Aβ deposition.

Recently, two new genes (presenilins) causing early-onset AD, one on chromosome 14 (presenilin 1) (Sherrington et al 1995) and one on chromosome 1 (presenilin 2) (Levy-Lahad et al 1995a,b, Rogaev et al 1995) have been identified. Both proteins have a 65% amino acid homology and hydrophobicity plots predict seven transmembrane regions, resembling the topology of a receptor, a channel or a structural membrane protein. In total, 10 different pathogenic missense mutations have been identified in the presenilin 1 (e.g. Sherrington et al 1995, Wasco et al 1995, Rogaev et al 1995) and two distinct mutations in the presenilin 2 gene of patients of the Volga German families (Levy-Lahad et al 1995a, Rogaev et al 1995). We sequenced the presenilin 1 cDNA from brain and lymphoblasts of patients belonging to two Belgian chromosome 14q24.3-linked AD families, AD/A and AD/B (Van Broeckhoven et al 1992). Two additional mutations were found. Single-strand conformational polymorphism (SSCP) and restriction enzyme digestions confirmed that the mutations occur in all patients and at-risk individuals possessing the disease haplotype and not in non-patients and 90 control individuals (Cruts et al 1995).

Fibroblasts from chromosome 14-linked patients seem to secrete more of the longer Aβ peptides. This observation implies that the presenilin gene is one of the factors interfering in the Aβ pathway, providing new evidence for the Aβ cascade hypothesis and the pivotal role of the Aβ peptide in the genesis of AD pathology. Presenilins display some similarity to the SPE-4 gene, which codes for a membrane-bound protein from sperm cells of the nematode *Caenorhabditis elegans* (reviewed by Barinaga 1995). Since SPE-4 is involved in cellular transport one can speculate that the human presenilins affect the cell sorting and trafficking of proteins, including APP. This in turn could lead to altered Aβ production. However, it is still possible that presenilins do not interfere with the APP processing pathway, implying that the Aβ amyloid cascade hypothesis has to be reconsidered. Studies aiming to unravel the function of these presenilin genes have to be conducted in order to give insight in the function of the presenilins and their involvement in AD pathophysiology. Since APP mutations and presenilin mutations account for 5.5% and about 75% of early-onset AD cases, respectively, other early-onset AD genes must exist.

Acknowledgements

The Alzheimer's disease research work in the laboratory of Neurogenetics (University of Antwerp, UIA) is funded by the Flemish Biotechnology Programme of the Ministry of Economy, the National Fund of Scientific Research, a concerted action of the Ministry of Education, Belgium, BIOMED (GENE-CT93-0015) and BIOTECH (BIO2-CT94-2065) programmes of the European Community and by the Alzheimer's Disease Research Programme of the American Health Assistance Foundation.

References

Barinaga M 1995 New Alzheimer's gene found. Science 268:1845–1846

Cai X-D, Golde TE, Younkin SG 1993 Release of excess amyloid β-protein from a mutant amyloid β-protein precursor. Science 259:514–516

Chartier-Harlin M-C, Crawford F, Houlden H et al 1991 Early-onset Alzheimer's disease caused by mutations at codon 717 of the β-amyloid precursor protein gene. Nature 353:844–846

Citron M, Oltersdorf T, Haass C et al 1992 Mutation of the β-amyloid precursor protein in familial Alzheimer's disease increases β-protein production. Nature 360:672–674

Citron M, Vigo-Pelfrey C, Teplow DB et al 1994 Excessive production of amyloid β-protein by peripheral cells of symptomatic and presymptomatic patients carrying the Swedish familial Alzheimer disease mutation. Proc Natl Acad Sci USA 91:11993–11997

Citron M, Teplow DB, Selkoe DJ 1995 Generation of amyloid β protein from its precursor is sequence specific. Neuron 14:661–670

Clements A, Walsh DM, Williams CH, Allsop D 1993 Effects of the mutations Glu^{22} to Gln and Ala^{21} to Gly on the aggregation of a synthetic fragment of the Alzheimer's amyloid β/A4 peptide. Neurosci Lett 161:17–20

Cras P, van Harskamp F, Stefanko SZ et al 1995 Amyloid angiopathy is associated with a large amyloid core type of senile plaques in the amyloid precursor protein 692Ala→Gly mutation. J Neuropathol Exp Neurol 54:431(abstr)

Cruts M, Backhovens H, Theuns J et al 1995 Genetic and physical characterization of the early-onset Alzheimer's disease Ad3 locus on chromosome 14q24.3. Hum Mol Gene 4:1355–1364

Felsenstein KM, Hunihan LW, Roberts SB 1994 Altered cleavage and secretion of a recombinant β-APP bearing the Swedish familial Alzheimer's disease mutation. Nat Genet 6:251–256

Goate A, Chartier-Harlin M-C, Mullan M et al 1991 Segregation of a missense mutation in the amyloid precursor protein gene with familial Alzheimer's disease. Nature 349:704–706

Haass C, Selkoe DJ 1993 Cellular processing of β-amyloid precursor protein and the genesis of amyloid β-peptide. Cell 75:1039–1042

Haass C, Schlossmacher MG, Hung AY et al 1992 Amyloid β-peptide is produced by cultured cells during normal metabolism. Nature 359:322–325

Haass C, Hung AY, Selkoe DJ, Teplow DB 1994 Mutations associated with a locus for familial Alzheimer's disease result in alternative processing of amyloid β-protein precursor. J Biol Chem 269:17741–17748

Haass C, Capell A, Citron M, Teplow DB, Selkoe DJ 1995 the vacuolar H^+-ATPase inhibitor bafilomycin A1 differentially affects proteolytic processing of mutant and wild-type β-amyloid protein precursor. J Biol Chem 270:6186–6192

Hardy JA, Higgins GA 1992 Alzheimer's disease: the amyloid cascade hypothesis. Science 256:184–185

Hendriks L, van Duijn CM, Cras P et al 1992 Presenile dementia and cerebral haemorrhage linked to a mutation at codon 692 of the β-amyloid precursor protein gene. Nat Genet 1:218–221

Hendriks L, Cras P, Martin J-J, Van Broeckhoven C 1995 Alzheimer's disease and haemorrhagic stroke: their relationship to βA4 amyloid deposition. In: Kosik KS, Christen Y, Selkoe DJ (eds) Alzheimer's disease: lessons from cell biology. Springer-Verlag, Berlin, p 37–48

Jarrett JT, Berger EP, Lansbury PT Jr 1993 The carboxy terminus of the β-amyloid protein is critical for the seeding of amyloid formation: implications for the pathogenesis of Alzheimer's disease. Biochemistry 32:4693–4697

Johnston JA, Cowburn RF, Norgren S et al 1994 Increased β-amyloid release and levels of amyloid precursor protein (APP) in fibroblast cell lines from family members with the Swedish Alzheimer's disease APP670/671 mutation. FEBS Lett 354:274–278

Kang J, Lemaire HG, Unterbeck A et al 1987 The precursor of Alzheimer's disease amyloid βA4 protein resembles a cell-surface receptor. Nature 325:733–736

Levy E, Carman MD, Fernandez-Madrid IJ et al 1990 Mutation of the Alzheimer's disease amyloid gene in hereditary cerebral hemorrhage, Dutch type. Science 248:1124–1126

Levy-Lahad E, Wasco W, Poorkaj P et al 1995a Candidate gene for the chromosome 1 familial Alzheimer's disease locus. Science 269:973–977

Levy-Lahad E, Wijsman EM, Nemens E et al 1995b A familial Alzheimer's disease locus on chromosome 1. Science 269:970–973

Mullan M, Crawford F, Axelman K et al 1992 A pathogenic mutation for probable Alzheimer's disease in the APP gene at the N-terminus of β-amyloid. Nat Genet 1:345–347

Murrell J, Farlow M, Ghetti B, Benson MD 1991 A mutation in the amyloid precursor protein associated with hereditary Alzheimer's disease. Science 254:97–99

Rogaev EI, Sherrington R, Rogeava EA et al 1995 Familial Alzheimer's disease in kindreds with missense mutations in a gene on chromosome 1 related to the Alzheimer's disease type 3 gene. Nature 376:775–778

Seubert P, Vigo-Pelfrey C, Esch F et al 1992 Isolation and quantification of soluble Alzheimer's β-peptide from biological fluids. Nature 359:325–327

Seubert P, Oltersdorf T, Lee MG et al 1993 Secretion of β-amyloid precursor protein cleaved at the amino terminus of the β-amyloid peptide. Nature 361:260–263

Sherrington R, Rogaev EI, Liang Y et al 1995 Cloning of a gene bearing missense mutations in early-onset familial Alzheimer's disease. Nature 375:754–760

Suzuki N, Cheung TT, Cai X-D et al 1994 An increased percentage of long amyloid β protein secreted by familial amyloid β protein precursor (βAPP_{717}) mutants. Science 264:1336–1340

Tamaoka A, Odaka A, Ishibashi Y et al 1994 APP717 missense mutation affects the ratio of amyloid β protein species (Aβ1–42/43 and Aβ1–40) in familial Alzheimer's disease brain. J Biol Chem 269:32721–32724

Van Broeckhoven C 1995 Molecular genetics of Alzheimer disease: identification of genes and gene mutations. Eur Neurol 35:8–19

Van Broeckhoven C, Backhovens H, Cruts M et al 1992 Mapping of a gene predisposing to early-onset Alzheimer's disease to chromosome 14q24.3. Nat Genet 2:335–339

van Duinen SG, Castaño EM, Prelli F, Bots GTAB, Luyendijk W, Frangione B 1987 Hereditary cerebral haemorrhage with amyloidosis in patients of Dutch origin is related to Alzheimer disease. Proc Natl Acad Sci USA 84:5991–5994

Wasco W, Pettingell WP, Jondro PD et al 1995 Familial Alzheimer's chromosome 14 mutations. Nat Med 1:848

Wisniewski KE, Dalton AJ, Crapper-McLachlan DR, Wen GY, Wisniewski HM 1985 Alzheimer's disease in Down's syndrome: clinicopathologic studies. Neurology 35:957–961

Wisniewski T, Ghiso J, Frangione B 1991 Peptides homologous to the amyloid protein of Alzheimer's disease containing a glutamine for glutamic acid substitution have accelerated amyloid fibril formation. Biochem Biophys Res Commun 179:1247–1254

Yoshikai S, Sasaki H, Doh-Ura K, Furuya H, Sakaki Y 1990 Genomic organization of the human amyloid beta-protein precursor gene. Gene 87:257–263

DISCUSSION

Masters: How many of the supposedly sporadic early-onset cases of Alzheimer's disease are caused by mutations?

Hendriks: We have looked at a couple of hundred, but we haven't found any mutations. However, we didn't sequence them all. We did single-strand conformational polymorphism (SSCP) and restriction enzyme analysis for the most common mutations, so we might have missed some. I don't think mutations are a major cause of these sporadic early-onset cases.

J. D. Buxbaum: What is the evidence that the VRSQ motif is a consensus for phosphorylation? Which protein kinases might be active on this sequence, in the context of the flanking sequences in presenilin?

Hendriks: The VRSQ sequence is part of two possible phosphorylation sites for protein kinase C (TVR) and casein kinase II (SQND).

Benson: The Phe717 mutation (chromosome 21) family show symptoms in the late 30s or the early 40s: if they make it to the early 50s they're probably beyond risk. Consequently I wouldn't compare this mutation with S182. Ile717 appears to have later onset. I don't know about Gly717.

Goldgaber: How many families with early-onset Alzheimer's disease do not show any mutations so far described?

Hendriks: We have DNA and lymphoblastic cells from six early-onset and four late-onset Alzheimer's disease families (Van Duijn et al 1994). One early-onset Alzheimer's disease family showed suggestive linkage with chromosome 14 DNA markers (Van Duijn et al 1994) and a mutation has been detected in the presenilin 1 gene (unpublished results). In the other families no mutation has been found so far. Screening has been done by SSCP and restriction enzyme analysis for the most common presenilin 1 and presenilin 2 mutations. Sequencing of the entire coding regions of these genes is underway. It is possible that other AD genes exist besides APP and presenilin 1 and 2, but at present we cannot say how many early- or late-onset AD families do not carry mutations in these three genes. Most research groups have only partially screened their AD families for mutations, especially in the two presenilin genes.

Kisilevsky: Where on chromosome 1 is the presenilin 2 gene?

Hendriks: 1q31–42.

Kisilevsky: The reason I ask is that the gene for the HSPG, perlecan, the one found in many amyloids, is also on chromosome 1, at p36.1.

Reference

Van Duijn CM, Hendriks L, Farrer LA et al 1994 A population based study of familial Alzheimer disease: linkage to chromosome 14, 19 and 21. Am J Hum Genet 55:714–727

Prion protein amyloid: separation of scrapie infectivity from PrP polymers

Holger Wille*, Michael A. Baldwin*, Fred E. Cohen†‡¶, Stephen J. DeArmond*§ and Stanley B. Prusiner*†

*Departments of *Neurology, †Biochemistry and Biophysics, ‡Molecular and Cellular Pharmacology, ¶Medicine and §Pathology, University of California, San Francisco, CA 94143, USA*

Abstract. The prion protein (PrP) undergoes a profound conformational change when the cellular isoform (PrP^C) is converted into the scrapie form (PrP^{Sc}). Limited proteolysis of PrP^{Sc} produces PrP27–30 which readily polymerizes into amyloid. To study the structure of PrP amyloid, we employed organic solvents that perturb protein conformation. 1,1,1,3,3,3-Hexafluoro-2-propanol (HFIP), which promotes α-helix formation, modified the ultrastructure of rod-shaped PrP amyloids, producing flattened ribbons with a more regular substructure. As the concentration of HFIP was increased, the β-sheet content and proteinase K resistance of PrP27–30 as well as prion infectivity diminished. HFIP reversibly decreased the binding of Congo red dye to the rods, whereas inactivation of prion infectivity was irreversible. In contrast to 10% HFIP, 1,1,1-trifluoro-2-propanol (TFIP) did not inactivate prion infectivity but, similarly to HFIP, TFIP did alter the morphology of the rods and abolished Congo red binding. Our studies separate prion infectivity from the amyloid properties of PrP27–30 and underscore the dependence of prion infectivity on PrP^{Sc} conformation. Our results also demonstrate that the specific β-sheet-rich structures required for prion infectivity are different from those needed for amyloid formation.

1996 The nature and origin of amyloid fibrils. Wiley, Chichester (Ciba Foundation Symposium 199) p 181–201

Prions cause neurodegenerative diseases such as scrapie in sheep, bovine spongiform encephalopathy in cattle, and Creutzfeldt–Jakob disease (CJD) in humans (Prusiner & DeArmond 1995). The only known component of the prion particle is the scrapie isoform of the prion protein, designated PrP^{Sc} (Prusiner 1991). Although prions multiply, there is no evidence that they contain nucleic acid (Kellings et al 1992). PrP^{Sc} is derived from the cellular protein (PrP^C) by a post-translational process during which PrP^C undergoes a profound conformational change.

Molecular modelling studies suggested that PrP^C might be a four-helix bundle protein. This prediction gained considerable support when spectroscopic studies of PrP^{C} demonstrated that the protein contains 42% α-helix and is devoid of β-sheet (Pan et al 1993). In contrast, PrP^{Sc} is dominated by β-sheets (43%) and has a lower α-helical content (20–30%) (Pan et al 1993, Safar et al 1993a). All attempts to date to identify a chemical modification that distinguishes PrP^{Sc} from PrP^{C} have been unrewarding (Stahl et al 1993). Procedures that denature proteins diminish prion infectivity (Prusiner 1982) and, more specifically, have been shown to diminish the β-sheet content of PrP^{Sc} (Gasset et al 1993, Prusiner et al 1993, Safar et al 1993a).

Limited proteolysis of PrP^{Sc} produces an N-terminally truncated protein designated PrP27–30 with retention of infectivity. Polymers of PrP27–30 form amyloids as demonstrated by staining with the dye Congo red and green–gold birefringence when examined under polarized light (Prusiner et al 1983). To date, all amyloids studied exhibit these tinctorial properties which result from their high β-sheet content and ordered, linear polymeric structures (Cohen et al 1982, Glenner 1980, Glenner et al 1972). The β-sheet content of PrP27–30 as measured by Fourier transform infrared spectroscopy, circular dichroism and X-ray diffraction is between 47 and 54% (Caughey et al 1991, Gasset et al 1993, Nguyen et al 1995, Pan et al 1993, Safar et al 1993b) and it forms linear polymers that are indistinguishable from amyloids ultrastructurally (McKinley et al 1991a, Prusiner et al 1983).

We compared the prion infectivity with the ultrastructure of PrP polymers prepared by different purification schemes. Fluorinated solvents were used to alter both the solubility and conformation of PrP27–30. These solvents were also used to dissociate the prion infectivity from both the amyloid properties and proteinase K resistance of PrP27–30. These findings extend earlier studies which showed that scrapie infectivity can be preserved when PrP amyloid is dispersed into detergent–lipid–protein complexes (DLPCs) (Gabizon et al 1987) and that PrP^{Sc} only forms amyloid polymers after it is converted into PrP27–30. The results presented here and those from earlier investigations argue that amyloid formation is not required for either PrP^{Sc} synthesis or prion propagation. This conclusion stands in opposition to the view of others that PrP^{Sc} formation occurs through amyloid polymers (Bessen et al 1995, Come et al 1993, Gajdusek 1987, 1994, Jarrett & Lansbury 1993, Kocisko et al 1994, 1995). While both scrapie infectivity and amyloid formation require PrPs with β-sheets, the specific β-sheet-rich structures required for prion infectivity are different from those needed for amyloid formation.

Pathogenesis of PrP amyloid

An early indication that PrP^{Sc} might be pathogenic was the finding that the amyloid plaques in human and animal prion diseases react specifically with PrP antibodies (DeArmond et al 1985, 1987, Kitamoto et al 1986, Roberts et al

1988, Snow et al 1989). However, amyloid plaques are not a constant feature of prion diseases. They are detected by standard haematoxylin and eosin stain, periodic acid–Schiff reaction or Congo red dye stain in only 5–10% of CJD and 50–70% of kuru cases (Masters et al 1981). By definition, all cases of Gerstmann–Sträussler–Scheinker disease (GSS) have amyloid plaques, since the diagnosis requires the triad of cerebellar and/or corticospinal tract degeneration, dementia and cerebral amyloidosis (Gerstmann et al 1936).

In experimental scrapie of rodents, amyloid plaques are found in some but not all instances. Amyloid deposition depends upon the prion isolate or 'strain' used to inoculate the animal and on the sequence of the PrP gene. In fact, amyloidogenicity has been one of the characteristics used to classify prion isolates (Bruce et al 1976). For example, the 87V prion isolate leads to the formation of well-defined PrP amyloid plaques in several inbred mouse strains, but 22A prions do not. Since the amino acid sequence of PrP in a given mouse strain is presumably the same regardless of the prion isolate, one would have to postulate that 87V confers amyloidogenic secondary and/or tertiary configurations (e.g. a different β-sheet configuration) to PrP which 22A does not possess.

In transgenic (Tg) mice expressing Syrian hamster (SHa) PrP, the *de novo* synthesis of prions is species specific and reflects the genetic origin of the inoculated prions (Prusiner et al 1990). Similarly, the neuropathology of Tg(SHaPrP) mice is determined by the genetic origin of prion inoculum. Mouse prions injected into Tg(SHaPrP) mice produced a neuropathology characteristic of mice with scrapie. A moderate degree of vacuolation in both the grey and white matter was found while amyloid plaques were rarely detected (Table 1). Inoculation of Tg(SHaPrP) mice with SHa prions produced intense vacuolation of the grey matter, sparing of the white matter, and numerous SHaPrP amyloid plaques characteristic of Syrian hamsters with scrapie.

The inherited prion diseases of humans demonstrate that formation of PrP amyloid is also related to the amino acid sequence of PrP. For example, patients with GSS (P102L) always develop PrP amyloid plaques which contain the mutant protein as determined by amino acid sequencing (Hsiao et al 1989, Kitamoto et al 1991). In contrast, patients with familial CJD (E200K) exhibit profound spongiform degeneration but do not show PrP amyloid accumulation (Gabizon et al 1993, Hsiao et al 1991). Although GSS patients always develop PrP amyloid plaques, only some Tg(MoPrP—P101L) mice which express a mouse PrP transgene mimicking the codon 102 mutation of GSS also develop amyloid plaques (Hsiao et al 1990, 1994). The deposition of PrP in Tg(MoPrP—P101L) mice was greatly increased when these animals were crossed with null Prnp°/° mice in which the MoPrP gene was disrupted, which eliminated the expression of wild-type PrP (G. C. Telling & S. B. Prusiner, unpublished results).

TABLE 1 Species-specific prion inocula determine the distribution of spongiform change and deposition of PrP amyloid plaques in transgenic mice

	SHa prions					*Mo prions*			
		Spongiform change[a]		*PrP plaques*[b]			*Spongiform change*[a]		*PrP plaques*[b]
Animal	*n*[c]	*Grey*	*White*	*Frequency*	*Diameter*[d]	*n*[c]	*Grey*	*White*	*Frequency*
Non-Tg	ND[e]			ND		10	+	+	–
Tg 69	6	+[f]	–	Numerous	6.5 ± 3.1 (389)	2	+	+	–
Tg 71	5	+	–	Numerous	8.1 ± 3.6 (345)	2	+	+	–
Tg 81	7	+	–	Numerous	8.3 ± 3.0 (439)	3	+	+	Few
Tg 7	3	+[g]	–	Numerous	14.0 ± 8.3 (19)	4	+	+	–
SHa	3	+	–	Numerous	5.7 ± 2.7 (247)	ND			ND

[a]Spongiform change evaluated in hippocampus, thalamus, cerebral cortex and brainstem for grey matter and the deep cerebellum for white matter.
[b]Plaques in the subcallosal region were stained with SHaPrP mAb 13A5, anti-PrP rabbit antisera R073 and trichrome stain.
[c]*n*, number of brains examined.
[d]Mean diameter of PrP plaques given in microns ± SEM with the number of observations in parentheses.
[e]ND, not determined.
[f]+, present; –, absent.
[g]Focal: confirmed to the dorsal nucleus of the raphe.
From Prusiner (1992).

Prion rod fine structure

Although prion rods are an artefact of limited proteolysis in the presence of detergent, they do possess the properties of amyloids and thus have a naturally occurring counterpart, i.e. the amyloid fibrils of PrP plaques in the brains of some animals with prion disease. When we examined the fraction P3 generated from scrapie-infected Syrian hamster brain by limited proteolysis in the presence of detergents (Prusiner et al 1983), we observed small rod-like aggregates and larger sheets (Fig. 1A). Further fractionation of P3 by sucrose gradient centrifugation produced rod-shaped aggregates often referred to as prion rods (Fig. 1B). To distinguish these rods from those prepared by another method, we refer to them as 'SG rods'.

An alternative method of preparation using ultrafiltration in the presence of Sarkosyl (Hecker et al 1992) also produces rod-shaped structures but these appear to be less tightly aggregated. These rods (termed 'UF rods') show a more detailed substructure with individual fibrils running parallel to the long axis (Fig. 1C). Dilution of the Sarkosyl followed by a precipitation and centrifugation led to a loss of UF rod ultrastructure. Residual detergents and lipids appear to form small vesicular structures and may contain some PrP27–30 molecules (Fig. 1D). When the UF rods were subjected to sucrose gradient centrifugation, small rods with the same ultrastructural features as the original SG rods (Fig. 1E) were found. The rods prepared by combining ultrafiltration and sucrose gradient centrifugation were designated 'UFSG rods'. The major difference between the SG rods and the UFSG rods is that the latter are smaller. If the residual Sarkosyl of the UF rod preparation was removed by repeated washing, all rods disappeared and only membranous vesicles were observed (data not shown). Since PrP27–30 was precipitated during these repeated washings, we conclude that the protein is associated with the membranes.

Morphology of prion rods exposed to HFIP

Negatively stained samples of untreated SG rods showed the typical prion rod structures (Fig. 2A). After addition of 10% 1,1,1,2,2,2-hexafluoro-2-propanol (HFIP), the rods began to disassemble into smaller units which exhibited a more regular substructure. The disassembly appeared more prominent at the ends of the rods (Fig. 2B). A few minutes after the addition of HFIP, all SG rods had disassembled into smaller particles which we then termed 'HFIP rods' (Fig. 2C). HFIP rods resemble sheet-like structures with curled-up edges, resulting in two light bands visible in the electron micrographs. Evaporation of HFIP led to a reaggregation into amorphous structures which showed no regular substructure or similarities to normal SG rods (Fig. 2D).

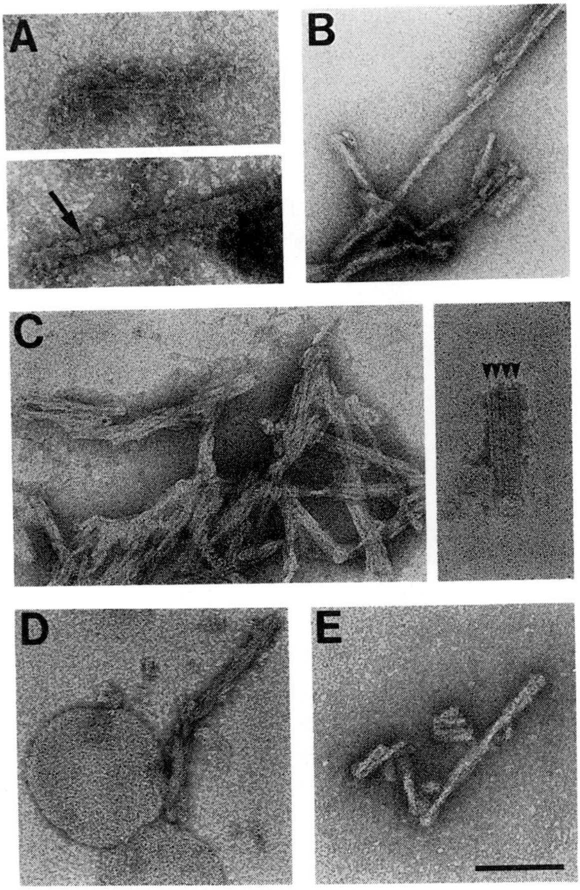

FIG. 1. Electron microscopy of prion rods. Purified fractions negatively stained with 2% ammonium molybdate. (A) The P3 fraction prepared by detergent extraction and limited proteolysis (Prusiner et al 1983) contained some small rod-shaped structures and larger sheets (arrow). (B) SG rods obtained by sucrose gradient centrifugation. Internal substructure is difficult to discern presumably due to the tightly packed aggregates of PrP27–30. (C) UF rods prepared by ultrafiltration. These rods in the retentate demonstrate more substructure suggesting that the aggregates are composed of less tightly bound PrP27–30 molecules. Arrowheads denote filamentous substructures. (D) UF rods after removal of Sarkosyl by dilution and precipitation (denoted P4) lose their regular substructure. Residual lipids and Sarkosyl seem to form membranous vesicles which most likely contain PrP27–30. (E) UFSG rods formed from P4 by sucrose gradient centrifugation These rods show no clear ultrastructure and resemble SG rods. Bar = 100 nm.

In contrast, UF rods (Fig. 2E) showed very few ultrastructural changes even at high concentrations of HFIP (50% HFIP, Fig. 2F). This behaviour parallels the resistance shown in bioassays of HFIP-treated UF rods described below (see Table 2). Furthermore, addition of sucrose does not allow the UF rods to form HFIP rods upon addition of the solvent (data not shown). UF rods subjected to sucrose gradient centrifugation (UFSG rods, Fig. 2G) treated with HFIP resembled those seen after addition of HFIP to SG rods (Fig. 2H).

Although up to 4% HFIP did not alter the morphology of the rods, 5% HFIP produced a marked increase in substructure. However, the SG rods still retained their overall shape. At 6% HFIP or higher, the ultrastructure of the rods underwent a profound change which was coincident with the decrease in prion infectivity (Fig. 3).

HFIP inactivates prion infectivity

Increasing the concentration of HFIP resulted in a progressive reduction in prion infectivity of the SG rods. Up to 2.5% HFIP did not alter infectivity, whereas 5% HFIP reduced the infectivity by more than a factor of 10. At 7% or higher concentrations of HFIP, infectivity of the SG rods was almost completely abolished (Fig. 2). In contrast, the UF rods showed little reduction in infectivity at concentrations of up to 10% HFIP (Fig. 3). However, sucrose gradient centrifugation of the UF rods rendered prion infectivity susceptible to inactivation by HFIP. The HFIP inactivation profile for the UFSG rods was similar to that of the SG rods. From these findings, we concluded that exposure to sucrose rendered prion infectivity susceptible to inactivation by HFIP.

Neither removal of HFIP by evaporation nor addition of acetonitrile (which promotes β-sheet formation) reversed the inactivation of prion infectivity by HFIP. Unexpectedly, the structurally related solvent 1,1,1-trifluoro-2-propanol (TFIP) had no adverse effect on infectivity at concentrations of up to 50% (Table 2). It is notable that TFIP seems to disperse the SG rods into smaller structures, perhaps increasing the efficiency of infection. A variety of solvents including 2,2,3,3-tetrafluoro-1-propanol (tetF1P) and 1-methyl-2-pyrrolidinone (NMP), similarly to TFIP, did not inactivate prion infectivity while 1,1,1,3,3,3-hexafluoroacetone (HFA) reduced SG rod infectivity at higher concentrations. The solvents perfluoro-tert-butyl alcohol (PFtBA) and 1,1,1,3,3,4,4,4-octofluoro-2-butanol (OFIB) reduced SG rod infectivity at low concentrations like HFIP. Control animals injected with diluted solvents showed no abnormalities (data not shown).

UF rods proved to be much more resistant to inactivation of prion infectivity by various solvents. Up to 10% HFIP reduced infectivity by a factor of about 10, which probably did not represent a significant change. The other solvents tested had no effect on infectivity (Table 2).

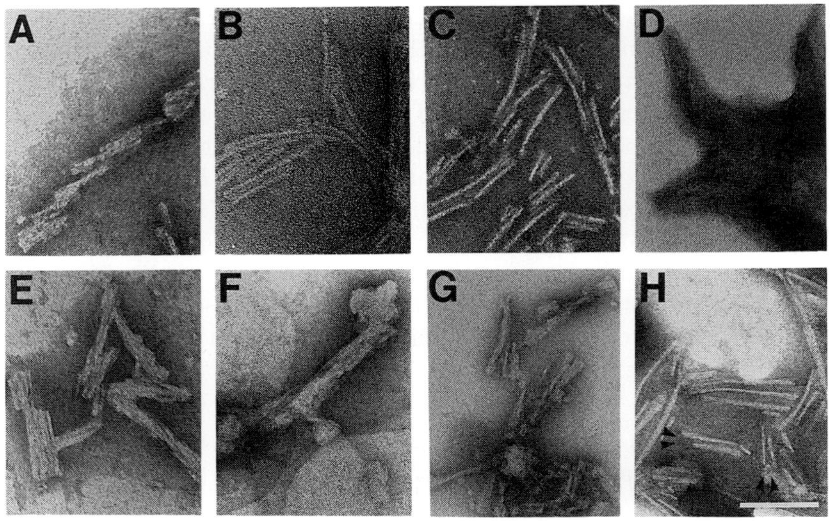

FIG. 2. Electron microscopy of negatively stained prion rods exposed to HFIP. (A) SG rods without HFIP. (B) SG rods examined immediately after exposure to 10% HFIP. Rods starting to break up into smaller particles and reveal a more regular substructure. (C) SG rods incubated with 10% HFIP for 20 min at room temperature. Rods are smaller and exhibit more regular sheet-like structures which were termed 'HFIP rods'. These HFIP rods showed two parallel, unstained bands which seem to originate from the curled edges of flattened sheet-like rods. (D) Removal of the HFIP by evaporation led to a reaggregation into amorphous aggregates. These aggregates showed no substructure. (E) UF rods without HFIP. (F) UF rods treated with 50% HFIP. The rods showed some loss of substructure. (G) UFSG rods showed the same lack of clear substructure as SG rods. (H) UFSG rods exposed to 10% HFIP resemble typical HFIP rods. Panels A, B, C, D, G and H stained with 2% uranyl acetate; E and F with 2% ammonium molybdate. Bar = 100 nm.

Proteinase K resistance and exposure to solvents

Since formation of the rods depends on the resistance of PrP^{Sc} to limited proteinase K digestion, we measured the resistance of the SG rods to proteolytic digestion after 20 min exposure to various solvents. Whereas 10% HFIP abolished the resistance to proteinase K, similar concentrations of TFIP, NMP and 2-propanol did not. Since both HFIP and TFIP inhibited the activity of proteinase K, we removed these solvents by evaporation prior to the digestion. Thus, proteinase K resistance could not be restored by the removal of HFIP. In contrast, NMP and 2-propanol did not inhibit proteinase K activity. At concentrations of HFIP up to 2.5%, it had no effect on the proteinase K resistance of SG rods but at 3%, the amount of PrP27–30 after proteinase K digestion was substantially reduced and at concentrations of 3.5% or higher, no PrP27–30 could be detected.

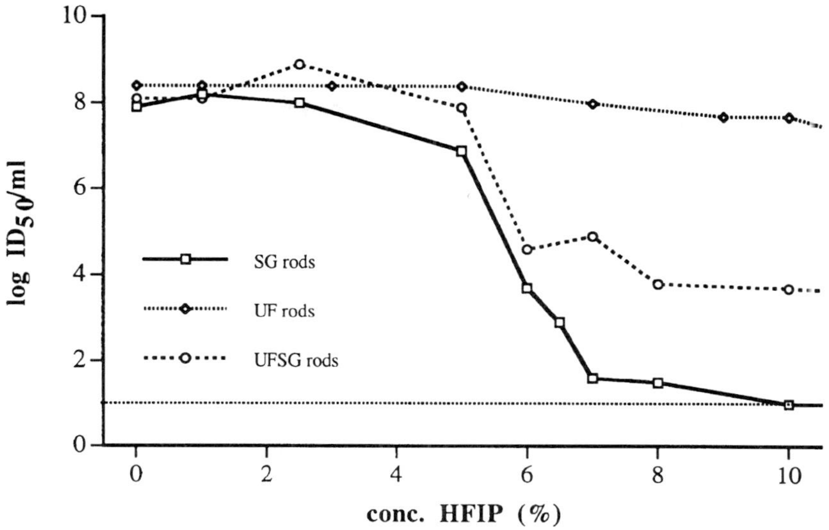

FIG. 3. Bioassays of prion rods exposed to HFIP. Prion rods were exposed to increasing concentrations of HFIP for at least 20 min at room temperature. SG rods (squares), UF rods (diamonds) or UFSG rods (circles) exposed to HFIP were diluted 100 times and aliquots (50 μl) thereof were inoculated intracerebrally into Syrian hamsters. Prion titres in ID_{50} units/ml were calculated from standard curves relating incubation times to prion dose.

Sucrose but not glycerol supports the HFIP changes

The profound changes in the induced ultrastructure of the SG and UFSG rods by HFIP were prevented if the sucrose from the gradient was diluted below 12.5% (w/v) (data not shown). Replacing the ~50% sucrose from the sucrose gradient centrifugation by 50% (w/v) solutions of di- and monosaccharides such as maltose, β-lactose, galactose or glucose did not interfere with the HFIP effect. Even polyalcohols, such as inositol, sorbitol or adonitol supported the HFIP effect. Erythritol, as a small polyalcohol, induced an intermediate response to HFIP with some SG rods being transformed into HFIP rods while others appeared unchanged (data not shown). The structure of the SG rods was unperturbed by HFIP when either 1,2,6-trihydroxyhexane or glycerol was substituted for sucrose.

Besides preventing the effects of HFIP on SG rod morphology, 50% glycerol also prevented the inactivation of prion infectivity (Table 4). Bioassays showed that the presence of co-solvents had a marked effect on the HFIP-induced reduction in infectivity of PrP27–30. While 50% glycerol does not support the formation of HFIP rods (see above), it protects the infectivity against HFIP (Table 4). Sarkosyl seems to provide modest protection of prion infectivity from inactivation by HFIP but it was not as effective as glycerol.

TABLE 2 Bioassays of solvent-treated prion rods

Protein	*Solvent added*	(n/n_0) [a]	*Log titre* $(ID_{50}/ml \pm SD)$
SG rods	none	5/8[b]	7.6 ± 0.6
	10% HFIP	0/4	< 1
	10% HFIP, −HFIP[c]	0/4	< 1
	50% HFIP, −HFIP[c]	0/8	< 1
	10% HFIP, +50% acetronitrile, −solvents[c]	0/8	< 1
	10% TFIP	4/4	8.4 ± 0
	50% TFIP, −TFIP[c]	4/4	8.4 ± 0
	10% tetF1P	4/4	7.9 ± 0.3
	50% tetF1P	3/4	7.9 ± 0.4
	10% 3TF1P	4/4	8.3 ± 0.1
	50% 3TF1P, −3TF1P[c]	4/4	7.5 ± 0.2
	10% HFA	4/4	7.7 ± 0
	50% HFA	0/4	< 1
	10% PFtBA	4/4	4.8 ± 0
	50% PFtBA	3/4[b]	4.8 ± 0
	10% OFIB	4/4	4.8 ± 0
	50% OFIB	3/4	5.3 ± 0.8
	10% NMP	4/4	7.9 ± 0.3
	50% NMP, −NMP[cd]	4/4	7.8 ± 0.2
	5% acetonitrile	4/4	8.1 ± 0
	10% acetonitrile	4/4	7.6 ± 0.3
	25% acetonitrile	4/4	7.8 ± 0.4
UF rods	none	4/4	8.4 ± 0
	10% HFIP	4/4	7.2 ± 0.6
	10% TFIP	4/4	8.3 ± 1.3
	10% 3TF1P	4/4	8.4 ± 0
	10% NMP	4/4	8.6 ± 0.1
Buffer control		0/8	< 1

[a]Number of animals with clinical scrapie/number of animals inoculated.
[b]Remaining animals died of causes other than scrapie.
[c]Organic solvents were removed by evaporation after incubation for at least 20 minutes.
[d]Incomplete removal of NMP.

TABLE 3 Ultrastructural effects of various solvents on prion rods

Solvent	SG rods	Solvent-induced structural changes	
		Rods with increased substructure[a]	*HFIP rods*
HFIP	−	−	+ + +
TFIP	−	+	+ +
PF1P	−	+ +	+
tetF1P	−	+ +	+
3TF1P	+	+ +	−
2-propanol	+ + +	−	−
HFA	−	+ + +	−
PFtBA	−	−	+ + +
OFIB	−	−	+ + +
TFE	−	+ +	+
HFB	+ +	+	−
NMP	+	+ +	−
acetonitrile	+ + +	−	−
n-butanol	+ + +	−	−

+ + +, close to 100% of all rods in this state; + +, around 60% of all rods in this state; +, around 30% of all rods in this state; −, no rods in this state.
[a]HFIP rods and rods with similar ultrastructure not included.

Congo red binding

Because prion rods bind Congo red dye and exhibit green–gold birefringence under polarized light (Prusiner et al 1983), we examined the effect of HFIP on Congo red dye binding. In the presence of 50% sucrose, Congo red alone showed an absorption maximum at 504 nm which shifted to a shorter wavelength of ~450 nm when bound to SG rods (Fig. 4A). Addition of 2.5% HFIP or more disrupted the protein–dye complex and the Congo red spectrum shifted back to its unbound state (data not shown). The presence of as little as 0.1% HFIP reduced the Congo red binding by >50% (Fig. 4B, triangles). Further addition of HFIP up to 1.2% had little impact on the residual Congo red binding with an apparent plateau between 0.4 and 1.2% HFIP. At 2.5% HFIP, Congo red binding was abolished even though prion infectivity remained unaffected at this concentration (Fig. 4B, triangles; Fig. 3). After incubation of SG rods with HFIP, the solvent was evaporated and the Congo red binding restored (Fig. 4B, empty squares). Reversing the sequence of addition of HFIP and Congo red gave virtually the same results, arguing that the results were unlikely to be due to interference between HFIP and

TABLE 4 Effects of glycerol and Sarkosyl on scrapie infectivity after addition to prion rod preparations

Protein	*Additions*	*(n/n_0)* [a]	*Log titre ($ID_{50}/ml \pm SD$)*
SG rods	(control)	4/4	7.7 ± 0.8
	+10% HFIP	0/4	<1
	in 50% glycerol, +10% HFIP	4/4	7.5 ± 0.4
	in 50% glycerol	4/4	7.9 ± 0.5
	+2% Sarkosyl, 10% HFIP	4/4	4.5 ± 0
	+2% Sarkosyl	3/4	8.1 ± 0
Buffer control		0/4	<1

[a]Number of animals with clinical scrapie/number of animals inoculated.

Congo red (data not shown). PrP^C did not bind Congo red under the conditions used here (Fig. 4B, closed square).

The closely related solvent TFIP had essentially the same effect on Congo red binding as HFIP. Congo red dye binding was substantially diminished at 0.8% and abolished at 10% (v/v) TFIP (Fig. 4C). As with HFIP, the inhibition of Congo red binding by TFIP was reversible (data not shown). NMP also inhibited Congo red binding but the effect was seen only at concentrations above 1.6% NMP (Fig. 4C).

Secondary structure conversions

Fourier transform infrared spectroscopy of SG rods in PBS with 0.12% Zwittergent 3-12 (PBSZ) showed a spectrum (Fig. 5) indicating a high amount of low frequency β-sheet (between 1641 cm^{-1} and 1613 cm^{-1}) and a small amount of α-helical and turn components at 1662–1650 cm^{-1} and 1682–1662.5 cm^{-1}, respectively. Occasionally, SG rods displayed a predominantly α-helical spectrum (data not shown). These preparations seemed to be contaminated with higher amounts of ferritin as determined by Western blotting α-ferritin antisera and electron microscopy; ferritin has a high α-helical content.

Transferring the SG rods from PBSZ in D_2O to 25% sucrose in D_2O shifted the infrared spectrum from low frequency β-sheet to one with more α-helical and high frequency β-sheet signals (Fig. 5). This shift from low frequency to high frequency β-sheet signals can be attributed to a shift from predominantly intermolecular to intramolecular β-sheet contacts (Byler & Susi 1986, Jackson & Mantsch 1992), during which the percentage of β-sheet decreases slightly (Table 5). The small increase in α-helix content could be explained by the helix-

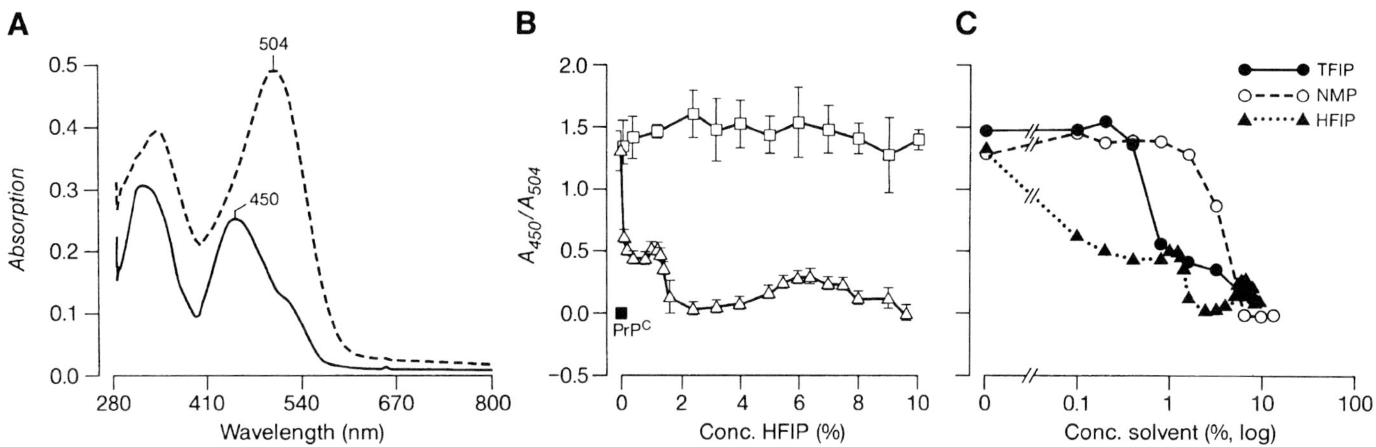

FIG. 4. Binding of Congo red dye to prion rods. (A) Absorption spectra of Congo red bound to SG rods in the presence of 50% sucrose (solid line) and Congo red alone (dashed line). (B) Disruption of the Congo red/SG rod complex as a function of HFIP concentration (open triangles) as measured by absorption at 450 and 504 nm. SG rods exposed to HFIP followed by evaporation of the solvent showed no significant decrease in the binding of Congo red (open squares). Data points for both curves represent the mean of three independent measurements, error bars indicate the standard deviation. PrP^C did not bind Congo red (closed square). (C) SG rods were exposed to HFIP, TFIP or NMP and absorption was measured at 450 and 504 nm.

promoting effect of polyols such as sucrose and glycerol that has been found in the model system melittin (Bello 1993).

Addition of 10% HFIP increased the amount of α-helix and decreased the β-sheet content to ~17% (Fig. 5), coinciding with a complete loss of infectivity (Fig. 3). The addition of 2.5% HFIP reduced the β-sheet content while increasing the content of α-helix and random coil, but did not alter infectivity. Addition of TFIP caused the infrared spectrum to increase its α-helix and random coil signals (Fig. 5, Table 5).

Perturbation of prion rod ultrastructure

As reported here, HFIP, which promotes α-helix formation and diminishes β-sheet content of polypeptides, decreased scrapie prion infectivity. HFIP also changed the morphology of the prion rods which are composed largely of PrP27–30. The rods acquired a more regular appearance and exhibited a better defined substructure after exposure to HFIP.

The precise mechanism by which solvents such as HFIP induce α-helical structure is still under debate, but it is likely that they disrupt internal hydrogen bond networks in folded proteins owing to the strong hydrogen bond donor characteristics of these solvents. This allows the formation of new and more stable secondary structure elements in the absence of well defined tertiary structures (Jackson & Mantsch 1992, Thomas & Dill 1993). It is interesting to note that HFA, which can only act as a hydrogen bond acceptor, is almost as effective as HFIP in diminishing prion infectivity (Table 1).

Limitations of spectroscopy

A comparison of the data reported for prion infectivity (Fig. 3; Table 2) and the secondary structure of PrP27–30 (Table 5) demonstrates the limitations of our attempts to correlate these parameters. While inactivation of scrapie infectivity seems to be associated with a change in secondary structure which is usually a decrease in β-sheet, such diminutions in β-sheet content are not necessarily accompanied by a decrement in prion titre. For example, 2.5% HFIP reduced the β-sheet content of PrP27–30 from ~45% to 21% (Table 5) without any change in infectivity (Fig. 3), whereas 10% HFIP produced no further decrement in β-sheet content but decreased infectivity by $>10^7$ ID_{50} units/ml. In contrast, 10% TFIP reduced β-sheet content from ~45% to 28% (Table 5) but no change in infectivity was observed (Table 2).

These comparisons suggest that spectroscopic measurements do not provide sufficient detail for precise correlations between protein structure and prion infectivity. While more precise assessments of PrP^{Sc} structure are desirable, the insolubility of this protein makes such measurements problematic. Neither the

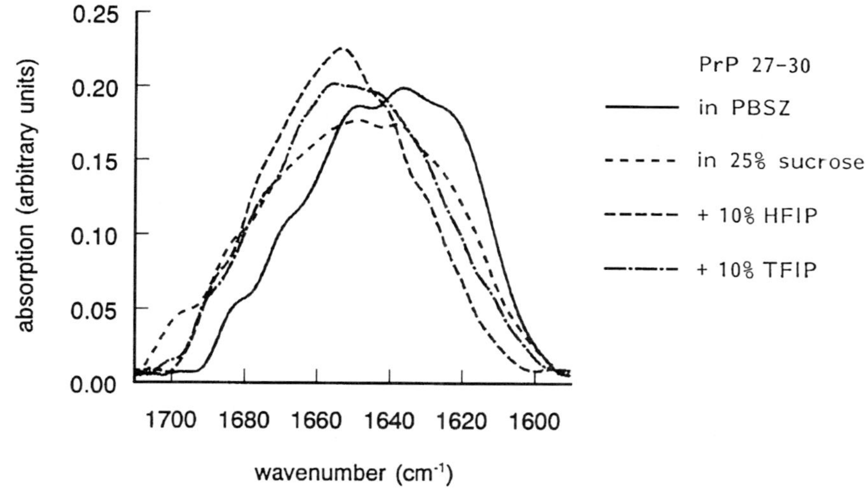

FIG. 5. Fourier transform infrared spectroscopy of SG rods exposed to HFIP or TFIP. SG rods in PBSZ (solid line) showed a broad maximum of absorption between 1650 cm^{-1} and 1610 cm^{-1}. HFIP surpassed the effect of TFIP increasing the α-helix and random coil signals even further. All curves were normalized to show equal areas.

binding of Congo red dye nor the rod ultrastructure provided better correlates with scrapie infectivity.

Prion propagation and PrP amyloid

Our attempts to identify structural parameters that correlate prion infectivity with amyloid had limited success. Although the formation of prion rods with

TABLE 5 Secondary structure content of PrP27–30 after exposure to HFIP and TFIP

		Secondary structure in %			
Protein	*Additions*	*α-helix*	*β-sheet*	*Turns*	*Coil*
SG rods in PBSZ		23	48	9	20
in 25% sucrose		27	43	13	17
	+2.5% HFIP	41	21	10	28
	+5% HFIP	36	25	15	24
	+10% HFIP	46	17	16	21
	+2.5% TFIP	34	33	11	22
	+5% TFIP	40	27	14	19
	+10% TFIP	40	28	12	20

the morphology and properties of amyloid has only been found associated with preparations exhibiting scrapie infectivity, such polymers are not obligatory for infectivity (Gabizon et al 1987, McKinley et al 1991b, Pan et al 1993). SG rods exhibited an altered morphology above 5% HFIP and infectivity diminished substantially; 10% TFIP also altered rod morphology but did not change prion titres.

The amyloid properties of the prion rods as measured by the binding of Congo red dye to PrP27–30 were clearly dissociable from scrapie infectivity. For example, 2.5% HFIP abolished Congo red binding to SG rods (Fig. 4) but did not alter prion titres (Fig. 3). With exposure to 10% HFIP, both Congo red binding and infectivity were abolished but Congo red binding could be restored by evaporation of the HFIP whereas infectivity was not.

This dissociation between PrP amyloid and scrapie infectivity is of significance since some investigators have argued that PrP^{Sc} synthesis proceeds through the addition of PrP^{C} molecules to PrP amyloid (Bessen et al 1995, Gajdusek 1987, 1994, Jarrett & Lansbury 1993, Kocisko et al 1994, 1995). Many lines of evidence argue against this hypothesis including many of the data presented here. First, fractions containing PrP^{Sc} purified from the brains of scrapie-infected Syrian hamsters contain only amorphous structures as judged by electron microscopy after negative staining (McKinley et al 1991b, Pan et al 1993). Second, limited proteolysis of PrP^{Sc} in the presence of detergent produced prion rods. Third, dispersion of the rods into DLPCs enhanced prion infectivity approximately 10-fold in many instances (Gabizon et al 1987). Fourth, Congo red dye binding did not correlate with scrapie infectivity (Figs 3 and 4).

Acknowledgements

We thank Hana Serban and the preparation team for the Pr27–30 and PrP^{Sc}, Keh-Ming Pan for the gift of PrP^{C}, Klaus Kellings for his samples of retentate material, Marilyn Torchia for help with the bioassays, Guo-Feng Zhang and Stephen D'Angelo for their help with some of the experiments for electron microscopy, Mei-Lie Wong for making available the darkroom facilities, and Dr Ronald Wetzel from SmithKline Beecham Pharmaceuticals for his advice on the Congo red binding assay. H. W. gratefully acknowledges postdoctoral fellowships from the Boehringer Ingelheim Fonds and Alexander von Humboldt-Stiftung. This work was supported by research grants from the National Institutes of Health and the Human Frontiers of Science program.

References

Bello J 1993 Helix promotion in polypeptides by polyols. Biopolymers 33:491–495

Bessen RA, Kocisko DA, Raymond GJ, Nandan S, Lansbury PT, Caughey B 1995 Non-genetic propagation of strain-specific properties of scrapie prion protein. Nature 375:698–700

Bruce ME, Dickinson AG, Fraser H 1976 Cerebral amyloidosis in scrapie in the mouse: effect of agent strain and mouse genotype. Neuropathol Appl Neurobiol 2:471–478
Byler DM, Susi H 1986 Examination of the secondary structure of proteins by deconvolved FTIR spectra. Biopolymers 25:469–487
Caughey BW, Dong A, Bhat KS, Ernst D, Hayes SF, Caughey WS 1991 Secondary structure analysis of the scrapie-associated protein PrP 27-30 in water by infrared spectroscopy. Biochemistry 30:7672–7680
Cohen AS, Shirahama T, Skinner M 1982 Electron microscopy of amyloid. In: Harris JR (ed) Electron microscopy of proteins, vol 3. Academic Press, New York, p 165–204
Come JH, Fraser PE, Lansbury PT Jr 1993 A kinetic model for amyloid formation in the prion diseases: importance of seeding. Proc Natl Acad Sci USA 90:5959–5963
DeArmond SJ, McKinley MP, Barry RA, Braunfeld MB, McColloch JR, Prusiner SB 1985 Identification of prion amyloid filaments in scrapie-infected brain. Cell 41: 221–235
DeArmond SJ, Mobley WC, DeMott DL, Barry RA, Beckstead JH, Prusiner SB 1987 Changes in the localization of brain prion proteins during scrapie infection. Neurology 37:1271–1280
Gabizon R, McKinley MP, Prusiner SB 1987 Purified prion proteins and scrapie infectivity copartition into liposomes. Proc Natl Acad Sci USA 84:4017–4021
Gabizon R, Rosenmann H, Meiner Z et al 1993 Mutation and polymorphism of the prion protein gene in Libyan Jews with Creutzfeldt–Jakob disease. Am J Hum Genet 33:828–835
Gajdusek DC 1987 The transmissible dementias and other brain disorders caused by unconventional viruses: relationship of transmissible to nontransmissible amyloidosis of the brain. In: Kurstak E, Lipowski ZJ, Morozov PV (eds) Viruses, immunity and mental disorders. Plenum, New York, p 3–22
Gajdusek DC 1994 Spontaneous generation of infectious nucleating amyloids in the transmissible and nontransmissible cerebral amyloidoses. Mol Neurobiol 8:1–13
Gasset M, Baldwin MA, Fletterick RJ, Prusiner SB 1993 Perturbation of the secondary structure of the scrapie prion protein under conditions associated with changes in infectivity. Proc Natl Acad Sci USA 90:1–5
Gerstmann J, Sträussler E, Scheinker L 1936 Über eine eigenartige hereditär-familiäre Erkrankung des Zentralnervensystems zugleich ein Beitrag zur Frage des vorzeitigen lokalen Alterns. Z Neurol 154:736–762
Glenner GG 1980 Amyloid deposits and amyloidosis. The β-fibrilloses. 1. N Engl J Med 302:1283–1292
Glenner GG, Eanes ED, Page DL 1972 The relation of the properties of Congo red-stained amyloid fibrils to the beta-conformation. J Histochem Cytochem 20:821–826
Hecker R, Taraboulos A, Scott M et al 1992 Replication of distinct prion isolates is region specific in brains of transgenic mice and hamsters. Genes & Dev 6:1213–1228
Hsiao K, Baker HF, Crow TJ et al 1989 Linkage of a prion protein missense variant to Gerstmann-Sträussler syndrome. Nature 338:342–345
Hsiao KK, Scott M, Foster D, Groth DF, DeArmond SJ, Prusiner SB 1990 Spontaneous neurodegeneration in transgenic mice with mutant prion protein. Science 250:1587–1590
Hsiao K, Meiner Z, Kahana E et al 1991 Mutation of the prion protein in Libyan Jews with Creutzfeldt–Jakob disease. N Engl J Med 324:1091–1097
Hsiao KK, Groth D, Scott M et al 1994 Serial transmission in rodents of neurodegeneration from transgenic mice expressing mutant prion protein. Proc Natl Acad Sci USA 91:9126–9130

Jackson M, Mantsch HH 1992 Halogenated alcohols as solvents for proteins: FTIR spectroscopic studies. Biochim Biophys Acta 1118:139–143

Jarrett JT, Lansbury PT Jr 1993 Seeding 'one-dimensional crystallization' of amyloid: a pathogenic mechanism in Alzheimer's disease and scrapie? Cell 73:1055–1058

Kellings K, Meyer N, Mirenda C, Prusiner SB, Riesner D 1992 Further analysis of nucleic acids in purified scrapie prion preparations by improved return refocussing gel electrophoresis (RRGE). J Gen Virol 73:1025–1029

Kitamoto T, Tateishi J, Tashima I et al 1986 Amyloid plaques in Creutzfeld–Jakob disease stain with prion protein antibodies. Ann Neurol 20:204–208

Kitamoto T, Yamaguchi K, Doh-ura K, Tateishi J 1991 A prion protein missense variant is integrated in kuru plaque cores in patients with Gerstmann-Sträussler syndrome. Neurology 41:306–310

Kocisko DA, Come JH, Priola SA et al 1994 Cell-free formation of protease-resistant prion protein. Nature 370:471–474

Kocisko DA, Priola SA, Raymond GJ, Chesebro B, Lansbury PT Jr, Caughey B 1995 Species specificity in the cell-free conversion of prion protein to protease-resistant forms: a model for the scrapie species barrier. Proc Natl Acad Sci USA 92:3923–3927

Masters CL, Gajdusek DC, Gibbs CJ Jr 1981 Creutzfeldt–Jakob disease virus isolations from the Gerstmann-Sträussler syndrome. Brain 104:559–588

McKinley MP, Taraboulos A, Kenaga L et al 1991a Ultrastructural localization of scrapie prion proteins in cytoplasmic vesicles of infected cultured cells. Lab Invest 65:622–630

McKinley MP, Meyer R, Kenaga L et al 1991b Scrapie prion rod formation *in vitro* requires both detergent extraction and limited proteolysis. J Virol 65:1440–1449

Nguyen JT, Inouye H, Baldwin MA et al 1995 X-ray diffraction of scrapie prion rods and PrP peptides. J Mol Biol 252:412–422

Pan K-M, Baldwin M, Nguyen J et al 1993 Conversion of α-helices into β-sheets features in the formation of the scrapie prion proteins. Proc Natl Acad Sci USA 90:10962–10966

Prusiner SB 1982 Novel proteinaceous infectious particles cause scrapie. Science 216:136–144

Prusiner SB 1991 Molecular biology of prion diseases. Science 252:1515–1522

Prusiner SB 1992 Molecular biology and genetics of neurodegenerative diseases caused by prions. Adv Virus Res 41:241–280

Prusiner SB, DeArmond SJ 1995 Prion protein amyloid and neurodegeneration. Amyloid: Int J Exp Clin Invest 2:39–65

Prusiner SB, McKinley MP, Bowman KA et al 1983 Scrapie prions aggregate to form amyloid-like birefringent rods. Cell 35:349–358

Prusiner SB, Scott M, Foster D et al 1990 Transgenetic studies implicate interactions between homologous PrP isoforms in scrapie prion replication. Cell 63:673–686

Prusiner SB, Groth D, Serban A, Stahl N, Gabizon R 1993 Attempts to restore scrapie prion infectivity after exposure to protein denaturants. Proc Natl Acad Sci USA 90:2793–2797

Roberts GW, Lofthouse R, Allsop D et al 1988 CNS amyloid proteins in neurodegenerative diseases. Neurology 38:1534–1540

Safar J, Roller PP, Gajdusek DC, Gibbs CJ 1993a Thermal-stability and conformational transitions of scrapie amyloid (prion) protein correlate with infectivity. Protein Sci 2:2206–2216

Safar J, Roller PP, Gajdusek DC, Gibbs CJ 1993b Conformational transitions, dissociation, and unfolding of scrapie amyloid (prion) protein. J Biol Chem 268:20276–20284

Snow AD, Kisilevsky R, Willmer J, Prusiner SB, DeArmond SJ 1989 Sulfated glycosaminoglycans in amyloid plaques of prion diseases. Acta Neuropathol 77: 337–342
Stahl N, Baldwin MA, Teplow DB et al 1993 Structural studies of the scrapie prion protein using mass spectrometry and amino acid sequencing. Biochemistry 32: 1991–2002
Thomas PD, Dill KA 1993 Local and nonlocal interactions in globular proteins and mechanisms of alcohol denaturation. Protein Sci 2:2050–2065

DISCUSSION

Masters: Have you identified the normal binding partner of PrP^C? How are you tackling this problem?

Prusiner: One way is simply to look for binding proteins. We have done this and have identified six different proteins, but none of them make any sense. One can use techniques such as the yeast two-hybrid system to try to find normal partners of PrP^C, but this is very difficult because we don't have a function for PrP^C. This is why it was so difficult to purify it by non-denaturing steps, because we had no way of checking to see whether it was really denatured or not. There are a couple of studies in the literature by John Collinge and his colleagues suggesting that PrP^C is important in synapse formation in the hippocampus (Collinge et al 1994), but when we tried to repeat these studies we were unable to find any defects in the null mice in terms of hippocampal synaptic transmission (Lledo et al 1996).

There is an interesting story evolving in yeast. It is thought that there are prions in yeast (Wickner 1994). A set of studies from the University of Chicago by Susan Lindquist, Sue Liebmann and Yuri Chernoff suggest that the key for one of the prion states (which they call [PSI] in yeast—these are not diseases but different metabolic states) can be transmitted not through Mendelian genetics but through an episomal element which is not a nucleic acid (Chernoff et al 1995). They suggest that this is a prion-like mechanism. The key is a molecular chaperone, HSP104. If this chaperone is expressed at either too low or too high level, you can't get the [PSI] state. HSP104 is present in yeast and some lower organisms, but its analogue is not present in humans or mice.

Masters: The crossing of the PrP101 mutation onto the null background is fascinating in terms of amyloidogenesis and differentiating amyloidogenesis from infectivity. Has this been published?

Prusiner: Not yet.

Masters: Could you summarize what this tells us in terms of amyloid production, rate of disease progression and infectivity?

Prusiner: I think we all thought from Dickinson's work (Bruce et al 1976, Bruce & Dickinson 1985) that if the mice lived long enough you would see more amyloid being produced. Our studies show exactly the opposite, because the animals with PrP amyloid plaques do not live as long as those without plaques. These results are due to a competition between wild-type and mutant PrP, which differ by a single amino acid. I don't understand exactly what that means in terms of amyloid deposition.

Masters: But it would suggest that in the null background, where you have no competition between the different forms, then it predisposes the brain to a higher rate of polymer formation of PrP^{Sc}.

Prusiner: Yes, that's exactly right. You may want to think about it in terms of wild-type PrP inhibiting this polymer formation, that it pairs up with mutant PrP^{Sc}. PrP^{Sc} of these animals is a little different from some of the PrP^{Sc} molecules that we've seen in that it is not protease resistant, but these diseases are transmissible. In more recent studies we have 100% transmission—in other words, every time we inoculate the brains of these animals into recipients, the inoculated mice develop disease.

Goldgaber: Which background?

Prusiner: It doesn't matter. The best animal for registering transmission is this animal that expresses the same transgene at a very low level, never gets sick spontaneously and has a null background so we don't have any interference or competition from wild-type PrP^{C}. Those animals live 600–700 days and do not develop neurological disease spontaneously, but if you inoculate them, then they become sick 180–190 days later.

Masters: This has direct relevance to the Alzheimer's disease (AD) problem, in getting a transgenic AD model. If you have an APP knockout, you may be able, by putting in a human mutation, to produce something far more authentic than what is currently available.

Prusiner: Investigators at Merck have produced an authentic APP knockout (Zheng et al 1995), unlike the one that Charles Weissmann and his colleagues published (Müller et al 1994). That animal might be an ideal substrate to begin with, but it eventually gets sick—it is not completely impervious to the knockout of APP.

Maeda: Is there any significant difference in the age of onset of the disease between the PrP-deficient and wild-type transgenic mice carrying the human mutant PrP gene?

Prusiner: If you introduce a human PrP gene with the codon 102 mutation in the wild-type mouse PrP background, those animals don't get sick spontaneously (Telling et al 1995). The same mutant human PrP gene in null mice is a control that is currently under observation. If you make a chimaeric PrP gene which is one-third mouse, one-third human and one-third mouse, and you also have the codon 102 mutation, then those animals become sick at about 350 days of age (Telling et al 1995). If you inoculate those animals with an extract prepared from human GSS brain, then they all become ill about 150 days after inoculation. If you inoculate them with wild-type prions from a sporadic case of CJD, the incubation time is prolonged by 100 days. With the wild-type chimaeric PrP transgene which lacks the mutation in the null background, if you inoculate these with human GSS prions carrying the codon 102 mutation, these mice don't get sick, but they're susceptible to the inherited CJD prions which carry the codon 200 mutation. Whether the recipient animals are resistant or susceptible depends on where this mutation is located in the PrP gene.

References

Bruce ME, Dickinson AG 1985 Genetic control of amyloid plaque production and incubation period in scrapie-infected mice. J Neuropathol Exp Neurol 44:285–294

Bruce ME, Dickinson AG, Fraser H 1976 Cerebral amyloidosis in scrapie in the mouse: effect of agent strain and mouse genotype. Neuropathol Appl Neurobiol 2:471–478

Chernoff YO, Lindquist SL, Ono B, Inge-Vechtomov SG, Liebman SW 1995 Role of the chaperone protein Hsp104 in propagation of the yeast prion-like factor [*psi*+]. Science 268:880–884

Collinge J, Whittington MA, Sidle KC et al 1994 Prion protein is necessary for normal synaptic function. Nature 370:295–297

Lledo P-M, Tremblay P, DeArmond SJ, Prusiner SB, Nicoll RA 1996 Mice deficient for prion protein exhibit normal neuronal excitability and synaptic transmission in the hippocampus. Proc Natl Acad Sci USA 93:2403–2407

Müller U, Cristina N, Li Z-W et al 1994 Behavioral and anatomical deficits in mice homozygous for a modified β-amyloid precursor protein gene. Cell 79:755–765

Telling GC, Scott M, Mastrianni J et al 1995 Prion propagation in mice expressing human and chimeric PrP transgenes implicates the interaction of cellular PrP with another protein. Cell 83:79–90

Wickner RB 1994 [URE3] as an altered URE2 protein: evidence for a prion analog in *Saccharomyces cerevisiae*. Science 264:566–569

Zheng H, Jiang M, Trumbauer ME et al 1995 β-amyloid precursor protein-deficient mice show reactive gliosis and decreased locomotor ability. Cell 81:525–531

General discussion IV

Cell-free conversion of protease-sensitive prion protein to the protease-resistant state: requirement for aggregates of scrapie-associated prion protein

Caughey: I would like to describe some work I have done in collaboration with D. A. Kocisko, G. J. Raymond and P. T. Lansbury Jr.

Scrapie and other transmissible spongiform encephalopathies (TSEs) are transmitted by an infectious agent that resembles a virus in that it replicates *in vivo* and has distinct strains (for review, see Pocchiari 1994). However, the agent has been proposed to contain only a neuropathogenic, protease-resistant form of the host's prion protein (PrP) (Prusiner 1991). The protease-resistant PrP (PrP^{Sc}) is derived post-translationally from normal, protease-sensitive PrP (PrP^C) (Borchelt et al 1990, Kocisko et al 1994). To simplify the analysis of the conversion mechanism and the relationship of PrP^{Sc} formation to TSE agent replication, we developed a defined cell-free system in which PrP^C is converted to protease-resistant forms similar to scrapie-associated PrP^{Sc} (Kocisko et al 1994). This conversion requires the presence of preexisting PrP^{Sc}, providing direct evidence that PrP^{Sc} derives from interactions between PrP^C and PrP^{Sc}.

The species specificity of this cell-free reaction has been tested using mouse and hamster PrP^{Sc}, and chimeric PrP^C molecules (Kocisko et al 1995). Species-specific conversions were observed which correlated with the relative transmissibilities of these strains of scrapie between mice and hamsters. Conversion experiments performed with chimeric mouse/hamster PrP^C precursors indicated that localized primary sequence differences between PrP^C and PrP^{Sc} strongly affected the conversion reaction. The species specificity in the conversion of PrP^C to protease-resistant forms may be the molecular basis for the barriers to interspecies transmission of scrapie and other TSEs *in vivo*.

We also tested whether scrapie-strain specific properties of PrP^{Sc} are transmitted to PrP^C during formation of new PrP^{Sc} (Bessen et al 1995). PrP^{Sc} isolated from the brains of hamsters with the HY and DY strains converted hamster PrP^C to two distinct sets of PrP^{Sc} species. This provided evidence that the self-propagation of PrP^{Sc} polymers with distinct 3D structures may be a molecular basis for scrapie strains.

The precise nature and mechanism of the activity within PrP^{Sc} preparations that converts PrP^C to PrP^{Sc}, i.e. the converting activity, is not well defined. Two theories for the mechanism of PrP^{Sc}-induced PrP^{Sc} formation have been proposed: (1) heterodimer (Prusiner 1991, Griffith 1967, Bolton & Bendheim

1988) and (2) nucleated (or seeded) polymerization (Brown et al 1991, Jarrett & Lansbury 1993). The first postulates that the converting activity is a PrP^{Sc} monomer that combines with PrP^{C} to form a heterodimeric complex. The PrP^{C} in the heterodimer then converts to PrP^{Sc} and dissociates from the complex to regenerate active PrP^{Sc} monomers. In contrast, the nucleated polymerization model asserts that the converting activity is an aggregate of PrP^{Sc} that propagates by recruiting PrP^{C} molecules into a growing PrP^{Sc} polymer. We have studied the properties of the converting activity and PrP^{Sc} in the cell-free reaction with particular consideration given to determining whether the converting activity is associated with monomeric or aggregated forms of PrP^{Sc} (Caughey et al 1995). Sedimentation and ultrafiltration analyses of the converting activity indicated that it was always associated with particles heterogeneous in size but at least several times larger than solubilized (presumably monomeric) PrP. These results indicate that converting activity requires a multimeric form of PrP^{Sc}. These results are inconsistent with the heterodimer model and consistent with the nucleated polymerization model of PrP^{Sc} formation.

Prusiner: There is an alternative interpretation of your results, which I favour and which might also explain why some people have had difficulty reproducing them. Intermediate levels of guanidine hydrochloride, for instance 3 M, partially denature PrP^{Sc}. The denatured PrP^{Sc} will go through the filter and will stay in the supernatant, and the non-denatured PrP^{Sc} will remain as the retentate. This is why you see the converting activity, although I would prefer to call it binding activity, because I don't see any evidence for conversion here. This is probably a more realistic explanation for these results, although by saying this I don't mean in any way to be disparaging about them because these are really important experiments.

Caughey: I should make it clear that guanidine treatment of PrP^{Sc} is not required for the overall conversion. Regardless of whether we treat with guanidine or not, all the converting activity goes with the pelletable or filterable material. That is, the aggregated material is active in this conversion, whereas you would expect that if only the monomeric form of PrP^{Sc} were active in this conversion assay, even in the absence of guanidine it would be exchanging off this aggregate and you would find it in the supernatant. There certainly isn't an obligate requirement for a monomeric or small oligomeric form of PrP^{Sc}. You are suggesting that what we are calling conversion is simply a binding phenomenon, and you are right in that a binding phenomenon may well be part and parcel to this conversion. But by 'conversion' we mean that in addition to binding, we are getting a conversion from a protease-sensitive form to a protease-resistant form, and this is protease-resistant in the same way that PrP^{Sc} is protease resistant. We are not saying that it is identical to PrP^{Sc}, but it is more than simply binding to the surface of an aggregate.

Prusiner: But I would argue that until you are able to isolate the PrP^C away from PrP^{Sc}, you can't call it conversion. It is bound to this aggregate. One of the problems is that no one knows how to make monomers of PrP^{Sc} that are still infectious. We only know that we have this material which is highly aggregated. We can disperse it in lipids, but this is an unsatisfactory situation for looking at interactions with other molecules because there is so much lipid present.

Caughey: We feel that the binding of PrP^C to PrP^{Sc} is the important event, so we wouldn't expect to separate the converted material from the PrP^{Sc} template and get a PrP^{Sc}-like molecule. If you reverse that binding you might get PrP^C back.

Prusiner: This sounds like one of those circular arguments from the early 1970s, when it was said that you could never purify an infectious scrapie agent because it was bound to membranes.

References

Bessen RA, Kocisko DA, Raymond GJ, Nandan S, Lansbury PT Jr, Caughey B 1995 Nongenetic propagation of strain-specific phenotypes of scrapie prion protein. Nature 375:698–700

Bolton DC, Bendheim PE 1988 A modified host protein model of scrapie. In: Novel infectious agents and the central nervous system. Wiley, Chichester (Ciba Found Symp 135) p 164–181

Borchelt DR, Scott M, Taraboulos A, Stahl N, Prusiner SB 1990 Scrapie and cellular prion proteins differ in the kinetics of synthesis and topology in cultured cells. J Cell Biol 110:743–752

Brown P, Goldfarb LG, Gajdusek DC 1991 The new biology of spongiform encephalopathy: infectious amyloidoses with a genetic twist. Lancet 337:1019–1022

Caughey B, Raymond GJ 1991 The scrapie-associated form of PrP is made from a cell surface precursor that is both protease- and phospholipase-sensitive. J Biol Chem 266:18217–18223

Caughey B, Kocisko DA, Raymond GJ, Lansbury PT 1995 Aggregates of scrapie associated prion protein induce the cell-free conversion of protease-sensitive prion protein to the protease-resistant stage. Chem & Biol 2:807–817

Griffith JS 1967 Self-replication and scrapie. Nature 215:1043–1044

Jarrett JT, Lansbury PT Jr 1993 Seeding 'one-dimensional crystallization' of amyloid: a pathogenic mechanism in Alzheimer's disease and scrapie? Cell 73:1055–1058

Kocisko DA, Come JH, Priola SA et al 1994 Cell-free formation of protease-resistant prion protein. Nature 37:471–474

Kocisko DA, Priola, SA, Raymond GJ, Chesebro B, Lansbury PT Jr, Caughey B 1995 Species specificity in the cell-free conversion of prion protein to protease-resistant forms: a model for the scrapie species barrier. Proc Natl Acad Sci USA 92:3923–3927

Pocchiari M 1994 Prions and related neurological diseases. Mol Aspects Med 15:195–291

Prusiner SB 1991 Molecular biology of prion diseases. Science 252:1515–1522

Ageing and amyloid fibrillogenesis: lessons from apolipoprotein AI, transthyretin and islet amyloid polypeptide

Per Westermark, Knut Sletten* and Kenneth H. Johnson†

*Department of Pathology I, Linköping University Hospital, S-581 85 Linköping, Sweden, *Department of Biochemistry and Biotechnology Center, University of Oslo, Oslo, Norway and †Department of PathoBiology, College of Veterinary Medicine, University of Minnesota, St Paul, Minnesota, USA*

Abstract. The age-associated (or senile) amyloidoses encompass a heterogeneous group of systemic or localized forms of amyloidosis. In this paper we present an overview of three age-associated amyloid forms derived from transthyretin, apolipoprotein AI and islet amyloid polypeptide. Mutations in the respective genes give rise to transthyretin and apolipoprotein AI forms of familial amyloidosis while senile forms of amyloid are associated with the wild-type proteins. Different mechanisms are probably of importance in the fibrillogenesis associated with these three amyloid types. It is also possible that different amyloidogenic pathways exist for a single amyloidogenic protein. Thus, limited proteolysis may be necessary in the fibrillogenesis in senile transthyretin amyloidosis but not in most familial transthyretin amyloidoses. Other factors in the pathogenesis of amyloidosis such as local concentration, nidus formation and glycation are also discussed.

1996 The nature and origin of amyloid fibrils. Wiley, Chichester (Ciba Foundation Symposium 199) p 205–222

Although almost all forms of amyloidosis increase in frequency with age, some amyloid types are more closely associated with the ageing process than others. Sometimes the association of amyloid with ageing seems to be secondary, i.e. the amyloid is a consequence of another disease that is age-dependent. In other age-related forms of amyloidosis, the age-associated factor or factors are not known (Table 1). In this paper, we have concentrated our interest on three different amyloid conditions in which the amyloid fibril protein is derived from transthyretin (TTR), apolipoprotein AI (apoAI) and islet amyloid polypeptide (IAPP), respectively. TTR- and apoAI-derived amyloidoses both occur in two main clinical forms: familial amyloidosis, associated with mutations in respective

TABLE 1 Human forms of senile amyloidosis in which the fibril proteins are known

Protein	*Distribution*	*Amyloid type*	*Associated disease*	*Wild-type precursor*	*Mutant precursor*
IAPP	Localized	Islet amyloid	NIDDM	Yes	No
ANF	Localized	Atrial	Miscellaneous cardiac diseases	Yes	No
Aβ	Localized	Cerebral	Alzheimer's	Yes	*
TTR	Systemic	Senile systemic	None	Yes	*
ApoAI	Localized	Aortic intima	Atherosclerosis	Yes?	*

*Mutant fibril proteins not found in the senile amyloid forms but are present in at least some familial forms derived from the same category of precursor protein.
IAPP, islet amyloid polypeptide; ANF, atrial natriuretic factor; Aβ, amyloid β-protein; TTR, transthyretin; apoAI, apolipoprotein AI; NIDDM, non-insulin-dependent diabetes mellitus.

genes, and 'senile amyloidosis' which is probably not associated with any gene abnormalities. IAPP gives rise to amyloid within certain endocrine tumours and within the islets of Langerhans. The latter is most common and severe in type 2 diabetes mellitus but also occurs as an ageing phenomenon without known association with other diseases. TTR is given most space in this paper due to the abundance of information on the TTR molecule and on TTR-related diseases.

TTR amyloidosis

In 1978, Costa and co-workers showed that the amyloid in the Portuguese familial amyloidotic polyneuropathy (FAP) is derived from TTR (Costa et al 1978). Shortly after, it was shown that FAP was associated with a point mutation in the TTR gene, leading to a methionine-for-valine substitution at position 30 of the 127 amino acid TTR monomer (Tawara et al 1983, Dwulet & Benson 1984, Saraiva et al 1984). Subsequently, in 1979 we showed by amino acid sequence analysis that the amyloid fibril in another amyloid syndrome, senile systemic amyloidosis (SSA), also contains TTR (Sletten et al 1980). In the following years numerous TTR mutations associated with amyloidosis have been described. Today more than 40 different substitutions, spread all over the TTR monomer (from Cys10 to Val122) are known to be associated with familial amyloid forms. Comparatively few substitutions not associated with amyloid deposition are also known.

Familial TTR amyloid forms

On a molecular basis the TTR amyloidoses can be divided into two main groups, the familial forms and the entity called SSA. The familial amyloid forms are heterogeneous and are associated with widespread systemic deposits in the peripheral nervous system, heart, lungs, kidneys, vitreous humour of the eye and other organs, but can be categorized into two main clinicopathologic groups. One group constitutes the syndromes in which polyneuropathy predominates, but which are clinically quite variable. The other main but smaller group of familial amyloidoses is associated with families having cardiomyopathy as a major manifestation. These latter diseases are also systemic, but the heart manifestations dominate the clinical picture. In these patients there is a progressive infiltration of amyloid in the myocardium which leads to enlargement of the heart. Infiltration of amyloid into the conduction system can give rise to arrythmias which may be lethal. The replacement of the muscle cells with amyloid often leads to heart failure, which is a major cause of death. This group is especially interesting in the context of amyloid and ageing since the pattern of amyloid deposition resembles that of SSA (see below).

Association of TTR variants with amyloid

Although the complex of symptoms may vary somewhat between different families carrying the same mutation, different amino acid substitutions usually lead to distinctive diseases. Thus, TTR amyloidoses with Leu111Met and Val122Ile (Jacobson et al 1990) always lead to cardiomyopathy and not polyneuropathy.

All of the familial TTR amyloidoses are associated with an amino acid substitution in the TTR molecule. The mode of inheritance is always autosomal dominant and most of the patients are therefore heterozygous, carrying one normal gene copy and one mutant. Since both alleles are expressed, both wild-type and mutant TTR are present in the circulation. Both forms can also be found in the TTR tetramer. Occurrence of mutant TTR alone does not explain development of amyloidosis. For example, homozygous individuals with Val30Met do not develop a more serious disease than heterozygous individuals (Yoshinaga et al 1992) and homozygous, non-affected elderly individuals have been identified (Yoshinaga et al 1992).

It has sometimes been claimed that the fibrils in familial TTR amyloidosis only contain mutant protein. However, we (Westermark et al 1987) and several other groups have found that wild-type TTR is also included. Surprisingly, we have found considerably more wild-type TTR than Val30Met mutant TTR (Westermark et al 1987) in amyloid of one individual with typical Swedish familial amyloidosis. The reason for this is unclear but one might speculate that fibrils from Val30Met TTR may act as a nidus for wild-type TTR fibrillogenesis.

Senile systemic amyloidosis

Senile systemic amyloidosis (Pitkänen et al 1984) is the most common form of TTR-derived amyloidosis. According to our experience this is a disease of advanced age and few affected individuals are below 80 years of age. It should be noted that in studies from other countries, SSA has been seen from the sixth decade (Olson et al 1987). In prevalence studies, up to 25% of the population over 80 were affected by this disease but, although the disease is a systemic one, the deposits are generally small and mainly affect vessels in different parts of the body. Thus it is usually a benign disorder but in some individuals, mainly men, it gives rise to severe cardiomyopathy (Pitkänen et al 1984), often with ultimate cardiac insufficiency. All sequence studies on the protein (Westermark et al 1990), cDNA (Christmanson et al 1991) and gDNA (Gustavsson et al 1995) levels have shown that no amino acid substitution exists in this form of amyloidosis. Thus, there is no TTR gene mutation in this disease. Instead, in addition to an intrinsic amyloidogenic property of wild-type TTR, some yet unknown age-associated factor is involved in the pathogenesis.

Amyloidogenicity of TTR: in vitro fibrillogenesis studies

TTR appears in the plasma as a stable tetramer, consisting of four identical monomers (Blake et al 1978). These monomers have almost 50% β-structure with two sheets, each consisting of four strands. Although it is not known why TTR makes amyloid, it is generally accepted that TTR has an intrinsic tendency to aggregate into fibrils, perhaps as an intermediate in a near-native state along the protein folding–unfolding pathway (Kelly & Lansbury 1994). *In vitro* fibrillogenesis studies with wild-type TTR and synthetic peptides corresponding to segments of TTR have shown that normal full-length TTR can form *in vitro* fibrils with dimensions and staining properties of amyloid fibrils (Gustavsson et al 1991). Also, small peptides corresponding to parts of TTR readily aggregate to amyloid-like fibrils, preferentially those corresponding to the β-strands (Gustavsson et al 1991) which would fit with the concept of the importance of the β-structure in the precursor protein (Glenner 1980a,b). However, two peptides corresponding to the DE loop and to the helix, respectively, departed from this principle: they both readily formed amyloid-like fibrils *in vitro* (Å. Gustavsson, U. Engström & P. Westermark, unpublished results). When the helix was included in a longer peptide that also contained the flanking regions, no fibrillogenicity was seen (Jarvis et al 1994). In this regard, it is interesting to note that in the fibrillogenesis of prion protein a transition from α-helix to β-sheet is believed to take place (Cohen et al 1994).

Post-translational modifications

TTR in amyloid fibrils, both in Val30Met familial amyloidosis and SSA, differs from normal plasma TTR in several ways. Disulfide bonds are constant findings in both forms whereas fragmentation is always seen in SSA and commonly in Val30Met TTR amyloid.

Disulfide bonds. Disulfide bridges are not seen in the normal TTR plasma molecule. However, we have found that in both Swedish Val30Met amyloid and in SSA amyloid most of the full-length TTR is bound by disulfide bonds as dimers or polymers (either homo- or heteropolymers) (Felding et al 1985)—a fact that we made use of for the separation of full-length amyloid TTR from fragments (Westermark et al 1990a). Whether this phenomenon reflects a post-fibril process or is of importance in fibrillogenesis is not yet known. Blake and co-workers (Terry et al 1993) have proposed a fibril model based on polymerization of near-native TTR tetramers by disulfide bridges. Opposing this idea is the fact that there is one TTR mutation associated with familial amyloidosis resulting in a substitution of Cys10 with Arg, making disulfide bonds impossible (McCutchen & Kelly 1993). However, this does not completely rule out the possibility of a crucial role for a disulfide bridge. If the basis for fibril formation is the tetramer, it is theoretically possible that in heterozygous individuals amyloid-forming tetramers contain both wild-type and mutant TTR. Theoretically, the mutant TTR could be the inducer while the wild-type TTR is the stabilizer. A crucial role for disulfide bonds in fibril formation or stabilization can be ruled out only if homozygous Cys10Arg (or any other position 10 mutants) occur.

Proteolytic cleavage. Pettersson et al (1987) have shown that TTR forms slightly truncated at the N-terminus exist normally in plasma. Such truncation is also commonly seen in amyloid TTR. In all cases of senile systemic amyloidosis so far studied, at least half of the fibril TTR has been cleaved. In SDS-PAGE, the amyloid fibril protein shows up as several closely located bands, smaller than native TTR monomers (Felding et al 1985). The split is not random but occurs regularly after position 45, 48 and 51, i.e. in the C strand or the CD loop (Westermark et al 1990a, Gustavsson et al 1995). Some other minor cleavage points have also been identified. Similar splits have been found in some familial TTR amyloids as well, reported by Hermansen et al (1995) in the Leu111Met amyloid and by Gorevic et al (1989) in the Val122Ile amyloid. This cleavage occurs in Swedish Val30Met amyloid, but to a more varying degree. Whether the fragmentation is a post-fibrillogenic event or is of importance in fibrillogenesis is still unclear. It has been proposed that the C and D strands are weakly interacting with the rest of the TTR β-sandwich and therefore an amyloidogenic folding intermediate could develop in which the C and D strand make a loop that is displaced from the rest of the molecule (Kelly & Lansbury 1994). According to this hypothesis, and as indicated by the fact that the TTR monomer is stable, the splits found in the TTR-monomer are a postfibril event. Some findings are, however, difficult to explain in this scenario. First, in several amyloid fibril materials, full-length TTR makes up a minor portion of the fibril protein, perhaps not more than 10–20% of amyloid TTR. In sequence analysis of the truncated products we have only been able to identify C-terminal fragments starting at positions 46, 49, 52 and 53 (Gustavsson et al 1995). An N-terminal fragment has not been identified. Second, in an analysis of fractions obtained from gel filtration of dissolved SSA fibrils, we used different antibodies in an ELISA system. C-terminal TTR fragments were present over the whole range of peptide sizes (M_r approximately 50 kDa and less) whereas there was a big peak corresponding to full length TTR monomer. Only a very small peak with immunoreactivity and size of a small N-terminal fragment was found (Gustavsson et al 1995).

Therefore, the possibility that cleavage occurs before fibrillogenesis and is important in amyloidogenesis in at least some amyloid syndromes has to be considered. The question as to whether proteolytic cleavage is of importance in fibrillogenesis is not unique to TTR amyloid, but is valid also for most other forms of systemic and some localized amyloids as well.

Antigenic epitopes in amyloid TTR

Studies with wild-type TTR have indicated that the number of antigenic epitopes in the normally folded tetramer is restricted (Sundelin et al 1985). A study of antigenic epitopes of TTR in (and purified from) SSA amyloid as well as plasma and pancreatic islet cell TTR gave interesting results (Gustavsson et al 1994). It was found that antibodies to normal TTR only label amyloid in which full-length TTR predominates; amyloid predominated by TTR fragments (46–127, 49–127 and 52–127) was not labelled, indicating a loss of all normal epitopes in the latter form. Moreover, an antiserum to residues 115–124 TTR labelled only amyloid and TTR extracted from amyloid, both in cases with full-length TTR and mainly TTR splice products. These findings indicate that there are major folding changes in the partially fragmented TTR. They also indicate a folding change in the H strand, which is of importance since this strand participates in the formation of the TTR dimer.

Tissue deposition: several amyloidogenic TTR forms?

Another fundamental unsolved question is why amyloid depositions occur at specific locations, especially with respect to the various TTR syndromes. Why does Val30Met TTR amyloidosis form deposits in both nerves and wild-type TTR, and Leu111Met TTR give rise to cardiac deposits? One possibility is that the different mutations and the amyloidogenic wild-type TTR lead to not one but several different partly unfolded forms (normal or abnormal) with amyloidogenic properties, perhaps by several mechanisms (i.e. slightly different partly unfolded variants may exist). These forms may behave differently and may interact differently with other components (amyloid P component, proteoglycans, ions like Ca^{2+}), giving rise to different clinical diseases. It could also be speculated that cleavage of TTR may result in amyloidogenic fragments which differ in behaviour from amyloidogenic full-length TTR. In this context, it is of interest to note that in amyloid from hearts of eight individuals with Swedish Val30Met amyloid, we have found that the cardiac tissue deposition pattern in individuals with full-length amyloid TTR differs from those in which the amyloid predominantly contains fragments. Therefore it seems possible that there is more than one amyloidogenic pathway for full-length TTR and also one pathway for fragmented TTR, the latter predominating in SSA.

Apolipoprotein AI

Apolipoprotein AI (apoAI) has been implicated as the fibril protein in several rare forms of familial systemic amyloidosis. ApoAI is the major protein component in the plasma high density lipoprotein (HDL) and is important in the transport of cholesterol from peripheral cells to the liver. Low plasma levels of apoAI, as occur in some familial disorders, are associated with atherosclerosis.

ApoAI is synthesized primarily by the liver and intestine as a 267 amino acid preproprotein and is secreted as proapoAI from which a N-terminal hexapeptide is removed to yield the mature 243 amino acid apoAI.

ApoAI familial amyloidosis

It has been shown that the amyloid in some rare familial forms of Ostertag-type systemic amyloidosis with progressive renal dysfunction is derived from mutant (Gly26Arg) apoAI with a 83 amino acid residue N-terminal fragment being the fibril protein (Nichols et al 1988). Further families with apoAI amyloidosis and who carry the same mutation have been identified (Vigushin et al 1994). Other apoAI gene mutations (Leu60Arg and Trp50Arg) associated with systemic familial amyloidoses have also been identified (Soutar et al 1992, Booth et al 1995). Interestingly, in all reported cases, the amyloid fibril protein has been an N-terminal fragment of 83–93 amino acid residues. Another interesting observation is that all reported amyloidogenic apoAI substitutions have made the molecules more basic (Booth et al 1995).

ApoAI as a fibril protein in senile amyloid forms

Amyloid deposits localized to pulmonary vessels occur commonly in dogs over 10 years of age (Roertgen et al 1995). This amyloid contains an approximately 80 amino acid residue N-terminal fragment of apoAI that, within the determined sequence (1–71), does not differ from normal canine apoAI (Johnson et al 1992). This is the first example of an apoAI-derived amyloid form in an animal and the first example of a non-systemic apoAI amyloidosis.

We have previously shown that the human aorta constantly develops amyloid deposits in association with ageing. These deposits are not homogeneous and one form, antigenically different from amyloid of the media, is restricted to atherosclerotic areas in the intima (Mucchiano et al 1992). Recently, we characterized the main amyloid fibril protein occurring in the intimal amyloid deposits as an N-terminal apoAI fragment (Westermark et al 1995a), constituting residues 1–69 of apoAI.

The high prevalence of the localized apoAI amyloid forms in canine pulmonary vessels and human atherosclerotic plaques is interesting in several ways. Given the high frequency of these amyloid forms and the absence of mutations in the N-terminally derived protein segments, a normal (non-mutated) gene product most probably gives rise to these amyloids. In this respect the situation is similar to TTR, where mutant forms are associated with familial amyloidoses and an amyloidogenic wild-type gives rise to SSA. Thus, a mutation may in some way increase the intrinsic amyloidogenicity of the protein, for example by facilitating formation of an amyloidogenic folding intermediate (Kelly & Lansbury 1994). Both localized forms of apoAI amyloid are associated with vessels, possibly implicating local production of apoAI or aberrant local processing of the fibril precursor. To date, all apoAI species identified in amyloid have been spliced products lacking more than 50% of the C-terminal part of the molecule. Interestingly, 192 amino acid apoAI N-terminal fragments still reconstitute to HDL but differ in some other important aspects from the native molecules, such as oligomerization (Ji & Jonas 1995).

Islet amyloid polypeptide

Islet amyloid polypeptide (IAPP) is the major amyloid fibril protein in insulinomas and in the islets of Langerhans in human and cats (Westermark et al 1986, 1987b). IAPP is a 37 amino acid polypeptide with strong sequence similarity to the neuropeptide calcitonin gene-related peptide (CGRP). IAPP is expressed normally by islet β-cells where it is stored within the same granules as insulin and is co-released with insulin during the process of exocytosis. The normal function of IAPP is not well understood but several effects on glucose metabolism, Ca^{2+} balance, food intake and gastric emptying have been proposed.

Islet amyloid develops in more than 90% of type 2 diabetic individuals, irrespective of ethnic group. In some but not all of these cases, a majority of islets are affected. In other individuals only relatively few islets contain amyloid deposits. Islets with amyloid have a reduced number of endocrine cells, and β-cells are typically most severely affected. Electron microscopic studies have indicated that the fibrils form on the plasma membrane, i.e. extracellularly (Westermark 1994). However, it is also possible that fibrils form within β-cells under certain circumstances (Yano et al 1981, Westermark et al 1995b).

Islet amyloid is also commonly seen as an ageing phenomenon in the absence of diabetes. The number of affected islets is generally lower than in type 2 diabetic patients (Bell 1959).

Fibrillogenesis of IAPP

From comparative studies it has been clarified that human and cat IAPPs have an intrinsic amyloidogenic sequence within a central segment of the molecule that differs from IAPP of species in which islet amyloidosis does not occur (Betsholtz et al 1989, Westermark et al 1990b). In addition to an amyloidogenic structure, overproduction of the polypeptide is believed to be important in amyloidogenesis. However, transgenic mice highly over-expressing human IAPP do not develop islet amyloid (de Koning et al 1994, Westermark et al 1995c), indicating that further factors must also be of importance in amyloidogenesis. Human IAPP has an unusually strong tendency to form amyloid-like fibrils *in vitro* and thus factors hindering fibril formation must be present *in vivo. In vitro* studies have shown that some islet β-cell granule components strongly affect fibril formation and a disturbance in the balance of fibril enhancers and inhibitors is suspected to be important (Westermark et al 1996). The association of islet amyloid with type 2 diabetes mellitus may depend both on overproduction (to be shown) and on this putatively disturbed balance of enhancing and inhibiting factors.

Fibrillogenesis and ageing

Very little is yet known regarding the factors associated with ageing *per se* that increase the risk of amyloid formation. From the three different examples discussed in this paper it can be concluded that several different mechanisms interact in the formation of amyloid fibrils but the presence of a protein in an amyloidogenic state is always a prerequisite. A mechanism has been proposed which implies that fibrils are formed from folding intermediates (Wetzel 1994, Kelly & Lansbury 1994) and also implies that proteins in their native state are not prone to form amyloid since their amyloidogenic (hydrophobic) determinants are buried in the core of the molecules. This hypothesis could at least be valid for complex amyloid precursor proteins such as TTR and immunoglobulin light chains. It is less clear whether such a mechanism could operate with a small precursor polypeptide. If an amyloid fibril is formed by aggregation of a folding intermediate, this intermediate must be present at the site of fibril formation. Lysosomes have been implicated in the fibrillogenesis of AA (secondary) amyloid (Shirahama & Cohen 1975) and the acidic lysosomal environment may denature proteins. However, evidence for participation of lysosomes in amyloidogenesis is lacking for other types of amyloidosis. Also, low level denaturation and renaturation of proteins takes place under normal conditions (Bai et al 1995).

Other possible age-associated amyloid-facilitating factors

Local concentration of a precursor protein. Among other factors of importance in amyloidogenesis is the concentration of the precursor protein. Fibrillogenesis *in vitro* certainly is partly concentration-dependent. Studies of the localized amyloids, among which are several common age-dependent forms, have reinforced the importance of concentration of the precursor protein. For example, these localized amyloids assemble close to the site of synthesis. Over-expression of the hormone is most probably of importance in the formation of the amyloid derived from atrial natriuretic factor (localized atrial amyloid) and IAPP (pancreatic islet amyloid).

In addition to increased synthesis, an impaired clearance of the fibril precursor seems to be of significance in some forms of amyloidosis. Studies with transgenic mice that markedly overexpress human IAPP have shown that overexpression alone does not give rise to amyloid (de Koning et al 1994, Westermark et al 1995c). On the other hand, islets from the same transgenic mice cultured *in vitro* rapidly form amyloid (de Koning et al 1994, Westermark et al 1995c). Amyloid deposits also occur in normal human islets transplanted to the subcapsular kidney region of nude mice (Westermark et al 1995b). Although not yet proven, these experimental conditions possibly lead to a disturbance in clearance of the released polypeptide. It should be emphasized that pancreatic interstitial fibrosis is a phenomenon related to ageing and that islet amyloid in the human pancreas often is most abundant in fibrotic areas.

Non-enzymic glycation. Non-enzymic glycation of a variety of proteins is seen in diabetes mellitus, but occurs also at normal blood glucose concentration. Glycation leads to changes in properties of proteins (Tarsio et al 1988) and to prolonged half-life. This latter fact is of special importance for the long-lived extracellular matrix proteins such as collagen, and may be one factor related to age-associated fibrosis, which secondarily may affect amyloid formation. Glycation has also been proposed to be of importance in making amyloid fibrils insoluble and glycation endproducts have been found in amyloid β-protein (Smith et al 1994). However, this glycation may only be a secondary reflection of the long life of amyloid fibrils.

Occurrence of precipitating factors (nidus). The possible importance of a nidus in amyloidogenesis has been discussed much during the last several years. This possibility has been inspired by the findings from studies of prion diseases (Cohen et al 1994). The shorter lag phase associated with the experimental induction of AA amyloidosis by amyloid-enhancing synthetic peptide fibrils may involve such a mechanism (Ganowiak et al 1994). Hypothetically, some age-related changes may act as enhancers of fibrillogenesis, e.g. fibrosis or perhaps lipofuscin. The latter is found predominantly in postmitotic cells, close to which some age-dependent amyloids develop.

Lag phase. A final possible explanation contributing to the common occurrence of some forms of amyloidosis specifically in old age is the requirement for a long lag phase. When many (perhaps all) amyloids develop, the predisposition has been present for a long time. AA amyloidosis is often seen after 10 years of inflammatory disease, and familial TTR amyloidosis usually takes decades to develop. 'Infection' with prions also gives rise to disease in humans only after a lag phase of several years. The first fibril that forms could act as a nidus (Jarrett & Lansbury 1993) and the development of some age-related amyloids only reflect the long time span for this fibril formation. The senile amyloidoses, therefore, may be examples of amyloid forms requiring an unusually long lag phase.

Acknowledgements

Work in our laboratories was supported by the Swedish Medical Research Council, the Swedish Diabetes Association, the Novo Nordic Insulin Fund, the Amyl Foundation, the Association against Familial Amyloidosis, the Norwegian Research Council, the National Institute of Diabetes and Digestive and Kidney Disease and the Mr and Mrs George W. Taylor Foundation.

References

Bai Y, Sosnick TR, Mayne L, Englander SW 1995 Protein folding intermediates: native-state hydrogen exchange. Science 269:192–197

Bell ET 1959 Hyalinization of the islets of Langerhans in nondiabetic individuals. Am J Pathol 35:801–805

Betsholtz C, Svensson V, Rorsman F et al 1989 Islet amyloid polypeptide (IAPP): cDNA cloning and identification of an amyloidogenic region associated with species-specific occurrence of age-related diabetes mellitus. Exp Cell Res 183:484–493

Blake CCF, Geisow MJ, Oatley SJ, Rerat B, Rerat C 1978 Structure of prealbumin: secondary, tertiary and quaternary interactions determined by Fourier refinement at 1.8 Å. J Mol Biol 121:339–356

Booth DR, Tan SY, Booth SE et al 1995 A new apolipoprotein AI variant, Trp50Arg, causes hereditary amyloidosis. Quart J Med 88:695–702

Christmanson L, Betsholtz C, Gustavsson Å, Johansson B, Sletten K, Westermark P 1991 The transthyretin cDNA sequence is normal in transthyretin-derived senile systemic amyloidosis. FEBS Lett 281:177–180

Cohen FE, Pan K-M, Huang Z, Baldwin M, Fletterick RJ, Prusiner SB 1994 Structural clues to prion replication. Science 264:530–531

Costa PP, Figueira AS, Bravo FR 1978 Amyloid fibril protein related to pre-albumin in familial amyloidotic polyneuropathy. Proc Natl Acad Sci USA 75:4499–4503

de Koning EJP, Morris ER, Hofhuis FMA et al 1994 Intra- and extracellular amyloid fibrils are formed in cultured pancreatic islets of transgenic mice expressing human islet amyloid polypeptide. Proc Natl Acad Sci USA 91:8467–8471
Dwulet FE, Benson MD 1984 Primary structure of an amyloid prealbumin and its plasma precursor in a heredofamilial polyneuropathy of Swedish origin. Proc Natl Acad Sci USA 81:694–698
Felding P, Fex G, Westermark P, Olofsson B-O, Pitkänen P, Benson L 1985 Prealbumin in Swedish patients with senile systemic amyloidosis and familial amyloidotic polyneuropathy. Scand J Immunol 21:133–140
Ganowiak K, Hultman P, Engström U, Gustavsson Å, Westermark P 1994 Fibrils from synthetic amyloid-related peptides enhance development of experimental AA-amyloidosis in mice. Biochem Biophys Res Commun 199:306–312
Glenner GG 1980a Amyloid deposits and amyloidosis. The β-fibrilloses. 1. New Engl J Med 302:1283–1292
Glenner GG 1980b Amyloid deposits and amyloidosis. The β-fibrilloses. 2. New Engl J Med 302:1333–1343
Gorevic PD, Prelli FC, Wright J, Pras M, Frangione B 1989 Systemic senile amyloidosis. Identification of a new prealbumin (transthyretin) variant in cardiac tissue: immunologic and biochemical similarity to one form of familial amyloidotic polyneuropathy. J Clin Invest 83:836–843
Gustavsson Å, Engström U, Westermark P 1991 Normal transthyretin and synthetic transthyretin fragments form amyloid-like fibrils *in vitro*. Biochem Biophys Res Commun 175:1159–1164
Gustavsson Å, Engström U, Westermark P 1994 Mechanisms of transthyretin (TTR) amyloidogenesis: antigenic mapping of transthyretin purified from plasma and amyloid fibrils and within *in situ* tissue localizations. Am J Pathol 144:1301–1311
Gustavsson Å, Jahr H, Tobiassen R, Jacobson DR, Sletten K, Westermark P 1995 Amyloid fibril composition and transthyretin gene structure in senile systemic amyloidosis. Lab Invest 73:703–708
Hermansen LF, Bergman T, Jörnvall H, Husby G, Ranløv I, Sletten K 1995 Purification and characterization of amyloid-related transthyretin associated with familial amyloidotic cardiomyopathy. Eur J Biochem 227:772–779
Jacobson DR, Gorevic P, Buxbaum JN 1990 A homozygous transthyretin variant associated with senile systemic amyloidosis: evidence for a late-onset disease of genetic etiology. Am J Hum Genet 47:127–136
Jarrett JT, Lansbury PT Jr 1993 Seeding 'one-dimensional crystallization' of amyloid: a pathogenic mechanism in Alzheimer's disease and scrapie? Cell 73:1055–1058
Jarvis JA, Munro SLA, Craik DJ 1994 Structural analysis of peptide fragment 71–93 of transthyretin by NMR spectroscopy and electron microscopy: insight into amyloid fibril formation. Biochemistry 33:33–41
Ji Y, Jonas A 1995 Properties of an N-terminal proteolytic fragment of apolipoprotein AI in solution and in reconstituted high density lipoproteins. J Biol Chem 270: 11290–11297
Johansson B, Westermark P 1991 Senile systemic amyloidosis: a clinicopathological study of twelve patients with massive amyloid infiltration. Int J Cardiol 32:83–92
Johnson KH, Sletten K, Hayden DW, O'Brien TD, Roertgen KE, Westermark P 1992 Pulmonary vascular amyloidosis in aged dogs. A new form of spontaneously occurring amyloidosis derived from apolipoprotein AI. Am J Pathol 141:1013–1019
Kelly JW, Lansbury PT Jr 1994 A chemical approach to elucidate the mechanism of transthyretin and β-protein amyloid fibril formation. Amyloid: Int J Exp Clin Invest 1:186–205

McCutchen SL, Kelly JW 1993 Intermolecular disulfide linkages are not required for transthyretin amyloid fibril formation *in vitro*. Biochem Biophys Res Commun 197:415–421

Mucchiano G, Cornwell GG III, Westermark P 1992 Senile aortic amyloid. Evidence of two distinct forms of localized deposits. Am J Pathol 140:871–877

Nichols WC, Dwulet FE, Liepnieks JJ, Benson MD 1988 Variant apolipoprotein A-I as a major constituent of a human hereditary amyloid. Biochem Biophys Res Commun 156:762–768

Olson LJ, Gertz MA, Edwards WD et al 1987 Senile cardiac amyloidosis with myocardial dysfunction. Diagnosis by endomyocardial biopsy and immunohistochemistry. N Engl J Med 317:738–742

Pettersson T, Carlström A, Jörnvall H 1987 Different types of microheterogeneity of human thyroxine-binding prealbumin. Biochemistry 26:4572–4583

Pitkänen P, Westermark P, Cornwell GG III 1984 Senile systemic amyloidosis. Am J Pathol 117:391–399

Roertgen KE, Lund EM, O'Brien TD, Westermark P, Hayden DW, Johnson KH 1995 Apolipoprotein AI derived pulmonary vascular amyloid in aged dogs. Am J Pathol 147:1311–1317

Saraiva MJM, Birken S, Costa PP, Goodman DS 1984 Amyloid fibril protein in familial amyloidotic polyneuropathy, Portuguese type: definition of molecular abnormality in transthyretin (prealbumin). J Clin Invest 74:104–119

Shirahama T, Cohen AS 1975 Intralysosomal formation of amyloid fibrils. Am J Pathol 81:101–116

Sletten K, Westermark P, Natvig JB 1980 Senile cardiac amyloid is related to prealbumin. Scand J Immunol 12:503–506

Smith MA, Taneda S, Richey PL et al 1994 Advanced Maillard reaction end products are associated with Alzheimer disease pathology. Proc Natl Acad Sci USA 91:5710–5714

Soutar AK, Hawkins PN, Vigushin DM et al 1992 Apolipoprotein AI mutation Arg-60 causes autosomal dominant amyloidosis. Proc Natl Acad Sci USA 89:7389–7393

Sundelin J, Melhus H, Das S et al 1985 The primary structure of rabbit and rat prealbumin and a comparison with the tertiary structure of human prealbumin. J Biol Chem 260:6481–6487

Tarsio JF, Reger LA, Furcht LT 1987 Decreased interaction of fibronectin, type IV collagen, and heparin due to nonenzymatic glycation. Implication for diabetes mellitus. Biochemistry 26:1014–1020

Tawara S, Nakazato M, Kangawa K, Matsuo H, Araki S 1983 Identification of amyloid pre-albumin variant in familial amyloidotic polyneuropathy (Japanese type). Biochem Biophys Res Commun 116:880–888

Terry CJ, Damas AM, Oliveira P et al 1993 Structure of Met30 variant of transthyretin and its amyloidogenic implications. EMBO J 12:735–741

Vigushin DM, Gough J, Allan D et al 1994 Familial nephropathic systemic amyloidosis caused by apolipoprotein AI variant Arg26. Quart J Med 87:149–154

Westermark P 1994 Amyloid and polypeptide hormones: what is their interrelationship? Amyloid: Int J Exp Clin Invest 1:47–60

Westermark P, Wernstedt C, Wilander E, Sletten K 1986 A novel peptide in the calcitonin gene related peptide family as an amyloid fibril protein in the endocrine pancreas. Biochem Biophys Res Commun 140:827–831

Westermark P, Sletten K, Olofsson B-O 1987a Prealbumin variants in the amyloid fibrils of Swedish familial amyloidotic polyneuropathy. Clin Exp Immunol 69:695–701

Westermark P, Wernstedt C, Wilander E, Hayden DW, O'Brien TD, Johnson KH 1987b Amyloid fibrils in human insulinoma and islets of Langerhans of the diabetic cat are derived from a neuropeptide-like protein also present in normal islet cells. Proc Natl Acad Sci USA 84:3881–3885

Westermark P, Sletten K, Johansson B, Cornwell GG III 1990a Fibril in senile systemic amyloidosis is derived from normal transthyretin. Proc Natl Acad Sci USA 87:2843–2845

Westermark P, Engström U, Johnson KH, Westermark GT, Betsholtz C 1990b Islet amyloid polypeptide: pinpointing amino acid residues linked to amyloid fibril formation. Proc Natl Acad Sci USA 87:5036–5040

Westermark P, Mucchiano G, Marthin T, Johnson KH, Sletten K 1995a Apolipoprotein A1-derived amyloid in human aortic atherosclerotic plaques. Am J Pathol 147:1186–1192

Westermark P, Eizirik DL, Pipeleers DG, Hellerström C, Andersson A 1995b Rapid deposition of amyloid in human islets transplanted into nude mice. Diabetologia 38:543–549

Westermark G, Arora MB, Fox N et al 1995c Amyloid formation in response to β cell stress occurs *in vitro*, but not *in vivo*, in islets of transgenic mice expressing human islet amyloid polypeptide. Mol Med 1:542–553

Westermark P, Li Z-C, Westermark G, Leckström A, Steiner DF 1996 Effect of beta cell granule components on human islet amyloid polypeptide fibril formation. FEBS Lett 379:203–206

Wetzel R 1994 Mutations and off-pathway aggregation of proteins. Trends Biotechnol 12:193–198

Yano BL, Hayden DW, Johnson KH 1981 Feline insular amyloid. Ultrastructural evidence for intracellular formation by nonendocrine cells. Lab Invest 45:149–156

Yoshinaga T, Nakazato M, Ikeda S, Ohnishi A 1992 Homozygosity for the transthyretin-Met30 gene in three Japanese siblings with type I familial amyloidotic polyneuropathy. Neurology 42:2045–2047

DISCUSSION

Masters: At what stage of atherosclerotic plaque formation can you see apoAI? For example, do you see it in the very earliest aortic streaks in a 16 year old?

Westermark: We are only at the beginning of these studies, so I can't answer that. The only stages we have studied are the very mature plaques, some of which have lots of amyloid.

Masters: Even in a common case of atherosclerosis, if you find an area of very limited plaque formation, can you still see apoAI there?

Westermark: We don't see amyloid; I don't know about apoAI.

Merlini: Non-enzymic glycation has been reported to occur in β_2-microglobulin haemodialysis-associated amyloidosis (Miyata et al 1993, Niwa et al 1995) and is thought to participate in its pathogenesis through the induction of a cellular inflammatory response leading to joint/bone destruction (Miyata et al 1994). There is evidence that islet amyloid is also glycated. Do you think that protein glycation may play a role in the pathogenesis of the pancreatic islet damage associated with diabetes?

Westermark: It is certainly present. Islet amyloid occurs in glycated form, but I don't know whether this is a primary or secondary phenomenon. Aβ amyloid has also been shown to be glycated.

Merlini: Have you seen any cellular reaction around pancreatic amyloid deposits?

Westermark: No.

J. N. Buxbaum: Because there is so much non-enzymic glycation in diabetes, if glycation were to be important in amyloidogenesis in general, I would expect to see more amyloid in patients with type 2 diabetes, and yet the only place we really see it is in the pancreas.

Westermark: I'm not aware of any epidemiological studies on other forms of amyloidosis in diabetics. There could be a small increase that is not immediately apparent.

Goldgaber: In your experiment where you transplanted normal human islets to the subcapsular region of nude mice, what actually provokes the formation of amyloid in the islets?

Westermark: It could be simply that there is a clearance problem, with these islets being in an unphysiological place and lacking their normal vascular support. This may lead to an unusually high concentration of IAPP outside islet β-cells; we know that IAPP amyloidogenesis is concentration dependent *in vitro*. However, there are many other factors that may affect IAPP fibrillogenesis, such as changes in the local concentrations of insulin C-peptide, Zn and Ca^{2+} (Westermark et al 1996).

Goldgaber: Could it be a response of the transplanted cells to the stimuli from the surrounding tissue?

Westermark: It could be.

Benson: I have a question that may tie into that. If insulin protects against the production of IAPP fibrils, do you find any temporal correlation between fibril formation and the phases of diabetes? That is, does fibril production vary with insulin production?

Westermark: These studies are very difficult to do in humans, but similar studies have been performed in cats (O'Brien et al 1986) and some monkey species (Howard 1978, de Koning et al 1993), where it is quite obvious that some degree of islet amyloidosis occurs quite early in the prediabetic phase. I don't think that the islet amyloid is an early cause of insulin deficiency, but when the deposits become pronounced, they may explain a drop in insulin production. I guess that this is what happens in some type 2 diabetic individuals when oral antidiabetic drugs fail after years of treatment.

Benson: But the ratio of the two hormones might be very important in fibril formation.

Westermark: It is quite possible that the ratio of insulin to IAPP is of importance in amyloid formation, since insulin is such a strong inhibitor of fibrillogenesis *in vitro*.

Maury: Ageing *per se* appears to be a risk factor for amyloidosis. Have you looked at elderly individuals with chemically different types of amyloid?

Westermark: It is very common to have atrial and islet amyloid in old age.

J. N. Buxbaum: This was looked at by Wright and Calkins in an autopsy study. If you look with increasing age, you find more people with more than one kind of amyloid. There is an increase in the frequency of all of these amyloids, but only a small number of people have more than one type. While there was a general trend, it didn't seem to be universal nor did it seem to be systematic.

Westermark: If you look carefully in people over 50, they all tend to have at least two forms of amyloid deposits: aortic and in the choroid plexus. Many individuals also have deposits in pancreatic islets, atria and seminal vesicles.

J. N. Buxbaum: I would like to comment on late-onset cardiac amyloid, where Per Westermark and I have somewhat different experiences, since we deal with different populations. We have been looking at African Americans with the Ile for Val substitution at position 122 in TTR. About 4% of African Americans are heterozygous for this amino acid substitution. We had access to the results of 53 000 autopsies that were carried out at the Los Angeles County Hospital and analysed for the presence of cardiac amyloid. If you plot the degree of deposition against age in all individuals with cardiac amyloid, you don't get a linear distribution. This is the opposite of what I expected. However, if you look at the Ile122 positives, there is a relationship between age and degree of deposition, but it only accounts for about a third of the variance. You cannot account for the accumulation of relatively isolated cardiac amyloid related to a late-onset mutation by age alone. In Caucasians, the story is somewhat different. We are clearly looking at a much more heterogeneous population than Per Westermark, because we've seen a number of patients in whom cardiac symptoms are severe and the onset of the disease is quite early in life, yet they have no mutations in their genes.

Maeda: Are there any results indicating that IAPP is overexpressed in patients with islet amyloid?

Westermark: In obese type 2 diabetics, there is a slight overproduction of IAPP, but this is completely parallel to that of insulin. There is no major overexpression.

Maeda: Is IAPP only expressed in the islet?

Westermark: On the whole, yes. There is a small production in the some endocrine cells of the gastrointestinal tract, but this is minor.

Maeda: If it is not overexpressed, we might need to cause diabetes in transgenic mice to get the disease model.

Westermark: We have crossed transgenic mice, over-expressing human IAPP in their islet β-cells, with the mouse models of diabetes, the Ob and Db mice. In this way we have created mice producing large quantities of human IAPP. In spite of this, the mice do not develop islet amyloidosis (Westermark et al 1995). Consequently, we believe that there is more to IAPP amyloidogenesis than simply overexpression of IAPP.

Lundgren: What happens to TTR Met30 individuals who do not develop FAP: do they get the senile manifestation of the same type as normal senile individuals or do they get it at a different rate? There is a low penetrance of this mutation in Swedes: not all of them develop FAP.

Westermark: That is an interesting question. I've not seen cases of this, but you have to look for senile amyloidosis to find it.

Benson: We argue about the cause of diabetes. Has anyone yet found amyloid in transplanted pancreas? We are now doing a lot of pancreas transplants to diabetic individuals.

Westermark: We have been looking at transplanted pancreata. There is islet amyloid in some of them. It is well known that islets transplanted into the portal circulation to treat type 1 diabetes only work for a short while. One explanation for this is an accumulation of islet amyloid.

Kisilevsky: What is the current thinking on the role of IAPP in the development of diabetes?

Westermark: It is a controversial issue. Directly after its discovery, IAPP was an attractive candidate molecule for the explanation of several phenomena in type 2 diabetes, since experimentally it inhibits insulin secretion and induces peripheral insulin resistance (for review see Westermark et al 1992). Now, most people do not believe that IAPP is the major factor in the development of type 2 diabetes. The main reason for this scepticism is that supra-physiological plasma levels are needed to obtain the peripheral effects and that no major over-expression of IAPP has been found in human diabetes. However, this does not exclude the possibility that IAPP has a physiological role in the modulation of insulin effects.

References

de Koning EJP, Bodkin NL, Hansen BC, Clark A 1993 Diabetes mellitus in *Macaca mulatta* monkeys is characterized by islet amyloidosis and reduction in β-cell population. Diabetologia 36:378–384

Howard CFJ 1978 Insular amyloidosis and diabetes mellitus in *Macaca nigra*. Diabetes 27:357–364

Miyata T, Oda O, Inagi R et al 1993 β_2-microglobulin modified with advanced glycation end products is a major component of haemodialysis-associated amyloidosis. J Clin Invest 92:1243–1252

Miyata T, Inagi R, Iida Y et al 1994 Involvement of β_2-microglobulin modified with advanced glycation end products in the pathogenesis of haemodialysis-associated amyloidosis. J Clin Invest 93:521–528

Niwa T, Miyazaki S, Katsuzaki T et al 1995 Immunohistochemical detection of advanced glycation end products in dialysis-related amyloidosis. Kidney Int 48:771–778

O'Brien TD, Hayden DW, Johnson KH, Fletcher TF 1986 Immunohistochemical morphometry of pancreatic endocrine cells in diabetic, normoglycaemic glucose-intolerant and normal cats. J Comp Pathol 96:357–369

Westermark P, Johnson KH, O'Brien TD, Betsholtz C 1992 Islet amyloid polypeptide—a novel controversy in diabetes research. Diabetologia 35:297–303

Westermark G, Arora BM, Fox N et al 1995 Amyloid formation in response to β cell stress occurs *in vitro*, but not *in vivo*, in islets of transgenic mice expressing human islet amyloid polypeptide. Mol Med 1:542–553

Westermark P, Li Z-C, Westermark GT, Leckström A, Steiner DF 1996 Effects of β cell granule components on human islet amyloid polypeptide formation. FEBS Lett 379:203–206

General discussion V

4′-Iodo-4′-deoxydoxorubicin for the treatment of AL amyloidosis

Merlini: One of the main rational aims of therapy in amyloidosis is to reduce or, if possible, eliminate the supply of amyloid fibril precursor proteins in the hope that disease progression will be retarded or halted. This goal is presently achievable in at least a percentage of patients with immunoglobulin light chain-related amyloidosis (AL) by attacking the amyloidogenic clone through cytostatic therapy (Merlini 1995). The melphalan-prednisone (MP) regime has been used as a first step for treating patients with AL. The Mayo Clinic group reported that the rate of response (defined as objective regression of renal, hepatic and cardiac clinical involvement associated with the disappearance of serum and urinary monoclonal immunoglobulin) was 18%, with the highest rate being observed among nephrotic patients (Gertz et al 1991). The latest update of the Italian AL study group reported that 35.5% of the patients treated with melphalan-prednisone for at least 6 months showed improvement in the function of involved organs (Merlini et al 1994). In both studies, responsive patients achieved long survivals. Although alkylating agent-based chemotherapy is an appropriate first step, it requires a long time (median ~1 year) to achieve a response, and unfortunately the prognosis of many patients with amyloidosis is less than one year. This stresses the need for earlier diagnosis and for more rapid and effective treatment. The final goal remains the suppression and possibly the annihilation of the amyloidogenic clone. In order to attain this goal, high-dose chemotherapy with bone marrow or, preferably, peripheral stem cell rescue has been attempted in a few patients. One of our patients with AL amyloidosis was chosen for this procedure and started the high-dose chemotherapy program before bone marrow transplantation by receiving a single high dose (100 mg/m^2) of an experimental anthracycline derivative: 4′-iodo-4′-deoxydoxorubicin (I-DOX). This drug is a derivative of doxorubicin in which the C′ 4-hydroxyl group is substituted by an iodine atom. This substitution significantly increases (by about 40 times) the hydrophobic and lipophilic character of I-DOX. The drug is absorbed orally and is rapidly metabolized to 4′-iodo-4′-deoxy-13-dihydrodoxorubicin (I-DOXOL). The patient (no. 1 in Table 1 [*Merlini*]) presented with severe skin involvement that made him unable to use his hands and seriously limited his gait, with macroglossia that impaired speech and with heart interventricular septum thickening (13 mm). Within 48 h of receiving I-DOX, the patient experienced

TABLE 1 ***(Merlini)* Effects of I-DOX treatment**

			Response to I-DOX		
Patient	*I-DOX dose (mg/m²)*	*Before I-DOX*	*Clinical*	*Instrumental*	*Survival (months)*
1	100	PS:2, severe skin involvement, gait impaired, IVS: 13 mm, macroglossia impairing speech	PS:1, skin improved, gait improved, speech improved	IVS: 11 mm, u. light chain fragments	10†
2	80 × 2	Serum creatinine 451 μmol/l	Stable	No	36†
3	80, 100	PS:2, diarrhoea (8–10/d)	PS:1, diarrhoea reduced	No	50
4	30 × 4, 80, 100	Massive hepatomegaly, sAP: 1225 U/l	Stable for 4 months	sAP: 395 U/l	4†
5	30 × 2, 15, 20	PS:2, severe nephrotic syndrome, u. protein 16 g/d	PS:1	u. protein 5–6 g/d for 6 months then 10–12 g/d	41
6	30, 15, 20	CHF (NYHA III), IVS 11 mm	No	IVS: 8 mm	12†
7	30 × 4	Severe nephrotic syndrome, u. protein 13 g/d	No	u. protein 7.5 g/d	20†
8	30 × 2, 20 × 2	Sacral amyloidoma (d. 10 cm), skin infiltration (11 × 1 cm), pain, [^{131}I]SAP uptake: liver, spleen, amyloidoma	Resolution of pain	Sacral amyloidoma: 8 cm, skin infiltration 5 × 0.6 cm, [^{131}I]SAP uptake: markedly reduced	35

I-DOX, 4′-iodo-4′-deoxydoxorubicin; PS, performance status (WHO); IVS, heart interventricular septum thickness; sAP, serum alkaline phosphatase; CHF, congestive heart failure; [^{131}I]SAP, labelled serum amyloid P component; †, died of disease-related complications.

polyuria, loss of 3 kg of body weight, dramatic amelioration of the severe skin involvement, and sudden improvement in general performance. He could again flex his fingers, walk long distances (2 km) and work full time. The rapid regression of macroglossia was concomitant with an important improvement in speech. The thickness of the interventricular septum decreased to 11 mm in two weeks. Western blot analysis with anti-λ antiserum of urine collected 48 h after the infusion of I-DOX showed the appearance of light chain fragments of the same size as those present in amyloid fibrils extracted from a small amyloidoma excised from the patient's left thigh. This finding suggested that the drug had induced resorption of amyloid deposits. Following this first observation we performed a phase I trial in seven additional patients with progressive light-chain related amyloidosis (Gianni et al 1995). None of those previously treated responded to therapy. Table 1 (*Merlini*) summarizes the clinical effects of I-DOX. A few administrations of the drug produced objective evidence of amyloid resorption in two more cases. In patient 6 a reduction in the interventricular septum thickness from 11 to 8 mm was documented, while in patient 8 there was a decrease in the size of the amyloidoma and of liver and spleen deposits, as documented 14 months after I-DOX therapy by imaging and kinetic studies with labelled serum amyloid P (SAP). A comparison of imaging with labelled SAP was performed in three more patients (5, 6 and 7): there was no significant change at 3 to 4 weeks after treatment with I-DOX, and a definite, although relatively modest, increase of amyloid deposits was documented after 18 months in patient 5. In three patients (2, 3 and 5) we observed clinical improvement which lasted for a median of 6 months. In patients 4, 6 and 7 the expected natural history of the disease was not affected despite objective amyloid resorption in patient 6 and a temporary reduction of urinary protein excretion in patient 7. The heterogeneity of the clinical effects mirrors the clinical heterogeneity of this type of amyloidosis. Overall, three patients are alive at 35, 41 and 50 months after starting treatment with I-DOX, whereas five have died of disease-related complications. The efficacy of I-DOX was not related to cytotoxicity. In fact, we did not observe any significant or persistent modification of the serum or urinary concentrations of the monoclonal protein in any of the patients, with the exception of patient 1 in whom the serum and urine monoclonal component only transiently decreased after I-DOX. Patients 2 and 3 agreed to cerebrospinal fluid (CSF) sampling; at 4 h (patient 2) and 5 h (patient 3) after I-DOX administration I-DOXOL concentrations in CSF corresponded to 18 and 15 nmol/l, respectively. The plasma pharmacokinetics of I-DOX was studied in two patients. The plasma concentrations of I-DOX during infusion, as well as those of I-DOXOL, were significantly lower than the mean concentration in the control group (Gianni et al 1995). This faster clearance in amyloidotic patients is likewise consistent with the concept that the drug avidly binds to a target easily accessible from the blood or interstitial fluid, which we presume to be the amyloid deposits. This specific targeting to amyloid fibrils was investigated by *in vitro* studies which showed that I-DOX at a therapeutic concentration of 10^{-7} M binds strongly to all five types of natural amyloid fibril tested: immunoglobulin light chains, reactive amyloid A, hereditary mutated Met30 transthyretin, β_2-microglobulin of chronic dialysis, and Alzheimer's amyloid β-protein (Merlini et al 1995). Similar results were obtained with the metabolite I-DOXOL. Quantitative binding studies showed that I-DOX and its metabolite I-DOXOL, but not doxorubicin, bind strongly to synthetic insulin amyloid fibrils. This binding is saturable and involves two apparently distinct binding sites with K_d values of 5.9×10^{-11} M and 3.4×10^{-9} M. The possible interference of I-DOX with amyloidogenesis was investigated in an animal model. In the mouse, incubation of amyloid enhancing factor (AEF) with I-DOX reduced the amount of amyloid deposited. The critical factor in these experiments was the AEF to I-DOX ratio; if AEF was injected in excess of I-DOX, no significant inhibition of amyloid formation was observed. This indicates that the effect of I-DOX is related more to its binding to the active component of AEF than to the host reaction to the AEF injection. This was further supported by the observation that I-DOX did not affect serum amyloid A (SAA) synthesis, thus ruling out the possibility that the reduction in amyloid deposits induced by I-DOX could be due to inhibition of SAA precursor synthesis by the drug (Merlini et al 1995). The binding of I-DOX to amyloid fibrils with different biochemical compositions strongly suggests that this drug specifically recognizes certain structural features common to all the amyloid fibrils tested. We believe that this specific targeting most likely plays a key role in the mechanism of action of I-DOX, which appears to be independent of its cytotoxicity. The demonstration that I-DOXOL can be found in the CSF after systemic administration of I-DOX may offer the possibility of targeting amyloid deposits within the CNS, as in the case of Alzheimer's disease. An obvious drawback to I-DOX is its toxicity, which prevents its use in patients with non-AL amyloidosis. Non-toxic analogues, presently under development, may make these therapeutic and diagnostic opportunities available for other forms of amyloidosis.

Lundgren: Does I-DOX compete with SAP?

Pepys: We did a preliminary experiment that gave very clear results, in mice with experimentally induced amyloid that we can quantify precisely by localization of intravenously injected radiolabelled human SAP. Administration of I-DOX did not reduce the amount of tracer localized to the amyloid, so we don't think it is a competitive inhibitor.

I heard lately that Mark Sherman at Merck has reported an anthracycline (the same family as I-DOX) as a fibrillogenesis inhibitor.

Merlini: I didn't show the data regarding the interference of I-DOX with insulin fibrillogenesis *in vitro* which are reported in our recent paper (Merlini et al 1995). However, it is not known how this interference translates *in vivo*.

Kelly: A number of molecules have been discovered by US pharmaceutical companies. It is interesting that they all have the same structures and it is not at all clear how they work.

Blake: I would have thought that they act by intercalation, that is, by inserting into the 'ladder' structure of the amyloid fibril and interacting with the hydrophobic core of the fibril.

Merlini: It should be possible to test this hypothesis by crystallographic studies. Pharmacokinetic studies of I-DOX do indeed suggest a specific targeting to amyloid deposits *in vivo.* This targeting is very reminiscent of Congo red. We expect to have radiolabelled I-DOX available in the near future so that we can perform imaging and kinetic studies of amyloid deposits.

Sipe: Does I-DOX treatment result in resorption of established AA amyloidosis in mice?

Merlini: It seems to be easier to prevent the amyloid than it is to remove it in mice. So far, experiments aimed at resorbing experimental AA amyloid in mice have provided controversial results.

Kelly: The amount of this drug that gets past the blood–brain barrier is phenomenally high: it is almost unprecendented. Is this because it binds to the amyloid?

Merlini: It is probably because the drug is highly lipophilic.

References

Gertz MA, Kyle RA, Greipp PR 1991 Response rates and survival in primary systemic amyloidosis. Blood 77:257–262

Gianni L, Bellotti V, Gianni AM, Merlini G 1995 New drug therapy of amyloidoses: resorption of AL-type deposits with 4′-iodo-4′-deoxydoxorubicin. Blood 86:855–861

Merlini G, Marinone MG, Anesi EF, Ascari E 1994 Report of an Italian study protocol on AL amyloidosis. Blood 84 (suppl 1):179A

Merlini G 1995 Treatment of primary amyloidosis. Semin Hematol 32:60–79

Merlini G, Ascari E, Amboldi N et al 1995 Interaction of the anthracycline 4′-iodo-4′-deoxydoxorubicin with amyloid fibrils: inhibition of fibrillogenesis. Proc Natl Acad Sci USA 92:2959–2963

FAP mutations destabilize transthyretin facilitating conformational changes required for amyloid formation

Wilfredo Colon, Zhihong Lai, Sandra L. McCutchen, Greta J. Miroy, Candace Strang and Jeffery W. Kelly

Texas A&M University, College Station, TX 77843–3255, USA

Abstract. Functional transthyretin (TTR) can be transformed into amyloid by partial acid denaturation yielding a monomeric amyloidogenic intermediate which self-associates. The amyloidogenic intermediate has substantial β-sheet structure with non-native but defined tertiary structure. pH-dependent proteolysis sensitivity studies have identified portions of TTR which become disordered and solvent-exposed in the amyloidogenic intermediate. These include the C-strand-loop D-strand portion of TTR which moves away from the core of the β-sandwich fold. Mutations that are associated with early onset-amyloid disease (familial amyloidotic polyneuropathy; FAP) function by destabilizing tetrameric TTR in favour of the monomeric amyloidogenic intermediate which has a rearranged C-strand-loop D-strand region. In most cases the FAP mutations do not significantly alter the native folded structure, but instead act on the denaturation pathway by a mechanism that is not completely understood. Interestingly, mutations have also been characterized which strongly stabilize tetrameric TTR and make amyloid formation very difficult at pHs accessible *in vivo*.

1996 The nature and origin of amyloid fibrils. Wiley, Chichester (Ciba Foundation Symposium 199) p 228–242

Amyloid fibril formation refers to a pathological process where one of 16 human amyloidogenic proteins abnormally self-assembles into a fibril 60–100 Å in width and of variable length having a characteristic cross-β structure. Although there is considerable evidence for a causal link between fibril deposition and amyloid disease, the pathological mechanism remains unclear (Kisilevsky 1983, Castaño & Frangione 1988, Benson 1989, Benson & Wallace 1989, Jacobson & Buxbaum 1991, Kelly & Lansbury 1994, Pepys 1994, Sipe 1994). Although the amyloidogenic proteins outlined in Table 1 exhibit little apparent sequence or structural homology, they are converted into amyloid fibrils of similar structure *in vivo* as discerned from analogous fibre X-ray

TABLE 1 Amyloid diseases caused by different amyloidogenic proteins

Clinical syndrome	*Precursor protein*	*Fibril component*
Alzheimer's disease	Amyloid β-protein (Aβ)	Aβ 1–40, 1–41, 1–42, 1–43
Primary systemic amyloidosis	Immunoglobulin light chain	Intact light chain or fragments thereof
Secondary systemic amyloidosis	Serum amyloid A	Amyloid A (76 residue fragment)
Senile systemic amyloidosis	Transthyretin	Transthyretin or fragments thereof
Familial amyloidotic polyneuropathy I	Transthyretin	Over 45 transthyretin variants
Hereditary cerebral amyloid angiopathy	Cystatin C	Cystatin C minus 10 residues
Haemodialysis-related amyloidosis	β_2-microglobulin	β_2-microglobulin
Familial amyloidotic polyneuropathy III	Apolipoprotein AT	Fragments of apolipoprotein AT
Finnish hereditary systemic amyloidosis	Gelsolin	71 amino acid fragment of gelsolin
Type 2 diabetes	Islet amyloid polypeptide (IAPP)	Fragment of IAPP
Medullary carcinoma of the thyroid	Calcitonin	Fragments of calcitonin
Spongiform encephalopathies	Prion	Prion or fragments thereof
Atrial amyloidosis	Atrial natriuretic factor (ANF)	ANF
Hereditary non-neuropathic systemic amyloidosis	Lysozyme	Lysozyme or lysozyme variants or fragments thereof
Injection-localized amyloidosis	Insulin	Insulin
Hereditary renal amyloidosis	Fibrinogen	Fibrinogen fragments

diffraction patterns, electron micrographs and spectroscopic features (Lansbury 1992, Kelly & Lansbury 1994). The unexpected result that unrelated proteins can form amyloid having a common tertiary and quaternary structure can be rationalized by considering the possibility that the similarity of the amyloidogenic proteins is not due to their normally folded structures. In fact, normally folded amyloidogenic proteins appear to be incapable of fibril formation, even at high concentrations. Instead, the amyloidogenic proteins appear to be related by their ability to undergo a conformational change affording a metastable amyloidogenic intermediate with a common structural element(s) allowing self-assembly into amyloid (Kelly & Lansbury 1994, Kelly 1996). The sequence requirements responsible for the formation of such a conformational intermediate during protein denaturation are not yet clear, although progress is being made in this area. In support of this amyloidogenic intermediate hypothesis, a number of amyloidogenic proteins, including transthyretin (TTR) (Colon & Kelly 1991, 1992, Gustavsson et al 1991) and variants thereof (McCutchen et al 1993, 1995), immunoglobulin light chains (Hurle et al 1994), and lysozyme (Pepys et al 1993), have been converted into amyloid by the induction of conformational changes in the normally folded proteins. Conformational changes also appear to be required for the conversion of soluble amyloid β-peptide (Aβ) into β-amyloid which putatively causes Alzheimer's disease. However, these changes are different in that the Alzheimer's intermediate is likely to be more structured than the normal solution conformation (Lee et al 1995). An amyloidogenic protein such as TTR and a small peptide like Aβ represent opposite extremes of a structural continuum whereby TTR must unfold to adopt the amyloidogenic conformation whereas Aβ must become more structured to adopt a conformation which is amyloidogenic (Fig. 1; Kelly 1996). Maggio and co-workers have demonstrated that the Aβ10–35 fragment exhibits pH-dependent fibril competence similar to the full length 1–40 peptide (Lee et al 1995). Comparisons of the fibril-incompetent 1–28 fragment with the competent 10–35 fragment reveal that both peptides are sampling multiple conformations at pH 2.1, i.e. they are largely unfolded. However as the pH is increased into range where 10–35 can add to preformed fibrils, the 10–35 polypeptide chain adopts a metastable structure best described as a 'turn-strand-turn' motif involving residues 13–24. This structure is not present in the plaque-

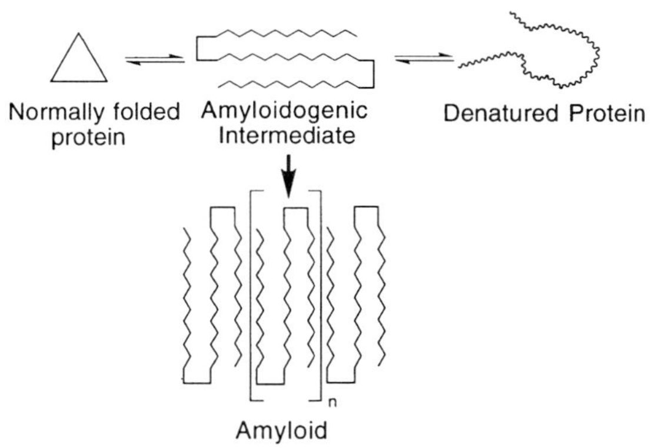

FIG. 1. The structural continuum in the fibrillogenesis pathways in several of the amyloidogenic proteins studied to date.

incompetent peptide implying that it is close to the structure of the amyloidogenic intermediate. Additional evidence in favour of the conformational change hypothesis in amyloid disease is provided by the striking conformational changes required for the conversion of the soluble cellular prion protein (PrP^C) into the scrapie form (PrP^{Sc}). Even though there are some significant differences between prion diseases and amyloid diseases, it is clear that they are similar in that they both involve the conversion of a normally soluble form of a protein into a prionogenic conformational intermediate which renders the PrP^C protein capable of forming the aggregated prion-like particle referred to as PrP^{Sc} characterized by a predominantly β-sheet structure (Caughey et al 1991, Pan et al 1993, Safar et al 1993, 1994, Come & Lansbury 1994, Baldwin et al 1995, Daggett 1995, Lansbury 1995, Nguyen et al 1995, Zhang et al 1995). This paper will focus on our current understanding of the biophysics of TTR amyloid fibril formation, which undergoes a conformational change affording an intermediate which self-assembles into amyloid

Twenty-five years ago Glenner and others demonstrated that lysosomal extracts or lysosomal enzymes under acidic conditions could convert the amyloidogenic Bence–Jones proteins into amyloid (Glenner et al 1971). Proteolysis catalysed by lysosomal proteases was thought to transform the soluble protein into a fragment that spontaneously formed amyloid. Undoubtedly, proteolysis plays a role in some amyloid diseases. However, the denaturing environment may be a more important factor. Purified TTR can be converted into amyloid fibrils via an acid-induced conformational change *in vitro*, suggesting that conformational changes alone are sufficient to produce an intermediate capable of amyloidosis in certain proteins (Colon & Kelly 1991, 1992, Gustavsson et al 1991). Invoking a conformational intermediate as the precursor to amyloid was a novel idea at that time; however, the concept that a conformational intermediate on the folding/denaturation pathway was capable of self-assembly was firmly established in the protein chemistry literature through the work of Goldberg, Jaenicke, Brems, Fink, Horowitz, King, Dill and others. The TTR result was not quickly accepted by the amyloid community, probably because the Alzheimer's literature at that time implied that proteolysis was required for Aβ fibril deposition. However, the discovery of soluble Aβ in healthy individuals by Seubert et al (1992) and Shoji et al (1992) forced investigators to reconsider the role of conformational changes in Aβ fibrillogenesis.

The predominantly β-sheet protein TTR adopts a tetrameric structure under normal physiological conditions as discerned from the crystal structure determined by Blake and colleagues and from solution analytical equilibrium ultracentrifuge data (Blake et al 1974, 1978, McCutchen et al 1995, Lai et al 1996). TTR functions as a transport protein by transporting both thyroxine and retinol. Thyroxine is bound in the central channel of TTR, whereas retinol is bound indirectly by binding to the retinol binding protein (RBP) which itself binds to TTR (Raz & Goodman 1969, Monaco et al 1995). In certain individuals wild-type TTR is converted into amyloid which appears to cause senile systemic amyloidosis (SSA) around age 80, sometimes characterized by heavy amyloid deposits in the heart leading to congestive heart failure (Cornwell et al 1988, Westermark et al 1990). In rarer examples of heterozygous individuals, one of over 40 single-site variants of TTR is found to predominate over wild-type TTR in the amyloid deposits of familial amyloidotic polyneuropathy (FAP) patients where the age of onset is generally earlier than SSA and is variant specific (Jacobson & Buxbaum 1991, Saraiva et al 1984, Benson 1989, Sakaki et al 1989, Saraiva 1995). FAP patients typically present with peripheral neuropathy in the location of amyloid deposits. Interestingly, certain FAP variants appear to deposit selectively in a given tissue. The basis of the variant tissue selectivity clearly harbours important clues concerning the physiological process of amyloid deposition but is currently not understood. Lastly, it is important to point out that the presence of a given amyloidogenic mutation does not necessarily lead to FAP. There are other genetic factors, perhaps chaperones (some of which have been postulated already) that protect certain individuals from the risk of disease associated with the amyloidogenic mutation. None the less, all of the early-onset TTR cases observed to date are associated with a mutation, which implies that the mutant TTR is necessary for disease onset, but is not the only factor.

We have shown that TTR will form amyloid *in vitro* when the protein is subjected to partial acid denaturation conditions and during pH mediated reconstitution from a mostly unfolded state, implying that an intermediate on the denaturation/reconstitution pathway is the amyloidogenic intermediate that leads to amyloid fibril formation (Colon & Kelly 1991, 1992, McCutchen et al 1993, 1995, Lai et al 1996). Extensive biophysical studies (far and near-UV circular dichroism, fluorescence, analytical equilibrium ultracentrifugation/ SDS-PAGE and fibrillogenesis assays) on both the wild-type and several FAP variants have led to an understanding of the denaturation pathway which is outlined in Fig. 2. As the pH is lowered, the tetrameric structure first rearranges, followed by dissociation to a monomeric amyloidogenic intermediate conformation characterized by near native-like secondary structure and an altered but partially defined tertiary structure. This intermediate rearranges further at lower pH affording an A-state like conformation (retains secondary structure but lacks tertiary structure) under physiological salt conditions. Neither the A-state, the rearranged tetramer nor the normal tetrameric structure are competent to form amyloid. All evidence accumulated to date points to a monomeric intermediate with altered structure as the subunit which self-assembles into amyloid. The structure of the monomeric amyloidogenic intermediate has been probed through proteolysis sensitivity studies and by fluorescence spectroscopy employing single-Trp-containing TTR variants to discern which portion(s) of the TTR structure rearrange in the

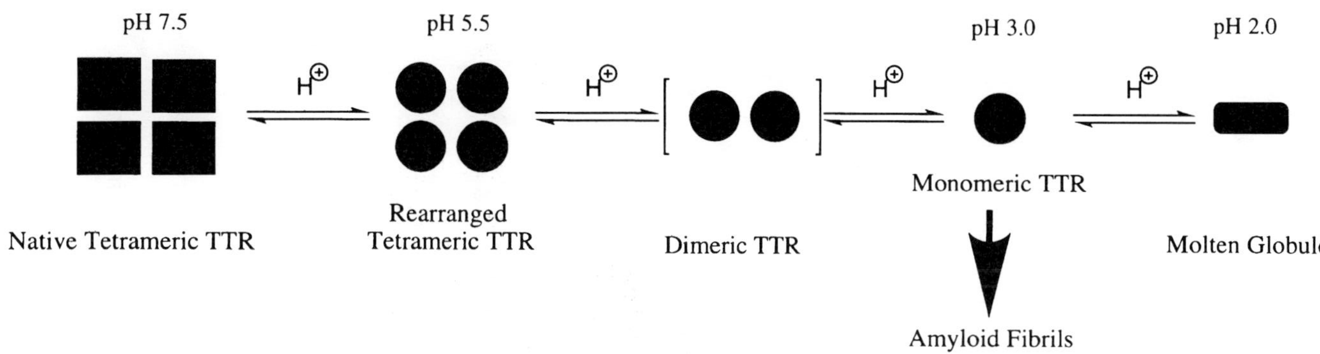

FIG. 2. An overview of the detailed acid-mediated denaturation pathway of transthyretin.

formation of this intermediate (Miroy & Kelly 1996, Lai et al 1996). These data, in combination with the location of the 40 generally conservative FAP-causing mutations allow us to propose a structure for the amyloidogenic intermediate shown in Fig. 3. Our assumption is that the FAP mutations cannot alter a region of the protein critical for quaternary structure (amyloid) formation. The structure of the amyloidogenic intermediate derived from our solution studies is consistent with the repeating subunit of TTR amyloid fibrils that has been proposed on the basis of oriented Met30Val TTR amyloid isolated from the eye and evaluated by X-ray diffraction and electron microscopy by C. Blake, P. Fraser and co-workers (personal communication). In further support of the structure of the amyloidogenic intermediate proposed in Fig. 3, A. Damas (personal communication) has reported a preliminary crystal structure of the Leu55Pro TTR variant which shows that this non-conservative mutation has converted the D-strand into a loop structure. This

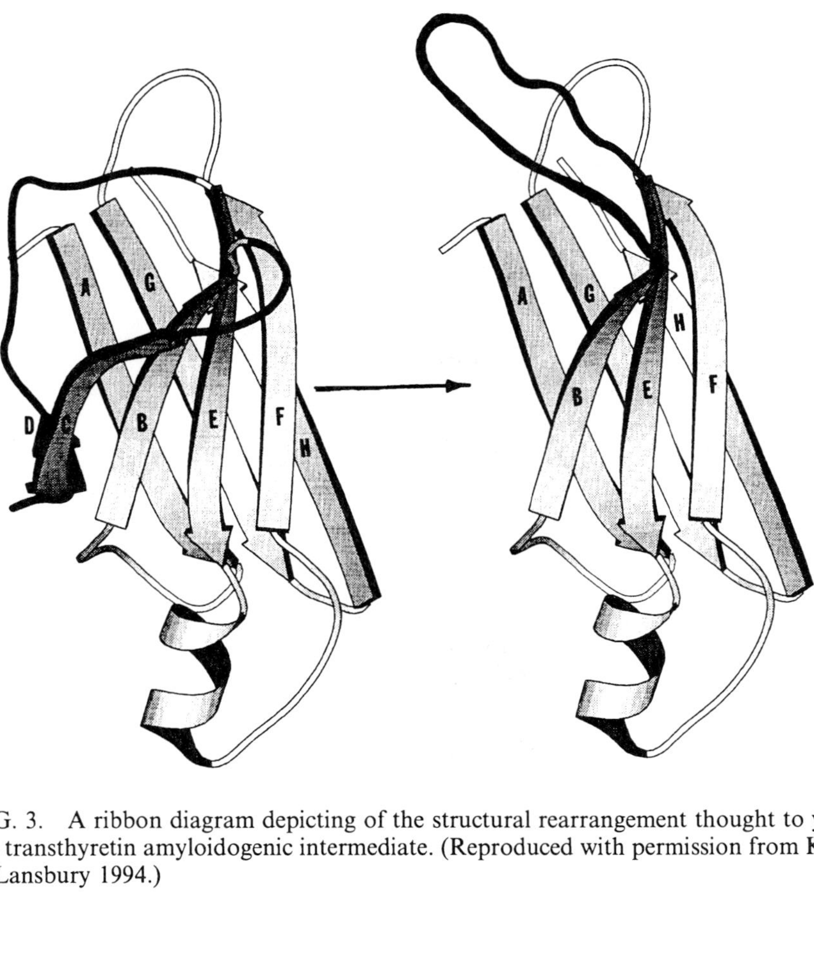

FIG. 3. A ribbon diagram depicting of the structural rearrangement thought to yield the transthyretin amyloidogenic intermediate. (Reproduced with permission from Kelly & Lansbury 1994.)

seems to explain the structural basis of the extreme amyloidogenicity of this variant in that it is already partially rearranged towards the structure of the amyloidogenic intermediate in its normally folded state, unlike the solid state structures of the other amyloidogenic variants solved to date which are virtually identical to wild-type TTR (*vide infra*).

We have shown that several of the single-site amyloidogenic variants that cause FAP behave similarly in that they destabilize tetrameric TTR in favour of the monomeric amyloidogenic intermediate (McCutchen et al 1993, 1995). In addition Atland and co-workers have recently examined the thermodynamic stability of numerous variants using a novel urea gradient gel electrophoresis system and have shown that nearly all of the FAP variants exhibit decreased tetramer stability relative to that of wild-type TTR (K. Atland, personal communication). Thus the amyloidogenic variants can form the amyloidogenic intermediate and self-assemble into amyloid under mildly acidic conditions where wild-type TTR is non-amyloidogenic (conformationally stable and tetrameric). The FAP variants studied thus far by Hamilton, Blake and Benson do not significantly alter the structure of the folded TTR tetramer, nor would they be expected to on the basis of the conservative nature of the mutations. The most common FAP variant, Met30Val, exhibits a structure that is very similar to that of the wild-type protein as discerned from a comparison of their X-ray crystal structures (Hamilton et al 1992, Terry et al 1993). The FAP mutations that have been characterized so far appear to function by destabilizing the native protein fold and/or by making the amyloidogenic intermediate more accessible relative to the folded state under mildly denaturing conditions, but not by altering the structure of the native fold (Kelly & Lansbury 1994, Kelly 1996, Miroy & Kelly 1996). The only exception to this general behaviour is the recent (unpublished) work of A. Damas, which shows that the non-conservative mutation Leu55Pro does significantly change the structure in a way that predisposes it to fibril formation. Interestingly, the more unstable the FAP variants are to acid denaturation *in vitro,* the earlier is the onset of FAP symptoms *in vivo*, consistent with the expectation that the destabilization will increase the steady state concentration of the monomeric amyloidogenic intermediate which increases the mass of amyloid formed by mass action (Table 2; McCutchen et al 1993, 1995). The most unstable TTR variant characterized to date is Leu55Pro TTR, which also exhibits the most aggressive pathology with onset in the second decade of life (Jacobson & Buxbaum 1991, McCutchen et al 1993). For the wild-type and several variant TTRs, the presence of and build-up in concentration of the amyloidogenic intermediate can be readily detected by the plateau exhibited by the Trp fluorescence over the pH range where amyloid forms (McCutchen et al 1995). A notable exception is the Thr119Met variant which has been shown to protect Met30Val heterozygotes from the onset of FAP. The Thr119Met variant is the most stable TTR variant studied to date and does not exhibit a fluorescence

TABLE 2 Correlation between Increasing pH_m *in vitro* and decreasing age of amyloid disease *in vivo*

Transthyretin variant	pH_m	*Age of disease onset*
Thr119Met	3.4	None reported
Wild-type	4.4	>80
Val30Met	4.7	30 (FAP)
Leu55Pro	5.4	Teens to early 20s (FAP)

plateau, consistent with the absence of a build-up in the concentration of the amyloidogenic intermediate. When the Thr119Met and Val30Met variant are introduced into the same subunit to serve as a model for the heterozygous situation where half the subunits are Val30Met and the others are Met119Val, the variant exhibits stability and amyloidogenicity between that of wild-type TTR and the most stable Val119Met variant, indicating that the role of the Met 119 variant is to stabilize the tetramer and reduce amyloidogenicity.

Current efforts are focused on understanding the means by which fibril formation can be inhibited. Agents that bind to and stabilize the tetramer in addition to peptidomimetics which bind to the amyloidogenic intermediate are being evaluated with very encouraging preliminary results. These will be reported in due time.

Acknowledgements

The author wishes to thank the National Institutes of Health (R29 DK46335-01) as well as the Alzheimer's Association for financial support of this research and Joel Buxbaum, Maria Saraiva and Per Westermark for many stimulating conversations throughout the years.

References

Baldwin MA, Pan KM, Nguyen J et al 1995 Spectroscopic characterization of conformational differences between PrP^C and PrP^{Sc}: an α-helix to β-sheet transition. Philos Trans R Soc Lond Ser B Biol Sci 343:435–441

Benson MD 1989 Familial amyloidotic polyneuropathy. Trends Biol Sci 12:88–92

Benson MD, Wallace MR 1989 Amyloidosis, the metabolic basis of disease. In: Scriver CP, Beaudet AL, Sly WS, Valles D (eds) The metabolic and molecular basis of inherited disease. McGraw-Hill, New York, p 2439–2460

Blake CCF, Geisow MJ, Rerat B, Rerat C, Swan IDA 1974 Structure of human plasma prealbumin at 2.5 Å resolution. A preliminary report on the polypeptide chain conformation, quaternary structure and thyroxine binding. J Mol Biol 88:1–12

Blake CCF, Geisow MJ, Oatley SJ, Rerat B, Rerat C 1978 Structure of prealbumin: secondary, tertiary and quaternary interactions determined by Fourier refinement at 1.8 Å. J Mol Biol 121:339–356
Castaño EM, Frangione B 1988 Biology of disease: human amyloidosis, Alzheimer disease and related disorders. Lab Invest 58:122–132
Caughey BW, Dong A, Bhat KS, Ernst D, Hayes SF, Caughey WS 1991 Secondary structural analysis of the scrapie-associated protein Prp 27–30 in water by infrared spectroscopy. Biochemistry 30:7672–7680
Colon W, Kelly JW 1991 Transthyretin acid induced denaturation is required for amyloid fibril formation *in vitro*. Applications of enzyme biotechnology. Plenum, New York, p 99–108
Colon W, Kelly JW 1992 Partial denaturation of transthyretin is sufficient for amyloid fibril formation *in vitro*. Biochemistry 31:8654–8660
Come JH, Lansbury PT Jr 1994 Predisposition of prion protein homozygotes to Creutzfeldt–Jakob Disease can be explained by a nucleation-dependent polymerization mechanism. J Am Chem Soc 116:4109–4110
Cornwell GC, Sletten K, Johansson B, Westermark P 1988 Evidence that the amyloid fibril protein in senile systemic amyloidosis is derived from normal prealbumin. Biochem Biophys Res Commun 154:648–653
Daggett V 1995 Theoretical studies of sequence effects on the conformational properties of a fragment of the prion protein: implication for scrapie formation. Chem Biol 2:305–315
Glenner GG, Ein D, Eanes ED, Bladen HA, Terry W, Page DL 1971 Creation of amyloid fibrils from Bence–Jones proteins *in vitro*. Science 174:712–714
Gustavsson A, Engström U, Westermark P 1991 Normal transthyretin and synthetic transthyretin fragments form amyloid-like fibrils *in vitro*. Biochem Biophys Res Commun 175:1159–1164
Hamilton JA, Steinrauf LK, Liepnieks J et al 1992 Alteration in molecular structure which results in disease: the Met-30 variant of human plasma transthyretin. Biochim Biophys Acta 1139:9–16
Hurle MR, Helms LR, Li L, Chan W, Wetzel R 1994 A role for destabilizing amino acid replacements in light chain amyloidosis. Proc Natl Acad Sci 91:5446–5450
Jacobson DR, Buxbaum JN 1991 Genetic aspects of amyloidosis. Adv Hum Genet 20:69–123
Kelly JW 1996 Alternative conformations of amyloidogenic proteins govern their behavior. Curr Opin Struct Biol 6:11–17
Kelly JW, Lansbury PT Jr 1994 A chemical approach to elucidate the mechanism of transthyretin and β-protein amyloid fibril formation. Amyloid: Int J Exp Clin Invest 1:186–205
Kisilevsky R 1983 Biology of disease amyloidosis: a familiar problem in light of current pathogenic developments. Lab Invest 49:381–390
Lai Z, Colon W, Kelly JW 1996 The acid-mediated denaturation pathway of transthyretin yields an intermediate which can self-assemble into amyloid. Biochemistry, in press
Lansbury PT 1992 In pursuit of the molecular structure of the amyloid plaque new technology provides unexpected and critical information. Biochemistry 31:6865–6870
Lansbury PT 1995 The chemistry of the scrapie infection: implications of the ICE 9 metaphor. Chem Biol 2:1–5
Lee JP, Stimson ER, Ghilardi JR et al 1995 H-1 NMR of Aβ amyloid peptide congeners in water solution-conformational changes correlate with plaque competence. Biochemistry 34:5191–5200

McCutchen S, Colon W, Kelly JW 1993 Transthyretin mutation Leu-55-Pro significantly alters tetramer stability and increases amyloidogenicity. Biochemistry 32:12119–12127

McCutchen SL, Lai Z, Miroy G, Kelly JW, Colon W 1995 Comparison of lethal and non-lethal transthyretin variants and their relationship to amyloid disease. Biochemistry 34:13527–13536

Miroy GJ, Kelly JW 1996 Working model of the structure of the transthyretin amyloidogenic intermediate based on proteolysis sensitivity and biophysical studies. Biochemistry, submitted

Monaco HL, Rizzi M, Coda A 1995 Structure of a complex of two plasma proteins: transthyretin and retinol-binding protein. Science 268:1039–1041

Nguyen J, Baldwin MA, Cohen FE, Prusiner SB 1995 Prion protein peptides induce α-helix to β-sheet conformational transitions. Biochemistry 34:4186–4192

Pan KM, Baldwin M, Nguyen J et al 1993 Conversion of α-helices into β-sheets features in the formation of the scrapie prion proteins. Proc Natl Acad Sci USA 90:10962–10966

Pepys MB 1994 Amyloidosis. In: Frank MM, Austen KF, Claman HN, Unanue ER (eds) Samter's immunologic diseases, 5th edn. Little, Brown & Co., Boston, MA, p 637–655

Pepys MB, Hawkins PN, Booth DR et al 1993 Human lysozyme gene mutations cause hereditary systemic amyloidosis. Nature 362:553–557

Raz A, Goodman DS 1969 The interaction of thyroxine with human plasma prealbumin and with the prealbumin-retinol-binding protein complexes. J Biol Chem 244:3230–3237

Safar J, Roller PP, Gajdusek DC, Gibbs CJ 1993 Thermal stability and conformational transitions of scrapie amyloid (prion) protein correlate with infectivity. Protein Sci 2:2206–2216

Safar J, Roller PP, Gajdusek DC, Gibbs CJ 1994 Scrapie amyloid prion protein has the conformational characteristics of an aggregated molten globule folding intermediate. Biochemistry 33:8375–8383

Sakaki Y, Yoshioka K, Tanahashi H, Furuya H, Sasaki H 1989 Human transthyretin (prealbumin) gene and molecular genetics of familial amyloid polyneuropathy. Mol Biol Med 6:161–168

Saraiva MJM 1995 Transthyretin mutations in health and disease. Hum Mutat 5:191–196

Saraiva MJM, Birken S, Costa PP, Goodman DS 1984 Amyloid fibril protein in familial polyneuropathy, Portuguese type: definition of molecular abnormality in transthyretin (prealbumin). J Clin Invest 74:104–119

Seubert P, Vigo-Pelfry C, Esch F et al 1992 Isolation and quantification of soluble Alzheimer's β-peptide from biological fluids. Nature 359:325–327

Shoji M, Golde TE, Ghiso J et al 1992 Production of the Alzheimer's amyloid β-protein by normal proteolytic processing. Science 258:126–129

Sipe JD 1994 Amyloidosis. Clin Lab Sci 31:325–354

Terry CJ, Damas AM, Oliviera P et al 1993 Structure of Met30 variant of transthyretin and its amyloidogenic implications. EMBO J 12:735–741

Westermark P, Sletten K, Johansson B, Cornwell GGI 1990 Fibril in senile systemic amyloidosis is derived from normal transthyretin. Proc Natl Acad Sci USA 87:2843–2845

Zhang H, Kaneko K, Nguyen JT et al 1995 Conformational transitions on peptides containing two putative α-helices of the prion protein. J Mol Biol 250:514–526

DISCUSSION

Kisilevsky: The contact points in the TTR tetramer are well known, and the proof of concept that you have indicated by using peptides for important sites in the fibril seems to work. Can you not therefore do the same sort of thing trying to mimic the contact points in the tetramer, to shift the equilibrium in favour of the monomer?

Kelly: That would be my interpretation of the results from the collaborative experiments that were shown earlier with deletions in the D strand. This is why I think Per Westermark's hypothesis is abundantly reasonable: if you go in and cut a protein, it lowers the kinetic barrier of structural transition enough to get the whole ball started. Once it is started, it propagates. Proteolysis and mutations could be critical in making those changes accessible. The bottom line answer is that I'm convinced that protein–protein interactions can do the same thing with the tetramer so that you can make the intermediate that will polymerize.

Blake: In relation to that, one interesting point is that the natural amyloidogenic mutants of TTR avoid the subunit interfaces, with one exception. This is the Asp18 variant, but it is the only one I can think of that would directly disturb the subunit interfaces. There may be resolution to this in terms of the need to maintain the normal function of TTR. The physiological function of TTR is to bind and transport thyroxine and vitamin A. Both these functions require TTR to be in the tetrameric state, and this may be the factor that opposes change in the subunit interfaces. Perhaps mutants in the subunit interface region that would destabilize the tetramer might be more amyloidogenic.

Kelly: We tried to be conservative and not make big changes, so we changed some of the residues to alanine. One of them definitely destabilizes it, but it doesn't make a monomer, so we are now using two. Jim Wells from Genentech saw the same thing in one of the interleukins, where he had to make several amino acid changes in the antiparallel β-sheet subunit to significantly change the dimer interface. Your point is well taken; these experiments are clearly worth doing.

Sipe: Have you tried to incubate TTR with cells to look for naturally formed amyloidogenic monomers?

Kelly: Initially we had the rather crazy idea that we could make amyloid in the periplasmic space of *Escherichia coli.* Our expression system expresses TTR in the periplasmic space, and we tried to change the pH in this compartment. These experiments are very hard to do without killing the cells, and although we have had some positive results, I don't believe them

Sipe: What about expressing TTR in a hepatoma cell or a macrophage cell line where you would expect to have physiologically acidic granules and organelles?

Kelly: I have a hard enough time growing *E. coli*! I think those experiments, particularly with macrophage-rich cells, would be very interesting.

Arvinte: Do you have experimental data on the pK of your monomer?

Saraiva: The pI for the monomer is 4.2.

Arvinte: This would be, by itself, a perfect explanation of the model.

Kelly: The pH maximum of fibre formation is very close to the pI, within 0.4 pH units.

Arvinte: Proteins aggregate in the vicinity of the isoelectric point. In the aggregated state conformational changes in the constituent peptides or protein can take place, i.e. through electrostatic or hydrophobic interactions.

Kelly: You are right. The difference in the amyloiodogenic proteins is that the aggregates they make are ordered. Most proteins form in an amorphous manner when they are precipitated isoelectrically. There are certainly common elements that make the protein insoluble, the difference being the structure.

Lundgren: Can your modified monomer exist in physiological pH? Does it then form dimers or tetramers?

Kelly: As I have said, we never see more that a few percent as a dimer and I believe that even this small quantity is an artefact of the gluteraldehyde cross-linking. There is some evidence for subunit exchange in the tetramer. This means that the tetramer has a dissociation constant such that there is an equilibrium at pH 7.5 which lies strongly in favour of the tetramer. We are trying to measure this now. It exists as 99.9% tetramer with traces of monomer. Many years ago it was published that if you put monkey and human TTR together you get subunit interchange. We haven't reproduced these results but they seem reasonable on a protein chemistry basis.

Saraiva: Experimentally, using wild-type and mutant TTR, we do not have evidence for subunit interchange. Thus, when we mix wild-type and Met30 TTR and evaluate thyroxine binding, no changes in the binding affinity of wild-type TTR are seen (after correction for dilution), indicating that subunit interchange has not occurred, otherwise a strong reduction in the affinity would have been detected because of the poor binding properties of heterozygotic Met30 TTR.

Kelly: We have no evidence for subunit interchange, but I would argue on a protein chemistry basis that it has to be possible.

Palha: In *in vivo* experiments with TTR Met30 transgenic mice, we have shown the existence of heterotetrameric species between mouse and human TTR (Palha et al 1994). *In vitro*, these heterotetramerics were only obtained after denaturation and renaturation. This suggests that in the Met30 transgenic mice heterotetrameric mouse–human species form in the liver prior to secretion and that subunit interchange is unlikely to occur.

Kelly: The complicating feature is whether there is an equilibrium. If there is, I think that the concentration of the monomer is so low that it is not terribly important.

Damas: You talked about a modified tetramer at pH 5.5, but we do not see these variations in the crystal structures we have of some of these variants.

Kelly: How were these crystallized?

Damas: The crystals were grown at pH 5 using ammonium sulfate.

Kelly: That is a problem. Ammonium sulfate stabilizes proteins incredibly. For all the data I showed in physiological salt, if you do the same denaturation curves in ammonium sulfate, the tetramer is stable all the way to pH 3 and you don't see those significant rearrangements. My point is that it isn't possible to compare crystals grown at a high pH in high salt with biophysical data where the protein is at physiological concentration in physiological salt.

Kisilevsky: In the context of your hypothesis, what do you think components like serum amyloid P (SAP) and apolipoprotein E might be doing?

Kelly: It really depends on where amyloid forms. If amyloid forms in a lysosome, they may do nothing; if amyloid forms extracellularly, they may play a role by binding to the amyloid that is not particularly stable yet. I think the idea of pathological chaperones is an intriguing one.

Blake: It would be interesting to know if the structure of the fibrils formed *in vitro* is similar to that of *in vivo* fibres. Perhaps the material formed *in vitro* is very simple material and is only related to the real material, but isn't the same as it.

Saraiva: Delipidating SAP fibrils doesn't change the cross-β structure (Damas et al 1995).

Kelly: It may be that *in vitro* the protofilament formation is absolutely normal, but the assembly is sometimes not. Most of the time *in vitro* fibrils resemble closely those taken from patients, but sometimes they are morphologically different: they still bind Congo red and have a cross-β type pattern, but they look different by electron microscopy.

Saraiva: When we examine TTR amyloid produced *in vitro* under the electron microscope, we have to search carefully on the grids to find fibrils morphologically resembling amyloid.

Kelly: It could be that what we are making is close but is not perfect.

Blake: It may be that aggregation of the protofilaments into fibrils, the second part of the fibril-forming process, is equally important in the long run.

Kelly: That's where the accessory molecules may play a huge role.

Pepys: It is unlikely to be merely trivial that every amyloid fibril isolated *ex vivo* has tightly bound glycosaminoglycans belonging to a very restricted set of species.

Kelly: Aβ is different in that it probably is associated with some protein *in vivo*, otherwise it would aggregate anyway. So the mechanism there is undoubtedly going to be more complicated than the case of lysozyme, TTR or immunoglobulin light chain.

References

Damas A, Sebastião MP, Domingues FS, Costa PP, Saraiva MJM 1995 Structural studies on FAP fibrils: removal of contaminants is essential for the interpretation of X-ray data. Amyloid: Int J Exp Clin Invest 2:173–178

Palha JA, Maeda S, Yamamura K, Shimada K, Gottesman ME, Saraiva MJM 1994 Analysis of thyroxine binding and heterotetramer formation in human transthyretin methionine 30 transgenic mice. Muscle & Nerve (suppl 1) A 21–8-72(abstr)

Index of contributors

Non-participating co-authors are indicated by asterisks. Entries in bold type indicate papers; other entries refer to discussion contributions.

Indexes compiled by Liza Weinkove

Subject index